PROMOTING THE HEALTH OF CHILDREN
a guide for caretakers and health care professionals

PROMOTING THE HEALTH OF CHILDREN

a guide for caretakers and health care professionals

SHEILA M. PRINGLE, R.N., M.S.Hyg., Ed.D.

Professor and Chairperson, College Misericordia,
Division of Nursing, Dallas, Pennsylvania

BRENDA E. RAMSEY, R.N., M.S.N.

Assistant Professor, College of Nursing, Villanova University,
Villanova, Pennsylvania

*With **46** illustrations*

The C. V. Mosby Company

ST. LOUIS • TORONTO • LONDON   1982

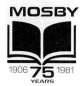

MOSBY

1906 **75** 1981
YEARS

A TRADITION OF PUBLISHING EXCELLENCE

Editor: Michael R. Riley
Editorial assistant: Susan R. Epstein
Manuscript editor: Sandra L. Gilfillan
Design: Susan Trail
Production: Stella Adolfson, Gail M. Hudson

Printed in the United States of America

The C.V. Mosby Company
11830 Westline Industrial Drive, St. Louis, Missouri 63141

Library of Congress Cataloging in Publication Data

Pringle, Sheila M.
　　Promoting the health of children.

　　Bibliography: p.
　　Includes index.
　　1.　Children—Care and hygiene.　2.　Child
development.　3.　Children—Diseases.　4.　Pediatric
nursing.　I.　Ramsey, Brenda E., 1928-
II.　Title.　[DNLM: 1.　Pediatric nursing.　WY 159
P957p]
RJ101.P66　　　613'.0432　　　81-14037
ISBN 0-8016-4048-2　　　AACR2

GW/VH/VH　9　8　7　6　5　4　3　2　1　　03/C/344

With love to my parents
Mr. and Mrs. Kenneth Rothermel
and my children
Susan, Jeffrey, and **Mark,**
his wife **Carol,** and their son **Mark, Jr.**

S. M. P.

To my friend with love
Edith and her husband **Rennard**
because of their love for each other,
their children, and families

B. E. R.

FOREWORD

The strength of a society or a community depends on the well-being of its children. We believe that early preventive health practices can achieve great gains in lifetime health status and play an important part in formulating positive attitudes toward health. Health promotion and disease prevention, recently identified at the highest levels of government as national health priorities, have always been consistent with the aims and goals of nursing practice. Focusing on these priorities, the authors of *Promoting the Health of Children: A Guide for Caretakers and Health Care Professionals* have developed a realistic guide for all who are concerned with the care of children. This book, with its emphasis on holistic health and consumer participation in health care, is a welcome addition to the literature on child health.

Evelyn R. Benson, R.N., M.P.H., Associate Professor of Nursing, Temple University, Philadelphia, Pennsylvania
Joan Q. McDevitt, R.N., M.S.N., Assistant Professor of Nursing, Rutgers University, Camden, New Jersey

A distinctive feature of the text is the way in which Pringle and Ramsey have organized essential information into easy-to-read columns. Drawing on their extensive knowledge and nursing expertise in child health, they have presented their topic in a practical and productive way. Their consistent use of the developmental cycle permits the reader to select that portion of the text which provides the kind of information and guidance needed at any period of the child's life cycle—infancy through adolescence.

In this book, substantive material has been presented in readable prose; at the same time a scholarly approach has been maintained. These two qualities combine to provide a useful tool for students and practitioners of the health professions as well as for parents and other caretakers. Pringle and Ramsey have created a climate in which the concepts of positive health promotion and disease prevention come alive for practical application in the day-to-day care of children.

PREFACE

As nurse educators we have often longed for a *single book* that would provide knowledge and directives useful to caretakers, nurses, and other professionals in promoting the health of children.

Nurses and other health professionals need specific knowledge bases about children: patterns of growth and development, common childhood illnesses, and factors that influence the maintenance of health or prevention of illness. Professionals use such knowledge in practice but often fail to translate or transmit the knowledge for caretaker use. Many childhood accidents and illnesses could be prevented if caretakers were taught and had ready access to information that could be easily understood and applied.

This book is designed as a handy reference tool for nurses and other professionals to use in counseling, guiding, and teaching caretakers those methods and strategies used to promote the health of children. The tabular approach in this text provides simplified explanations for caretakers alongside the information provided for the health professional.

The book comprises five units for specific ages (infancy, toddler, preschool, school age, and adolescence) and one unit devoted to procedures for the care of children in the home. Each unit has three major divisions: growth and development, health maintenance, and health problems.

The growth and development chapters focus on the major biological, psychological, and social milestones the professional uses to assess a child's progress. Each milestone has suggestions for anticipatory guidance for caretakers.

The health maintenance chapter of each unit speaks to those landmarks of development and achievement which warrant concern for safety, health protection, and health supervision. The rationale for each health maintenance measure is presented concurrently in lay terminology.

The health problem division of each unit focuses on common health problems for each age period. In these chapters material is presented in three columns. In the first column the health problem is defined and described. In the second column signs and symptoms, usual management and treatment, sequelae of the illness, and health care guidelines are presented for each health problem. The third column clarifies the health problem for caretakers in language they can understand. Helpful hints are also provided to assist caretakers in the home management of health problems. Incorporated throughout the chapter are suggested questions caretakers should ask or information they should provide when medical advice is sought.

The last chapter presents those procedures often needed by caretakers to maintain the healthy child or care for the sick child at home. Each procedure includes the purpose, essential materials, and necessary step-by-step directions to perform the task. It is hoped that this chapter will allay anxieties caretakers may have when performing these procedures.

We believe this book will prove to be a handy and beneficial reference for nurses, health professionals, and caretakers.

We would like to give special tribute to Evelyn N. Behanna, R.N., B.S.N., M.S.N., Director of Graduate Programs, College Misericordia, Dallas, Pennsylvania, for her support, encouragement, and contributions throughout the development of this book. In particular, we wish to thank Lynne for collaborating with us in writing Unit Two, Toddlerhood.

We would like to express our gratitude to Dorothea Ellis for her time and valuable suggestions at the onset of this endeavor; to Kay Bolger for her helpful comments; to the late Reverend Donald Kaufmann for his sermons on love; to Kelly Finnegan for her help with illustrations; to Susan Pringle for helping us see situations from a caretaker's point of view; to Dorothy Marlow for her faith in our abilities; and to Mary Eastburn for her availability for typing.

A special appreciation to Cathy Haas, superb typist, whose efficiency, availability, and secretarial skills proved invaluable. We also wish to acknowledge the staff of The C.V. Mosby Company and Jeanne Robertson, our illustrator, for consistent helpful assistance.

Thanks also to all of our relatives, professional colleagues, and friends who contributed knowledge and time, kept us motivated, and encouraged us in the completion of our book.

Sheila M. Pringle
Brenda E. Ramsey

CONTENTS

INTRODUCTION

Maintenance and promotion of health in children need greater emphasis in our society. This book will assist health professionals and caretakers in assessing, maintaining, and promoting the health status of their children from infancy through adolescence.

Anticipation of the expected growth and development changes within each stage of life provides for the identification of teachable moments, prediction of the knowledge needed, and institution of the appropriate health practices necessary to foster and maintain health.

Caretakers and health professionals, as they become more knowledgeable, will anticipate and prepare for those moments when teaching principles of health and safety can best occur as children progress through the various stages of life.

LANDMARKS OF GROWTH AND DEVELOPMENT

Landmarks of growth and development are explored for each of the following periods of life: infancy, toddlerhood, preschool, school age, and adolescence. The landmarks are those identifiable aspects of physical change, emotional behavior, and social adaptation which occur within each period.

Periods of life

Infancy is the period from birth through 12 months. During this period, many physical and physiological changes occur rapidly, and the socialization process begins.

Toddlerhood is that period from 1 through 3 years. During this period, many major changes occur, both in physical size and the complexity of newly developing abilities. The toddler will demonstrate curiosity, investigate the environment, and relate easily with others.

The *preschool* period includes 4- and 5-year-old children. This period is characterized by a reduction in the rapidity of physical change, but an increase in the ability to perform more complex mental and physical skills. This child has energy to spare, is assertive, is developing a conscience, and loves to explore an everexpanding world. The child may fail as a result of attempting tasks that are beyond the limits attainable at this point.

School age is the period from 6 through 12 years. It is characterized by involvement, investment, and cooperation in those tasks and activities which lay the groundwork for future roles and endeavors. School-age children will be encouraged in their attempts to achieve if they meet the expectations of parents, teachers, and friends. However, if the expectations of those whom the child wishes to please are greater than those which can be accomplished, a sense of inferiority may result.

The period of *adolescence* is from 12 through 18 years of age. It is characterized by a developing sense of security related to sex, capabilities, and limitations. The major struggles of this period center around "Who am I?" and "Where am I going?"

The specific changes in growth and development that occur in each of these stages of life will be covered in greater depth throughout the book. However, certain principles of growth and development should be kept in mind.

PRINCIPLES OF GROWTH AND DEVELOPMENT

Normal ranges of growth are established for each age that may vary from high to low or early to late. When comparing children's physical growth with the ranges of normal, an important precept to remember is: *Children develop at their own rates.* No two children grow or develop at precisely the same rate, although their patterns of growth and development will be similar.

Growth refers to a change or increase in physical size. *Development* refers to an increased capacity to function and is usually the outcome of maturation and learning. *Maturation* refers to the inborn capacity of the individual to progress. *Learning* is the process of gaining new knowledge and skills. Maturation and learning are interrelated in that individuals cannot learn unless they are mature enough to be able to understand and change their behavior.

1

When evaluating a child's developmental progress, the following are important principles to remember:
1. Large muscle control develops before fine muscle control.
2. Motor control develops from the midline of the body to the periphery.
3. Muscle development proceeds from head-to-toe (cephalocaudal development).
4. Voluntary muscle control proceeds from general to specific movements.

Infants exemplify these principles through the demonstration of their improved abilities. For example, in the first months, infants will grasp an object with both hands and hold it close to the body. Later, infants will grasp an object with one hand and hold it away from the body. These skills become further refined as infants pick up objects using only the index finger and thumb of one hand. In another example, head control precedes the ability to roll over or sit up. Infants will sit before they stand and usually creep before they walk.

Patterns of development enable health professionals and caretakers to identify particular landmarks that should be attained at each age level. Guidelines for health maintenance and safety practices of children can be formulated from the identified landmarks.

HEALTH MAINTENANCE

Emphasizing the maintenance of health can reduce the incidence of health problems that occur within each period of life. Teaching, reinforcing, and using sound health practices are major tasks that must be viewed as continuous responsibilities to be shared by caretakers, health professionals, and children. Certain topics pertaining to health should be taught, reviewed, and reemphasized throughout every individual's life in the home, school, and community. Although the following list is not exhaustive, major areas of concern to be addressed include nutrition, rest, sleep, exercise, energy levels, immunization, and safety.

Health professionals and caretakers often need assistance in teaching health practices and reorganizing opportunities where teaching can take place. To teach others, it is necessary to keep in mind the following fundamental principles of teaching and learning:

1. *Ascertain the learner's knowledge base.* New information should not be introduced until the amount of knowledge the learner possesses has been ascertained. Frequently, misinformation exists that must be clarified before new information is taught.

2. *Prepare a basic teaching plan.* Identify the content to be taught (the important points) and the behaviors to be learned (the activities or skills).

3. *Determine the readiness of the learner.* Learners give clues that they need information (often referred to as the teachable moment).

4. *Introduce small amounts of new material at any one time.* Consider the number of opportunities available to teach new skills or health practices. Often information (teaching) can be dispensed while the teacher performs the tasks.

5. *Permit the learner to actively participate.* Involvement in the new task, opportunities to try the new skill, raise questions, and to receive positive feedback enhance the learning process and alleviate doubts.

6. *Validate that learning has occurred.* A return demonstration by the learner of the new skill or correct answers to questions posed by the teacher are two examples of validation of learning.

7. *Avoid teaching when the learner is under stress or in pain.* Learning ability diminishes when pain or stress exists.

Despite efforts to maintain, promote, and teach health practices, health problems do occur.

COMMON HEALTH PROBLEMS

The common health problems for each period are described with suggestions for home care management and helpful hints. Knowledge of the causes, signs, symptoms, and courses of illnesses assists health professionals in the management and treatment of health problems. Sharing knowledge and assisting caretakers through guidelines and helpful hints on the management of healthy and sick children can reduce anxiety and reassure caretakers about their own competency.

Further assistance in specific techniques and procedures when giving care and treatments are described in Chapter 18.

TECHNIQUES FOR CARE

Health professionals and caretakers often need instruction to be able to perform certain procedures and techniques when maintaining and promoting the health of children. The methodology and rationale for the procedures and/or techniques are listed. Helpful hints are provided for each procedure.

It is our hope, with this body of knowledge related to growth and development, health maintenance, and the management of common health problems, that health professionals and caretakers will be able to better work together to foster and maintain sound health practices.

UNIT ONE

INFANCY *establishing trust*

The development of a healthy individual requires much more than a physically sound body. Equally important is the development of a sound personality.

As individuals travel through life, certain biological, psychological, and social changes do occur at rather predictable points in time. Important though the changes are at each stage of life, perhaps even more critical is the need to realize that these changes, as well as the environment, have a great impact on personality development.

Trust is the major cornerstone of personality development. This is the foundation on which all future experiences will be built. It is a learned behavior. It can be fragile. It can be destroyed. It can be strong, and it can be enduring. Trust is solidified through love and trusting relationships within the environment. In a relatively short period of time, that first 12 months of life, the foundation of trust must be developed.

At the time of birth the newborn must rely totally on others to meet needs for comfort and safety. The newborn has left a secure, comfortable environment and suddenly is thrust into harsh reality. Successful adaptation of the newborn to this environment highly depends on the sincere love and intent given by the caretaker. The term *caretakers* refers to natural parents, adoptive parents, or those individuals caring for children.

To foster a loving relationship with their newborn, caretakers must feel at ease with their present role, financial resources, and relationship with others who care. Husband and wife must remain mutually supportive and able to communicate openly their stresses to each other in order to decrease those frustrations in their new roles as father and mother. Likewise, the single individual, on becoming a parent, also needs to feel at ease and should have a strong support system to reduce tensions.

The ability of parents to foster and maintain an environment for their infant to develop trust depends on their own physical and psychological health. Mothers, for example, frequently experience a period of "baby blues" when their infants are about a week to 10 days old. This period of depression is easy to understand, but difficult to deal with. Whereas the mother had assistance in the care of the infant in the hospital and often some assistance the first few days at home, suddenly she and the newborn are alone. The totality of the responsibility, arriving at a time when her fatigue level is high and her emotional reserve very low, leads to depression. Meanwhile, the father is trying to make up for time lost at his job and is more aware of the need for additional money and space. The new demands come at a time when his support system (his wife) seems to be giving all her love and attention to someone else (the baby). To complicate the situation, this family may already have other children, each at his/her own stage of development and with different needs and problems. The neonate further adds to the confusion through needs for attention that seem to occur at the most inopportune times.

A sense of humor and the ability to view the situation objectively are essential. Parents should know that this pattern of confusion and bombardment of senses when a new member is added to the family is normal and to be expected. This cannot be overstressed.

The natural bond that occurs between mother and child during pregnancy must be recreated after birth. This bond is strengthened with continuing contact. Observations of mothers alone with their newborn for the first time reveal a pattern of exploration and identification that attempts to recreate the symbiotic relationship (bonding) which existed prior to birth. The mother's initial pattern of bonding reveals a thorough scrutiny of every minute detail of the infant. Mothers repeatedly examine and inspect all parts of their newborn as if to make sure they are all there and intact. Patterns of bonding have also been noticed with fathers in their exploration and identification of their infant. This is an area of study that must be further researched.

However, for trust to be developed in the newborn, caretakers other than the mother must be assisted in developing their own pattern of "symbolic bonding." This symbolic bonding could be described as that method by which others explore, identify, and create a unity with the newborn. A typical pattern of symbolic bonding observed in fathers and grandparents differs from that of the mother. Their manner of inspection is usually less detailed and tends to focus on comparison of the newborn's features with those of siblings and other relatives. The bonding process develops through continued relationships of the newborn with the caretaker and others.

Trusting relationships are facilitated as the infant matures and is able to respond. In the first 3 months of life the infant is becoming a more social being who now smiles and coos in response to others. This responsiveness stimulates a desire on the part of the caretaker and others to spend more time with the infant. The periods of wakefulness are longer and provide an increasing number of opportunities for caretakers and infants to be together.

As infants progress from the third to sixth months of life, they are able to differentiate the caretaker from siblings or relatives. The recognition factor further reinforces the infant's desire to repeat behaviors and precipitate pleasurable responses from others.

The 6- to 12-month-old infant has increased motor abilities and will search for others with whom to communicate, thus furthering a mutuality of relationships.

By the end of the first year, if a relationship of trust has been developed with caretaker, siblings, and other relatives, the infant will be ready to step out into the toddler stage of development with a sense of security.

CHAPTER 1

NEWBORN *birth through 28 days*

Birth through 28 days of life is referred to as the neonatal period of infancy. Never again in an individual's life will so many changes in behavior occur in such a short period of time. The internal and external adjustments to which a newborn is expected to adapt precipitate numerous physiological and psychological responses. The caretaker also experiences rapid changes: periods of sheer excitement and joy and periods of extreme frustration and discouragement. Although the caretaker may have planned and looked forward to the infant's birth with great expectation, there may now be feelings of awe, helplessness, and insecurity. Defenseless, yet strong willed, lovable, but demanding, are but a few of the phrases that caretakers begin to use to describe their newborn.

Meeting the physical needs of dressing, feeding, and cleansing the infant throughout every 24-hour period frequently overwhelms the caretaker, not because these are the most difficult of the many tasks to perform, but because they are the most time consuming. Organization of the many tasks required is difficult because the newborn's patterns of eating, eliminating, and sleeping are not yet established. As a result, the caretaker becomes tired, irritable, and anxious. Caretakers become so involved in the physical nature of these tasks that they often lose sight of the importance of the quality of their performance in developing that basic sense of trust in this new individual.

The caretaker will be unable to determine the specific strands of growth that weave through this neonatal period if he or she does not know the pattern of development for the newborn. However, if the caretaker is informed regarding the changes that will occur and when they should occur, the anxiety accompanying the unknown should be relieved.

In the remainder of the chapter, landmarks of growth and development in the newborn period are presented. Accompanying the landmarks are suggestions directed to the caretaker for determining the growth status of the newborn as a basis for anticipatory guidance.

GROWTH AND DEVELOPMENTAL LANDMARKS	**ANTICIPATORY GUIDANCE**

Biological

WEIGHT

The average weight range is 6 to 8½ pounds (2.7 to 3.85 kg).

Special scales for weighing infants at home are not necessary and should be discouraged because they are a source of anxiety and an unnecessary expense.

Birth weight, although important, is not the only criterion on which to base future expectations of the infant's growth and abilities.

Girls frequently fall in a lower weight range than boys.

The weight range for girls continues to be lower than for boys from infancy through the school-age years.

Variations in weight above and below the normal range can be expected.

The neonate who weighs more than 10 pounds (4.5 kg) may exhibit a hypoglycemic reaction (low blood sugar) within the first few days after birth. Signs of hypoglycemia may include difficulty with breathing, periods of cyanosis, involuntary tremors (twitching) of extremities, lethargy, and even convulsions. Mothers of infants weighing 10 pounds or more at birth and those who have a history of large babies should be encouraged to seek screening for diabetes.

When the weight of newborns exceeds 10 pounds, mothers should be screened for diabetes.

Neonates weighing less than the average birth range may require closer supervision and attention until a consistent pattern of weight gain and adjustment is established.

Adjustments to postuterine life bring about an initial weight loss of about 10% of the birth weight.

Weight loss is directly related to physiological adjustments such as ingestion and digestion of food and loss of excess body fluids.

Newborns lose weight as a result of their bodies adjusting to eating and digesting foods.

A gain of approximately 2 pounds (0.9 kg) above birth weight is typical during the newborn period.

HEIGHT

The average range for height is 18 to 21½ inches (45.7 to 54.6 cm).

Accurate measurement of length is best obtained when the infant's back is straight and the legs are extended (Fig. 1-1).

Infants do not appear to be as tall as they are because of the flexed position they assume at rest.

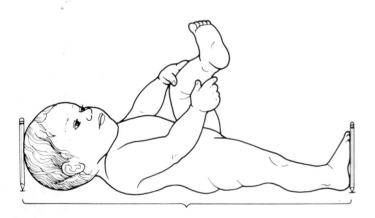

Fig. 1-1. Length measurement throughout infancy. Place pencil mark on surface at top of head and at sole of foot of extended leg and measure distance between these two points.

HEART RATE

The average range for heart rate is 120 to 150 beats per minute.

Heart rate must be evaluated in regard to the circumstances in which the neonate is found. The immaturity of the regulatory centers of the brain is a primary factor for irregularities. Irregularities in the rhythm may also be related to a change in breathing patterns. As the respiratory rate increases or decreases, the heart rate may likewise increase or decrease.

GROWTH AND DEVELOPMENTAL LANDMARKS

When the neonate cries or becomes irritable, the heart rate may rise as high as 170 beats per minute, and during sleep it may be as low as 80 to 90 beats per minute.

Heart rates are best obtained at the apex of the heart (Fig. 1-2).

Pulsations of the heart and some of the great blood vessels may be visible and palpable just below the midline of the chest (sternum).

ANTICIPATORY GUIDANCE

Caretakers may notice a throbbing (pulsations) at the sides of the head (near the eye) or just below the breastbone. Pulsations are especially evident at the soft spot at the top of the head when the infant is straining or crying.

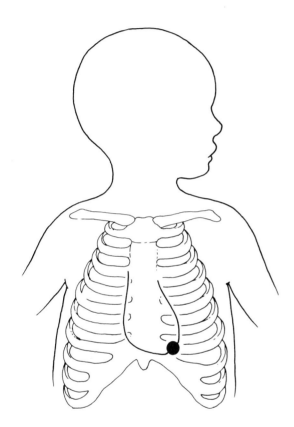

Fig. 1-2. Heart rate. Heart rates are best obtained at apex of heart.

RESPIRATION

The respiratory rate ranges between 35 to 50 breaths per minute.

Evaluate respirations in regard to the circumstances in which the neonate is found.

Respirations are clearly visible at the abdomen. Diaphragmatic and abdominal muscles are primarily used, and there is little thoracic movement.

Irregularities exist in rhythm, rate, and depth. The immaturity of the regulating mechanism is one factor for the wide variations in rate, rhythm, and volume.

An increased rate of 80 or 100 breaths per minute is not unusual if infection is present or if there is an obstructed air passage.

Brief periods of apnea are normal during this period.

Newborns breathe more rapidly when they cry or are startled, hungry, or otherwise uncomfortable. Short periods of crying are beneficial.

7

GROWTH AND DEVELOPMENTAL LANDMARKS

ANTICIPATORY GUIDANCE

Biological—cont'd

TEMPERATURE

The average range of body temperature for a neonate is 94° to 99° F (34.4° to 37° C).

The body temperature may fall to as low as 92° F (33.3° C) within minutes after delivery.

The neonate's temperature will fall or rise as variations in the environmental temperature occur.

The newborn's body temperature is likely to be slightly higher than the mother's.

The heat-regulating system of the newborn is immature and unable to make up for heat loss or exposure to the environment.

Change in behavior, such as restlessness, crying, or increased muscular activity, may indicate that the infant is either too cold or too warm.

Caretakers should realize that if the newborn's crib is near a radiator or in bright sunlight, the body temperature will rise.

If the crib is placed by an open window, cool air may cause chilling and a decrease in body temperature.

Removing or adding clothing or covers helps the newborn's body temperature adjust to the environment.

A body temperature higher than normal may indicate infection.

Subnormal temperatures may be due to an existing pathological condition.

Axillary temperature readings are quite reliable and are less traumatic to the infant than those taken rectally.

Caretakers can take their newborn's temperature safely by placing the thermometer directly under the armpit, pressing the arm firmly against the chest, and holding it there for 5 to 10 minutes. (See Chapter 18, Taking Temperatures With a Glass Thermometer.)

Due to the fluid loss in the first few days of life, the neonate's body temperature may rise to as high as 104° F (40° C). This is known as *transitory fever,* or dehydration fever.

Reduction of fever due to fluid loss can be accomplished by increasing the fluid intake. Feedings of water can be given to the baby between the regular feeding times to increase the amount of fluid taken within each 24-hour period. (See Chapter 4, Fluid Requirements.)

HEAD

The head circumference is usually between 13 and 14 inches (33 to 35.6 cm).

Measurement of head circumference must be accurate (Fig. 1-3).

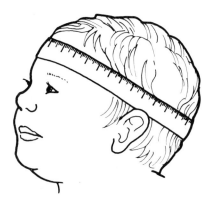

Fig. 1-3. Head circumference. Measurement of head circumference with cloth or paper tape measure. Encircle head at frontal and occipital bones for accurate measurement.

Normally the head is larger than the chest; it is about one fourth the total body length. This proportion will change as the child grows into adulthood, when the head will be about one eighth the body length.

Suture lines of the skull are visible, molding of bony structure is evident, and the fontanels (soft spots) are palpable.

The head often appears very large in proportion to the newborn's (neonate's) body. As the infant grows, the head will assume more adult proportions.

The space between the bones of the head (suture lines) becomes less apparent as the head assumes a more normal shape, hair covers the scalp, and the facial contour becomes more delineated.

GROWTH AND DEVELOPMENTAL LANDMARKS	ANTICIPATORY GUIDANCE

Fontanels are unossified spaces or soft spots between the cranial bones.

The anterior fontanel is diamond shaped, approximately 1 inch (2.5 cm) in width and 2 inches (5 cm) in length, and located at the juncture of the frontal and parietal bones (crown of the head). Pulsations are evident and frequently palpable at the anterior fontanel.

The posterior fontanel is triangularly shaped and much smaller than the anterior fontanel. The width is about ½ inch (1 to 1.5 cm), and the length is less than ½ inch (0.5 to 1 cm) and located at the juncture of the occipital and parietal bones (just above the nape of the neck) (Fig. 1-4).

Soft spots (fontanels) are protected by a tough membranous covering that is not easily damaged. The soft spots are easily palpable and are usually depressed (slightly concave) unless the infant is crying or straining to have a bowel movement. Pulsations at the soft spot on top of the head (the anterior fontanel) may be noticed, particularly at feeding times.

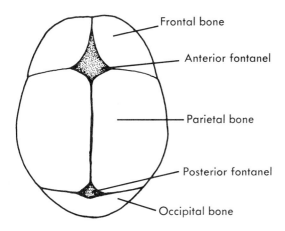

Fig. 1-4. Fontanels. Anterior and posterior fontanels (soft spots) between cranial bones.

Molding is the overriding of the bones of the skull at the suture line to accommodate the head through the birth canal. Molding may make the head distorted and/or elongated. Molding is most noticeable in infants who are born head first and may not be evident at all in the very small baby, the breech delivery (feet first), or the baby delivered by caesarian section.

A swelling or bulging appearance on the scalp may be indicative of caput succedaneum or cephalhematoma (Chapter 5).

The contour of the head will assume a more normal appearance within 24 to 48 hours as molding (a temporary distortion-elongation of the head caused during the birth process) disappears.

HAIR

The amount of hair to be found on a head ranges from almost none to a very large amount. Color will also vary. The texture is soft and downy.

The uniqueness of each newborn is often best characterized by the amount or lack of hair on the head.

Shampooing the hair and cleansing the scalp are discussed in Chapter 18, Bathing an Infant.

FACE

The facial contour for each neonate will be unique.

The facial contour is symmetrical. If asymmetry is present, it may be due to a birth injury such as facial paralysis (Chapter 5).

The eyes usually appear wide apart due to the somewhat large bridge of the flattened nose.

The mouth is small, and the tongue at times will protrude.

The skin of the face may be pink to red. There may be reddened or darkened areas along the cheeks and over the ears caused by pressure of the forceps used during delivery.

Facial features of the newborn are small compared to the size of the head, and caretakers initially may be surprised at how far apart the eyes seem to be, the flattened appearance of the nose, and the smallness of the mouth.

Caretakers should be informed that facial features become more distinct as the infant develops.

The facial skin color will change to a deep red when the newborn cries or strains.

Bruised areas on the cheeks and ears (forceps marks) are temporary and require no treatment.

GROWTH AND DEVELOPMENTAL LANDMARKS	ANTICIPATORY GUIDANCE

Biological—cont'd

FACE—cont'd

The cheeks are rounded and bulge because of sucking pads located on the inner surface.

The rooting reflex is present.

Lips and cheeks are highly sensitive to touch. Newborns will turn their head in the direction of stroked cheeks and will start sucking on an object that touches the lips. To encourage the newborn to suck, caretakers should stroke only the cheek on the side they wish the newborn to turn.

Facial features may be blurred because of additional tissue perfusion and the trauma of birth.

The puffy appearance of the newborn's face will disappear within 2 to 3 days after birth.

Across the bridge of nose there are frequently small white pinpoint lesions known as *milia,* which are caused by retention of sebaceous gland secretion.

EYES

At birth the eyes are usually bluish in light-skinned infants and brown in dark-skinned infants. The eyes will assume their permanent color sometime later in infancy.

The bluish color of the light-skinned newborn's eyes may range from slate to almost inky black. Dark-skinned infants usually have brown eyes. Although most newborns may have eyes of a particular color at birth, this may not be the permanent color.

The shape of the eyes can vary from oval to round.

Gestational age will influence whether the eyes appear somewhat prominent or sunken within the facial contour.

In some neonates, eyebrows and eyelashes may be very prominent.

Vision is present, but visual acuity is lacking.

Ocular movements frequently lack symmetry.

The newborn's eyes are highly sensitive to light.

Newborns often appear cross-eyed. As the infant matures, the eyes move together.

The neonate's ability to focus on an object will be evident within a few weeks.

Pupil size varies. Pupils should dilate and constrict equally.

Blinking is a common reflex that is highly evident during this period.

Tears are noticeable toward the end of the neonate period.

Normally there is no discharge from the eyes. Discharge from the eyes within the first 2 or 3 days of life could be due to irritation from silver nitrate instilled at birth.

Newborns tend to keep their eyelids tightly closed. They will blink in response to noise, light, and touch.

Newborns cry, but tears do not appear until after the first month.

NOSE

The nose is small and somewhat flattened.

Neonates are obligatory nose breathers.

The sneezing reflex is present and enables the neonate to clear the nasal passages.

Cilia are not visible.

Neonates frequently have a thin white mucous discharge. If nasal discharge persists or the character of it changes, it may be indicative of a health problem. (See Chapter 5, Rhinitis/Pharyngitis/Coryza.)

Normally there is a thin white mucous discharge from the nose. Dried mucus at the nostrils may be present when the newborn awakens in the morning. Cleansing of nose is discussed in Chapter 18, Bathing an Infant.

MOUTH

The mouth is small, and the tongue tends to protrude when the mouth is opened.

Reflexes present include sucking, swallowing, gagging, coughing, and yawning.

Full-term newborns will be able to suck vigorously. Sucking stimulates the swallowing reflex, which enables the newborn to eat.

The gag and cough reflexes are protective mechanisms. Gagging enables the newborn to rid the mouth of excessive food. Coughing enables the newborn to clear the air passages.

GROWTH AND DEVELOPMENTAL LANDMARKS

The mucous membrane of the mouth is reddish pink.
Tooth buds, and sometimes teeth, may be present.
Salivation is minimal.

In some neonates the maxillary and palatal processes may not close during uterine life, thus cleft lip and/or cleft palate may be present at birth (Chapter 5).

EARS

The ears seem to be set low on the head. The top of the ear will be level with the eye.
The outer ear is primarily made up of cartilage, which accounts for the flabby texture.
Hearing is present at birth.

Normally there is no discharge from the ear. A discharge that is present over a prolonged period of time may indicate a health problem (See Chapter 5, Otitis Media.)
Skin irritation behind the ear may occur where two skin surfaces rub together. (See Chapter 5, Intertrigo.)

SKIN

Skin color varies according to racial background, pigmentation of the skin, and physiological changes.

A white neonate's color tones will range from light pink to dark red. At birth the color of the extremities may be deep red with a bluish tinge.
Soft downy hair, called *lanugo*, is found over the entire body to some degree, although it may be more noticeable on certain parts of the body. Lanugo is more prevalent in premature infants.
Physiological jaundice (a yellowish tint to the skin) usually appears on the second day and disappears by the seventh day. Physiological jaundice is caused by the destruction of an excessive number of blood cells (bilirubin) that is not excreted by the kidney and thus appears in the tissues, giving the skin a yellow color.
Skin surfaces are frequently covered with a protective, creamy white cheeselike coating known as *vernix caseosa*. Large amounts are frequently found in the skin folds.
The skin is very sensitive during the neonatal period.

ANTICIPATORY GUIDANCE

Some drooling may occur because of the immaturity of the swallowing reflex. As this reflex becomes voluntary, the newborn will automatically swallow the saliva.

The appearance of the ears is unique for each newborn. Some newborns have larger ears than others.

Sudden loud noises will elicit a generalized muscular activity known as the *startle reflex*. The ability to hear may be tested by ringing a bell a short distance from an infant at rest; generalized activity will result.
As hearing becomes more acute, the newborn will be able to differentiate the caretaker's voice from others by the end of the first month.

Many newborns develop a skin irritation behind the ears, which can be prevented by keeping the area clean and dry.

Skin coloring at birth will be different for each newborn, and caretakers may need reassurance that color tones will change as the infant grows.
Bluish discoloration of the hands and feet may be due to immaturity, but tends to disappear without treatment.

The soft downy hair (lanugo) found on the newborn's skin will disappear within the first few weeks.

A yellowish tinge to the skin (jaundice) appearing on the second day of life usually disappears without treatment. If the jaundice remains or increases after the seventh day, the physician should be notified.

Some newborn's skin is covered with a cheeselike substance (vernix caseosa). No special attention need be given to this cheesy coating. It usually dries and flakes off within a few days.
Because the newborn tends to assume a flexed position at rest, the elbows, knees, and cheeks can develop pressure points. These reddened areas can quickly open and become sore. The infant's positions of rest should be alternated to reduce pressure spot formation.

GROWTH AND DEVELOPMENTAL LANDMARKS	ANTICIPATORY GUIDANCE

Biological—cont'd

CHEST AND ABDOMEN

The chest and abdomen are circular and almost equal in size. Both are smaller in circumference than the head.

Abdominal and diaphragmatic muscles are used more than thoracic muscles to maintain respiration.

Normally, the umbilical cord becomes blackened and dries and falls off within a few days (7 to 10). Inspection of the umbilical cord at the tip and point of attachment should be done daily until the cord falls off.

The abdomen tends to appear larger than the chest. This may be due to the activity of the muscles of the abdomen during breathing or the bulging of the stomach following feedings.

Newborns will often be discharged from the hospital with the birth cord still in place. Caretakers should inspect the cord daily to determine if there is any bleeding or seepage of fluid at the belly button area (umbilicus).

Daily cord care should be instituted until the cord falls off. Alcohol (70% solution) or witch hazel may be applied with a cotton-tipped applicator at the tip and base of the cord to shrink tissue and prevent infection.

After the cord falls off, applications of alcohol or witch hazel should be continued once or twice a day to the belly button area (umbilical site) until it is totally healed.

Some neonates may have a seepage of clear fluid at the base of the cord. Most cords dry without seepage. However, if bright red blood is seen, notify the physician because this indicates that the cord is not yet sealed off and can become a portal for bacteria.

If seepage of the cord occurs, the skin surface may become irritated. Cleansing and thorough drying of the irritated area are usually all that is necessary to aid in healing. If seepage continues or increases, the physician should be notified.

If bright red blood is noticed at the cord site, notify the physician.

The chest contour is symmetrical. The transverse diameter is greater than the anterior-posterior diameter.

Breasts may seem swollen (engorged) on both male and female neonates due to increased hormone levels of the mother. A few drops of yellow fluid (witch's milk) may be expressed from the breast.

The swollen breasts (engorgement) often seen in newborns will disappear within a few days.

ARMS

The arms are equal in size and length and are usually held close to the body in a flexed position.

When startled, neonates will suddenly fling both arms up in an outward motion away from their bodies, then back together toward the midline of their chests as if to embrace an object (startle reflex).

The Moro reflex (similar to the startle reflex) is triggered when the infant is suddenly jarred or equilibrium is changed.

The arms should be easily abducted and adducted. Asymmetry of motion may be an indication of a birth injury such as brachial paralysis (Erb's palsy) or a broken clavicle (Chapter 5).

Both arms should move equally and freely. When startled, the newborn's arms reach out as if to embrace a large object and then come back to rest against the chest (startle reflex).

HANDS

The fingers and thumb are usually held in a clenched fist, even when the neonate is sleeping.

The skin of the hands is delicate, and flaking (peeling) occurs.

Occasionally, extra digits (fingers) may be present on one or both hands at birth.

The grasp reflex is present throughout the neonatal period. When the examiner places one or two fingers in each palm of the neonate, the grasp reflex, being so strong, will permit the examiner to momentarily lift the neonate's head and shoulders a few inches from the bed surface.

The fingernails are very thin and tear easily.

The fingers and thumb will open, exposing the palm of the hand during the startle reflex.

Newborns will momentarily grasp a rattle or hold a finger when it is placed in their hand (grasp reflex).

Fingernails may have to be trimmed to protect the newborn from self-inflicted scratches. (See Chapter 2, Hands.)

GROWTH AND DEVELOPMENTAL LANDMARKS	ANTICIPATORY GUIDANCE

LEGS

The legs will be equal in size and length.

The legs tend to be bowed and appear shorter than the arms.

The neonate tends to assume a flexed position even at rest.

The legs can be easily extended, abducted, and adducted. Resistance to abduction, adduction, or lack of symmetrical movement may indicate a health problem. (See Chapter 5, Dislocated Hip.)

FEET

The sole of the foot is flat. When the sole is stroked with a blunt object, the toes will extend up and out (Babinski reflex).

The Babinski reflex will be present until the infants are about 12 to 18 months old. At this time, the reflex will be adultlike, whereby the toes curl downward when the sole of the foot is stroked with a blunt object.

Neonates held in an upright position with the toes touching the edge of a table surface will pull the leg upward in a stepping motion (dance, or stepping, reflex). The stepping reflex usually disappears by the end of the first month.

Both feet can be easily extended, flexed, inverted, and everted.

Occasionally, a neonate may have a foot that is twisted out of normal position. This may be bilateral or unilateral. (See Chapter 5, Clubfoot.)

The toenails are thin and tear easily.

BACK AND BUTTOCKS

The back is straight.

In response to a firm stroke along the spinal column, a neonate will arch the upper torso laterally (trunk incurvation).

The back muscles are immature.

The skin surface of the back and buttocks is smooth and unbroken.

Bluish green discolorations called *mongolian spots* evident at the lumbosacral area are seen most frequently in blacks, Orientals, or southern Europeans.

Dimples may be present bilaterally at the lumbosacral area.

The buttocks are uniform in size and shape.

Extra gluteal folds on one side may indicate a common health problem. (See Chapter 5, Dislocated hip.)

GENITALIA

Female genitalia may be swollen. A small amount of blood may be present at the vaginal orifice. The bloody discharge is a result of the influence of the increased hormone level of the mother on the infant during pregnancy.

Separation of the labia will usually reveal a creamy white substance known as smegma. Smegma is epithelial tissue that has flaked off and is seen chiefly at the external genitalia.

The bowed appearance of the newborn's legs will decrease as the infant grows.

The sole of an infant's foot is sensitive to touch. If the sole is tickled, the infant pulls the foot back quickly.

Newborns pull their legs up in a stepping motion when their toes touch the edge of a table surface (stepping reflex). This reflex is not an indication that the infant will walk early.

If the infant's foot or feet are unusually twisted out of position, treatment may be necessary.

See Chapter 2, Feet, for nail trimming procedures.

Good body alignment and support for the head, neck, and spine are essential.

A firm crib mattress is highly recommended. *Do not* use pillows to support infant's head. Suffocation may result should the newborn's head become buried in the pillow.

The head, back, and buttocks must be supported when lifting a newborn. (See Chapter 18, Lifting and Holding the Infant.)

Bluish discolorations at the small of the back (mongolian spots) will disappear without treatment.

Discolorations that may be present on the hips because of birth trauma will also disappear without treatment.

Swelling of the female external genitalia is quite common, requires no treatment, and will disappear within a few days.

Cleansing is recommended during bath time and with each diaper change to prevent accumulation of discharge or fecal material that may irritate or contaminate urinary tract and vaginal openings. (See Chapter 18, Bathing an Infant.)

GROWTH AND DEVELOPMENTAL LANDMARKS	ANTICIPATORY GUIDANCE

Biological—cont'd

GENITALIA—cont'd

Male genitalia characteristically consist of a large scrotum and very small penis. The scrotal sac should contain two testes that are equal in size.

Occasionally, the testicles may not be present in the scrotum. The absence of the testicles will give the scrotum a flattened appearance. An undescended testicle can be both unilateral and bilateral. (See Chapter 5, Undescended Testicle(s).)

In male infants who are not circumcised, the foreskin of the penis extends beyond the tip of the penis and can be retracted. Smegma often accumulates under the foreskin.

The urethral orifice should be visible at the tip of the penis. Occasionally, the urethral opening may not be at the normal location. When the urethral opening is located on the undersurface of the penis, it is known as *hypospadias,* and when it is located on the upper surface of the penis, it is known as *epispadias* (Chapter 5).

The scrotal sac of male newborns is extremely large, and the penis is very small. These features change as the infant grows.

Ordinarily the testicles are located in the scrotal sac at birth. An undescended testicle(s) requires treatment before the child reaches 6 years.

In males who are not circumcised, retraction of the foreskin daily is necessary for cleansing to prevent obstruction of the urinary tract opening. (See Chapter 18, Bathing an Infant.)

Circumcision is recommended for all male newborns to facilitate cleanliness.

Occasionally, the urinary tract opening is not at the proper location (tip of the penis). This condition requires surgery, and circumcision may be delayed.

Psychological

DEPENDENCY

Newborns totally depend on others for all their needs for food, comfort, love, and a safe environment.

Newborns will alert caretakers to their needs. Hunger is the primary need that newborns will communicate. Many infants cry only when they are hungry. Some also cry and are fretful or irritable when they are uncomfortable. Offering a feeding is not always the answer.

Before taking any action, caretakers must assess the infant's behavior by checking the following:
1. Diaper (wet or soiled)
2. Infant's position
3. Temperature of room
4. Length of time since last feeding
5. Type and duration of cry

It is logical to assume that the newborn is hungry if more than 2 hours have elapsed since the last feeding.

If the infant is crying or fretful, but has been fed and is dry, a position change may be all that is necessary.

Meeting needs as they arise will assist in establishing a firm base of trust in the newborn.

Social

Socialization begins to take place when the infant is held.

Newborns are content and appear to thrive on just being held, fed, and permitted to sleep. Prolonged periods of holding and rocking are not usually necessary.

VOCALIZATION

Neonates vocalize by crying.

The cry is unique for each neonate.

The cry is high pitched initially, then gradually changes in pitch, volume, and forcefulness.

Newborns cry to expand and add more air to their lungs as well as to signal their needs.

Crying, although not pleasant to hear, should be permitted for short intervals (2 or 3 minutes) to facilitate lung expansion.

Caretakers quickly learn to differentiate their newborn's unique cry from the cry of other newborns.

Once the newborn is at home, the caretaker can identify a variety of needs based on the character of the cry.

14

CHAPTER 2

EARLY INFANCY *1 through 6 months*

The period of early infancy, 1 through 6 months, continues to be a period of rapid growth and development. Although the infant remains a dependent being, awareness of the environment, awareness of others, and the socialization process begin to evolve.

Between the first and third month of an infant's life, the caretaker has become more confident in performing those repetitive tasks of feeding, cleansing, and dressing. The caretaker now becomes aware of the infant's pattern of behavior and can anticipate the infant's needs. The amount of time spent in meeting the infant's needs is now well delineated. Tasks that once were a cause of frustration now become enjoyable. Infants sleep longer, particularly at night, and a long-awaited full night's rest for the caretaker becomes a reality.

By 6 months mealtime is quite pleasant because most infants are not only willing, but eager, to try new foods. The infant also eats well for both caretakers and strangers.

Crying continues to be the tool of communication for infants, but it may become an effective tool for manipulating the environment. Discipline (limit setting) begins even at the early months of infancy when caretakers are able to differentiate distress cries from cries for attention. Infants develop a sense of trust from the consistent manner in which their distress needs are met. Infants begin to learn limits of behavior expected of them and a rudimentary sense of authority.

As the infant progresses through the first 6 months, muscle control becomes more developed. New motor skills permit infants to change position deliberately, thus reducing some of their dependency on others.

Infants from 3 to 6 months enjoy sitting in a propped position. Some infants will be able to assume and maintain a sitting position on their own by the end of the sixth month.

In the first few months infants learn to differentiate caretakers from other people. By the time infants are 6 months old, they are able to differentiate fathers from mothers, siblings from parents, and strangers from people often seen. The 6-month-old is still receptive to new people. The young infant enjoys a variety of toys, especially those which are bright colored, make noise, and can be easily held.

Whereas caretakers felt most comfortable keeping the newborn at home, now excursions into the outside world become commonplace. In nice weather, caretakers enjoy taking their infants for walks, visiting relatives and neighbors, or going on short shopping trips. Many infants are also introduced to the religious community through services of dedication or baptism.

The biological, psychological, and social landmarks of growth and development of the average 1- through 6-month-old infant are described. Concomitant suggestions for anticipatory guidance to be shared with caretakers by health care workers are provided. Opportunities for guiding and counseling should be developed and used by health personnel at every meeting, such as well-baby conferences, home visits, or hospitalization.

| GROWTH AND DEVELOPMENTAL LANDMARKS | ANTICIPATORY GUIDANCE |

Biological

WEIGHT

The average range is 8 to 16 pounds (3.6 to 7.3 kg).

The weight gain averages between ¼ and ½ pound (0.14 to 0.23 kg) per week through the third month.

The weight gain is approximately 1 pound (0.45 kg) per month from the fourth through sixth month.

By the fifth month, infants will usually have doubled their birth weight. An infant weighing 7 pounds (3.15 kg) at birth will now weigh approximately 14 pounds (6.3 kg).

A weight gain is most visible in the changing contour of the infant's face and extremities, since the skin surface becomes less wrinkled due to development of underlying tissue and deposits of fat.

A basic rule to remember is that infants will usually double their birth weight by 5 months and triple their birth weight by the end of the first year.

The weight gain appears to slow down about the sixth month, but this is no cause for alarm.

HEIGHT

Approximately 20 to 27 inches (50 to 68.6 cm) is the range for height.

During the first 6 months infants will grow about 1 inch (2.5 cm) per month.

Infants frequently grow 6 inches (15 cm) during the first 6 months.

If at birth the infant was 21 inches (52.5 cm) long, by the end of 6 months the height will be approximately 27 inches (68.6 cm).

Height is measured when infants are lying on their backs on flat surfaces. Measure from the top of the head to the base of the heel, with the knee extended and the foot flexed (Fig. 1-1).

HEART RATE

120 to 150 beats per minute.

The typical heart sound is a double sound: lub-dub, lub-dub, lub-dub.

Heart rates must be reviewed in relation to the activity and circumstance in which the infant is found. Slight irregularities, *arrhythmias*, of the heart sounds may still be present.

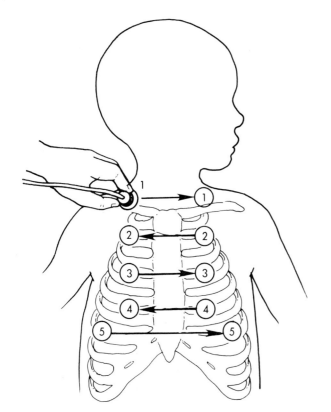

Fig. 2-1. Breath sounds. Accurate assessment of breath sounds is best obtained by uniform systematic pattern from upper to lower chest.

GROWTH AND DEVELOPMENTAL LANDMARKS	**ANTICIPATORY GUIDANCE**

Heart rates are best obtained at the apex of the heart (Fig. 1-2).

Heart rates above 150 beats per minute may be due to a recent feeding, crying, or fear.

Heart rates under 120 beats per minute may be due to deep sleep.

RESPIRATIONS

Infants take 30 to 40 breaths per minute.

The chest cage rises equally on both sides during inspiration.

Normal breath sounds should be inaudible.

Abnormal breath sounds are usually audible and can be more carefully distinguished with a stethoscope. When listening to breath sounds with a stethoscope, begin at the infant's anterior upper right chest area, then systematically move the stethoscope to the same position on the left side and progress downward, moving from side to side (Fig. 2-1).

An infant at rest will have a slower respiratory rate than the infant who is crying or frightened. Respiratory rates during crying may exceed 40 breaths per minute.

Colds or other illnesses influence heart and respiratory rates, as well as body temperature.

The respiratory rate must be reviewed in relation to conditions and circumstances in which the infant is found.

Ordinarily, a baby breathes evenly and quietly.

Infants may have noisy breathing when sleeping due to mucous accumulation in the nostrils or the position of the tongue in the mouth. Normally, noisy breathing disappears when the infant coughs, sneezes, or changes position.

TEMPERATURE

Temperatures range from 96.8° F to 99.6° F (37° C to 37.6° C)

Axillary or rectal temperatures may be taken.

Some newer measurement devices are sensitive to changes in temperature of skin and mucous membranes and can be used orally for small infants.

Body temperature must be viewed in relation to conditions and circumstances in which the infant is found.

Variations in body temperature may be due to decreased fluid intake, long periods of crying, temperature changes within the environment, as well as impending infection.

Body temperature normally fluctuates each day, being low in the morning, rising in the afternoon, and then decreasing in the evening.

Body temperature higher than normal also may be due to decreased fluid intake or impending infection.

Body temperature change can easily be detected by the touch (tactile) method. The skin may feel warm, very hot, moist, or dry. A truer reflection of body heat can be ascertained by placing the palm of the hand at the infant's neck and shoulder, rather than the forehead. Skin color change may also be an indication of body temperature. The infant's skin may be blue when cold and flushed or red when the temperature is elevated. For greatest accuracy, use a thermometer to determine temperature. (See Chapter 18, Taking Temperatures with a Glass Thermometer.)

HEAD

The head circumference is approximately the same as the chest circumference; by 1 year the measurements will become equal.

The posterior fontanel closes at approximately 2 months of age.

The anterior fontanel is still open and palpable and about the size of a nickel, although size will vary with each infant.

Infants 3 months old are able to hold their heads steady in a midline position when held with their backs supported. In a prone position, infants can easily turn their heads from one side to the other.

When lying on the abdomen, the infant is able to lift the head from the surface for short periods of time.

Head support is desirable when the infant is being held because the infant's muscle control is limited. The infant tires and loses head control without warning.

Provide play periods with the infant on the abdomen and place toys in the line of vision. This will permit natural development of head control as the infant lifts the head to view objects.

17

| **GROWTH AND DEVELOPMENTAL LANDMARKS** | **ANTICIPATORY GUIDANCE** |

Biological—cont'd

HEAD—cont'd

By 3 months, infants are able to keep their heads in a midline position when lying on their backs. The *tonic neck reflex* disappears between 2 and 4 months of age.

HAIR

Infants have much more hair than neonates.

A pattern of growth is evident and the texture becomes more coarse.

Secretions become noticeable on the scalp due to maturity of hair follicles and sebaceous glands.

Shampooing the infant's hair and scalp is recommended on a daily basis to prevent drying of oily secretions and the formation of cradle cap. (See Chapter 18, Bathing an Infant.)

EYES

Usually by 3 months of age, the eyes will move together (binocular coordination).

Initially an infant will notice an object, but be unable to focus or maintain the object in the line of vision. Infants can locate, focus, and maintain an object in their field of vision through a 180-degree arc by the end of their third month.

Binocular coordination becomes more refined. Infants can follow all moving objects with ease by the sixth month.

Infants from 3 to 6 months recognize familiar objects, maintain them in their field of vision, and are able to relocate dropped objects.

Tears are present by 2 months of age. Excessive tearing may indicate a correctable health problem, blocked tear duct. (See Chapter 5, Conjunctivitis.)

The eyes normally have no discharge. The presence of discharge may be indicative of conjunctivitis. (See Chapter 5, Conjunctivitis.)

To foster eye coordination and head movements, infants can be placed on their backs or in infant seats with mobiles or bright objects placed in their line of vision.

Sensory stimulation that appeals to visual, auditory, and tactile senses should also be encouraged. This can be accomplished through use of toys such as "busy boxes" as well as mobiles and music boxes.

Between 2 and 3 months of age the crying infant will display tears.

EARS

Hearing is more acute, as evidenced by the infant's response to a voice. The infant's head turns in the direction of the sound.

If drainage or a discharge is present, see Chapter 5, Otitis Media.

The infant's startle response to a loud noise does not always mean that the infant can hear, but may only a reaction to a concomitant vibration.

While the infant is distracted and focusing on a toy, the examiner should stand behind the infant and produce a noise with a rattle or bell. If the infants can hear, they will turn their heads in the direction of the sound.

Cleansing of the ear is not necessary. Cleansing of the external canal of the ear takes place naturally. Earwax is not usually present before 3 months of age.

By the sixth month infants recognize caretakers' voices and familiar sounds and will turn their heads in the direction of the sound.

GROWTH AND DEVELOPMENTAL LANDMARKS	**ANTICIPATORY GUIDANCE**

NOSE

A rudimentary sense of smell is present.

Infants are obligatory nose breathers until approximately 3 months of age.

Infants will sneeze to clear nasal passages.

Large amounts of drainage, ranging from clear to a green color, may indicate the presence of infection or allergies.

See Chapter 5, Rhinitis/Pharyngitis/Coryza, for further descriptions of abnormal respirations. See Chapter 18, for instillation of nosedrops and additional methods for clearing the nasal passages.

Nasal drainage in the early morning is normal. If sneezing does not clear the nasal passages, a gentle pinching pressure with the finger and thumb to the nostrils from the midpoint of the nose toward the nostril will often be adequate to clear the passages. A cotton cone moistened with water may also be used to assist in the removal of dried mucus and nasal discharge (Fig. 2-2).

Nasal congestion may lead to noisy, snoringlike breathing.

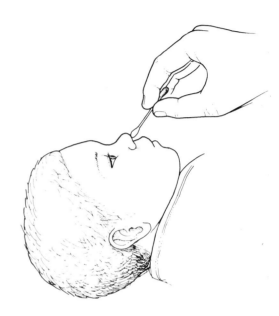

Fig. 2-2. Removal of nasal discharge. Use moistened cotton cone pledget.

MOUTH

The lips are still highly sensitive to touch.

The sucking reflex is very well developed.

Swallowing is no longer merely a reflex, but is deliberate and becoming controlled.

Dentition usually begins during this period. The dental arch is more formed and teeth will begin to appear.

By the end of the third month, budding of the teeth may be noticeable on both the upper and lower gums. (See Chapter 4, Dentition.)

Mucous membranes are dark pink and evenly colored.

White patches on the roof of the mouth, tongue, mucous membrane of the cheek, or on the gums may be indicative of infection.

The infant may still have a slightly protruding tongue through the third month, but this is usually self-correcting by 6 months of age.

Dry lips and/or a coated tongue may indicate dehydration. Drooling may occur because of incomplete control of swallowing, involuntary tongue movements, and the teething process.

The mouth continues to be the major route through which the infant achieves satisfaction and learns about the environment.

Oral hygiene for this age is best achieved by offering water between feedings.

Reassure caretakers that not all infants will have teeth appear before 7 months.

During the teething process infants frequently drool. Discomfort during teething may also be a problem. (See Chapter 4, Dentition.)

Because of immature control of the tongue's movement, introduction of solid foods may be difficult. (See Chapter 18, Feeding Techniques.)

ARMS

The arms are equal in length, size, and shape.

The infant is able to flex and extend the arms without difficulty. The infant will reach out with both arms to grasp an object by the end of the third month. Voluntary control of arm movements has begun. The *startle* or *Moro reflexes* have diminished. (See Chapter 1, Arms.) Muscle development is increasing. The infant becomes better able to use the arms in lifting the head and trunk when lying on the abdomen.

It is desirable to place the infant in positions where stretching and reaching activities can be encouraged and developed.

GROWTH AND DEVELOPMENTAL LANDMARKS	ANTICIPATORY GUIDANCE

Biological—cont'd

HANDS

The infant should begin noticing the hands by the end of the first month and be able to focus and maintain the hands in the line of vision for extended periods by the third month.

Infants 4 to 6 months old will reach out and securely grasp objects with the whole hand. They continue to investigate objects by putting them in their mouths.

By 6 months of age the infant will be able to grasp and hold a small toy in each hand.

The *grasp reflex* has disappeared by the third month. Voluntary control of grasp is being developed.

The skin of the hands is very sensitive and easily irritated and penetrated.

Nails are soft, break easily, and can be the cause of inadvertent, self-inflicted scratches.

Hand-eye coordination and muscle development are not mature enough for the infant to reach out and grasp objects consistently before the third month, but this skill develops quickly from the fourth to sixth month.

Caution caretakers in regard to placement of small objects within the infant's reach.

Toys such as rattles, blocks, small balls, and cuddly toys will provide an opportunity for infants to learn textures as well as develop motor skills.

Large, bright-colored toys, rattles, mobiles, and musical toys are all excellent for the development of fine motor coordination.

Skin irritation between the fingers can be prevented by careful bathing and drying. Lint from bedding frequently lodges between the fingers. (See Chapter 18, Bathing an Infant.)

Fingernails should be kept short and trimmed carefully. The use of manicure scissors is recommended; the use of nail clippers or large scissors should be avoided.

Hangnails occur frequently. Hangnails should be clipped carefully, using manicure scissors and avoiding pulling or tearing the skin.

LEGS

The legs are equal in length, size, and shape. They can be flexed and extended easily at the hips, knees, and ankles. Abduction of both legs should permit the knees to almost touch the table when the infant is in a supine position with the knees and hips flexed.

The legs are still slightly bowed, the stepping reflex is no longer present, and muscle control and coordination are developing.

The infant is able to push up into a standing position when held on the lap or supported in an erect position.

The infant is unable to sustain body weight or an erect position without support.

Increased muscle control enables the infant to pull the knees up and under the abdomen and to push forward when lying on a flat surface.

Caution: Do not leave the infant unattended on a dressing table, bed, or couch. When the infant is in a crib, have the side rails up.

FEET

The infant is developing control and coordination in the lower limbs. The infant can bring the foot within the line of vision and will place the foot into the mouth.

The sole of the foot is still flat; no arch is evident. Plantar resistance is noted when firm pressure is applied to the sole of the foot.

The toenails are soft and break easily.

Strengthening the leg and foot muscles is best achieved through play periods when the infant is being held on the lap and during bath time.

Shoes are not necessary at this stage in development, and leaving the feet bare is desirable. In cold weather, socks and booties provide adequate warmth.

Toenails should be trimmed straight across and not with the contour of the toe; this prevents ingrown nails. The use of manicure scissors is recommended; *avoid* using clippers or large scissors.

CHEST AND ABDOMEN

The chest contour is even, but barrel shaped. The anterior-posterior diameter is still less than the transverse diameter. Although breathing may still be through the use of abdominal muscles rather than the chest and diaphragm, the chest will move equally on both sides during inspiration and expiration.

Air passages as compared to lung size are larger, thus permitting great amounts of air to enter and exit easily.

Maximum mucous production has not yet occurred, and, as a result, the air passages are not adequately warmed or humidified.

Immaturity and limited function of the air passages are contributing factors to respiratory tract infections occurring in infancy.

The abdomen still seems more prominent than the chest in infants through the sixth month.

GROWTH AND DEVELOPMENTAL LANDMARKS	ANTICIPATORY GUIDANCE

The abdomen is round and equal on both sides, except immediately after feeding.

Positioning the infant on the abdomen after feeding is not harmful; in fact, it is beneficial for bubbling of air following the feeding. This position prevents choking or obstruction to the air passage if vomiting should occur.

The abdomen and umbilicus still tend to protrude.

Abdominal binders are no longer used for protrusion of the navel (umbilicus). As the abdominal muscles become strengthened, the belly button becomes flatter and recedes inward, appearing more adultlike.

Continued protrusion of the umbilicus more than ½ inch (1.3 cm) above the abdominal contour beyond 3 months of age may be indicative of an umbilical hernia. (See Chapter 5, Hernia.)

BACK AND BUTTOCKS

The spinal column is straight with no lateral curvatures. The contour of the trunk is equal on both sides.

Periods of exercise should be provided for infants. Strengthening of back muscles can be achieved by placing the infant on the back for some periods and on the abdomen for others.

The Landau reflex appears about the third month of age. When held in a prone horizontal position, with the head allowed to fall forward, the infant will pull the legs toward the abdomen.

The back muscles are becoming more developed; thus the infant will be able to maintain a sitting position with less support.

The buttocks contour will be equal in shape and size.

Any change in the contour, size, and/or shape of the buttocks may indicate the presence of a dislocated hip. (See Chapter 5, Dislocated Hip.)

With increased strength of the back muscles, the infant is now able to flip from the back to the abdomen. (See Chapter 4, Safety.)

MOBILITY

Infants 4 to 6 months old will propel themselves forward when on the abdomen by pulling the knees up to the chest and pushing with the legs.

By the end of 6 months the infant will be able to roll completely over from the back to the stomach to the back.

The 4-month-old infant will enjoy sitting with support and by 6 months will sit momentarily without support.

As infants grow older, caretakers may have to move furniture away from the crib to prevent infants from reaching objects that may be harmful to them.

Do not leave the infant unattended when on the bed, couch, dressing table, or any flat surface from which the infant can roll.

Caretakers may prop infants in sitting positions using infant seats for short periods each day. Infant seats and propping should never take the place of being held.

At first the infant will need assistance in assuming a sitting position, but by 6 months will attain this position without assistance.

The increasing motor ability of infants now enables them to move toward objects either by rolling over or pushing the body forward when on the abdomen.

Once infants are able to assume a sitting position without assistance, some may develop the ability to move backwards by pushing with the feet and hands, which is sometimes referred to as "hitching."

As infants continue to develop muscle control and coordination, reflexes such as the *Moro and tonic neck* reflexes will disappear.

This increased mobility requires additional precautions for a safe environment for the infant.

Psychological

DEPENDENCY

The infant remains dependent on caretakers for all needs.

As the infant's needs are anticipated and met, a sense of trust develops.

The consistency and manner in which needs are met contribute to the development of trust.

SELF-CENTEREDNESS

Although dependent on others, infants are totally consumed in themselves. They are aware of the physical presence of others, but are unaware of others' needs.

The typical position assumed by infants with flexed arms and legs held close to their bodies reflects self-centeredness.

| **GROWTH AND DEVELOPMENTAL LANDMARKS** | **ANTICIPATORY GUIDANCE** |

Psychological—cont'd

SELF-CENTEREDNESS—cont'd

Self-centeredness is in relation to the basic psychological needs such as eating, sleeping, elimination, and comfort.

Self-absorption can be recognized by the infant's immediate need for satisfaction, especially in regard to feeding. Infants want what they want, when they want it.

Self-centeredness is seen in infants' awareness now of their own body parts such as hands, fingers, and movements of arms.

Infants become fascinated with the movement of their fingers, hands, toes, and feet. This begins when the infants, for a fleeting moment, see their fingers and hands move; as muscle control develops, they will hold hands in their line of vision for long periods.

Social

SOCIAL AWARENESS

Infants are becoming more aware of others. By the end of the third month, the infant will consistently recognize the caretaker's voice and touch. At 6 months the infant is able to differentiate between caretakers, siblings, and strangers.

Infants' increasing awareness of people and objects makes it possible for them to be distracted for a few minutes or even longer periods of time before their needs are met.

Infants of this age are beginning to demonstrate a desire to be held and loved. They tend to cling closely to the caretaker's body when held and give the impression of not wanting to let go.

Infants should be held, fondled, and loved other than just at feeding time. Caretakers should not only hold the infants, but talk to them as well.

Infants should be introduced to other adults such as grandparents, relatives, and friends as long as these individuals are free of upper respiratory tract infection or other contagious illnesses.

Between 4 and 6 months infants become much more sociable than in earlier periods of infancy.

Infants enjoy social contact, and their enthusiastic responses encourage caretakers to spend more time with them.

Infants are now differentiating between various members of the household and definitely recognize the caretaker. By 6 months they may show anxiety in the presence of strangers.

Introduction of strangers to the infant should be done while the infant is held by the caretaker to decrease the infant's anxiety.

It is recommended that small children should not be permitted to hold the infant unless the caretaker supports the infant as well.

INVESTIGATIVE

Infants' increased hand-eye coordination and increased dexterity of the fingers and thumb permit infants to more readily pick up small objects and place them in their mouths.

By the end of the third month, infants will have enough voluntary muscle control to direct objects to their mouths.

Infants tend to pull small pieces of fuzz from blankets and twirl them in their fingers, brush them across their cheeks, as well as put them into their mouths.

Toys must be selected with the following criteria in mind, not only for safety, but for sensory stimulation:
1. Free of small loose parts
2. Unbreakable
3. Nontoxic
4. Smooth, free of sharp edges
5. Bright and colorful
6. Musical

Examples of toys include mobiles, rattles, music boxes, soft animals, and soft blocks.

Vision and hearing are still rudimentary.

TESTERS

The infant begins early to test people in the environment. Crying becomes the tool through which the infant gets attention.

As caretakers become tuned in to the cry of their infant, they soon are able to differentiate a cry of hunger from a cry of discomfort or pain.

Through loving, consistent attention to the infant's needs, a trusting relationship soon develops between the infant and the caretaker.

Establishment of this basic sense of trust in the infant prepares a firm foundation on which future personality traits will be built.

GROWTH AND DEVELOPMENTAL LANDMARKS	ANTICIPATORY GUIDANCE

RELATIONSHIPS

Infants have the ability to relate differently to people in their environment. This is most noticeable in the infant's facial expressions and the position assumed when being held. The infant will assume a relaxed position when held by someone known from previous contact. However, when infants are held by someone they do not know, they will tend to become fretful, pull away, and hold themselves rigid.

Relationships are best developed when the infant's needs are met in a calm, deliberate, quiet, and loving manner. Loud noises, bright lights, and abrupt movements will startle the infant.

Opportunities for developing relationships with other small children, such as siblings, should be encouraged. Siblings should be involved in the infant's care by bringing articles to the caretaker, such as clothing and diapers. Permitting small children to hold infants should not be encouraged.

VOCALIZATION

Crying is the infant's first method of vocalization and is used to express needs such as discomfort and distress.

Infants cry much less by the third month, developing an additional method of vocalization, that of cooing, especially when content.

When the infant is awake and cooing, respond to this attempt to communicate with you by talking back. Consistent chatter will encourage further communication and diminish the period of crying. Refrain from the use of baby talk to facilitate appropriate word usage as the infant develops future verbal communication patterns.

Infants cry to communicate needs and to control the environment. Although distress cries need to be responded to immediately, caretakers must learn to feel comfortable in delaying the immediate gratification of some of the infant's needs. Caretakers can prevent infants from controlling the environment.

Infants progress from cooing and babbling to vocalizing with pleasure and displeasure by the sixth month.

A softly played radio or record player will provide sounds and different voices. The volume of sound to which infants are exposed today causes some concern.

Vocalization becomes a repetitive use of syllables that have no specific meaning but are used by the infant when in contact with people and toys.

Encourage caretakers to provide opportunities for socialization and play periods.

CHAPTER 3

LATE INFANCY   *7 through 12 months*

During the seventh through the twelfth month of life the infant evolves from a passive, receptive being to a sociable, giving individual. Dependency of the infant on the caretaker still exists, but infants will now venture out to try new experiences.

The curiosity of infants encourages use of newly acquired skills as they investigate and explore everything within the environment. Infants 7 to 12 months old delight in new experiences and are challenged by new things and people. Caretakers find this age infant enjoyable but also in need of close supervision from dangers both inside and outside the home.

Sociability and eagerness to be with others make this age infant a delight to be with. They are more receptive to overtures of attention and love. Their imitated responses make for pleasurable relationships between themselves and others. Infants in the second half of the first year will also initiate social contact by babbling, reaching out, handling toys, and playing simple social games.

These late infancy babies sleep all night, requiring only one nap a day. Awaking happy, they will content themselves in self-play, no longer needing immediate attention for a diaper change or feeding. The infant is settling into predictable routines. During this period, infants begin to learn expected behaviors for many new situations. Although infants adapt to the household patterns better than in earlier months, new points of frustration occur.

Mealtime will often be the time infants become assertive and thus begins the battle of the wills between the infant and caretaker. Infants can control a mealtime. Eating patterns do change. The infant is often more interested in skill development than in eating. Consistency in the way in which caretakers react to trying situations helps infants learn limits and permits a sense of trust to become more firmly established.

Anticipatory guidance is provided for caretakers for each of the expected new biological, psychological, and social developmental landmarks.

| GROWTH AND DEVELOPMENTAL LANDMARKS | ANTICIPATORY GUIDANCE |

Biological

WEIGHT

Weight gain continues to approximate 1 pound (0.45 kg) a month (3 to 5 ounces; weekly) from 7 to 12 months of age.

Infants usually triple their birth weight by 1 year of age. For example, if an infant weighed 7 pounds (3.15 kg) at birth, at 1 year the infant's weight will be approximately 21 pounds (9.45 kg).

Although infants double their birth weight by 5 months, they will have tripled their weight by 1 year of age.

Increased mobility and interest in surroundings begin to decrease the infant's preoccupation with food and mealtimes.

Remind caretakers that a decreased appetite is normal.

HEIGHT

Infants increase in height by approximately ½ inch (1.25 cm) per month.

Infants height will increase to approximately one and a half times their birth length. For example, if an infant at birth was 21 inches (52.5 cm) long, by 1 year the infant's height will be 30 to 31 inches (75 to 77.5 cm).

Infants continue to appear taller when lying relaxed in bed because the extremities are extended and not held in the flexed position maintained when the infant is awake.

HEART RATE

The heart rate continues to have a wide range of normal, between 100 to 140 beats per minute.

The cardiac rate and rhythm are unique for each infant.

The cardiac rate is still best attained at the apex of the heart with a stethoscope (Fig. 1-2).

Cardiac rates must be evaluated in relation to the circumstances in which the infant is found.

Caretakers may need assurance in regard to the readily felt pulsations of the heart against the chest wall.

RESPIRATIONS

The respiratory rate decreases and begins to stabilize but continues to have a wide range of normal.

It is not unusual for an infant to have a respiratory rate as high as 36 to 40 breaths per minute or as low as 20 to 25 breaths per minute.

Respirations continue to be primarily abdominal.

Respiratory rates must be evaluated in relation to the circumstances in which the infant is found.

Infants develop their own unique patterns and rates of breathing.

TEMPERATURE

Temperatures for the 7- to 12-month-old infant continue to range between 96.8° to 99.6° F (36° to 37.5° C).

Alterations in body temperature occur as a result of changes in environmental temperature, fluid intake, activity, and metabolic changes.

Dress infants appropriately for the climate and activity. The 7- to 12-month-old infant is more active than a newborn, thus requiring fewer clothes.

Offer clear fluids to infants between feedings, especially during hot weather, to make up for fluid loss from perspiration. Gelatin and gelatin and water are excellent clear fluids.

HEAD

The head and chest circumferences are equal.

MOUTH

Teeth usually become visible about the sixth month, beginning with the central incisors (upper and lower).

Teeth erupt on an average of one per month from 6 to 12 months of age. The average 1-year-old will therefore have from six to eight teeth.

The teething process involves long periods of mouthing, biting, chewing, and gumming objects.

The gums may appear red and swollen and be tender to touch. (See Chapter 4, Dentition.)

Some infants may not have any teeth by 1 year of age.

Oral hygiene continues to involve offering water between feedings. If an infant is accustomed to going to bed with a bottle, fill it with water, because the sugar residue found in other liquids predisposes to dental caries.

GROWTH AND DEVELOPMENTAL LANDMARKS	ANTICIPATORY GUIDANCE

Biological—cont'd

HEAD—cont'd

Health workers must be alert to the environmental dangers of lead poisoning. (See Chapter 8, Poisoning.)

Objects on which infants chew should be inspected carefully to prevent them from swallowing small pieces of substances that may be injurious.

Counsel caretakers in regard to possible sources of lead poisoning. For example, in the past, lead-base paints were used to paint furniture and homes. It is possible that lead-base paints may still be in the infant's environment.

EYES

Increased binocular coordination is evident at this age. Infants actively participate in games of peek-a-boo and follow objects easily.

A simple game of peek-a-boo helps prepare the infant for future periods of separation from the caretaker. The awareness and knowledge that the object will reappear strengthen the bond of trust between the infant and caretaker.

MOBILITY

A rapid increase in the motor abilities of infants is seen between 7 and 12 months of age.

Motor activities include creeping, crawling, standing, cruising, and walking.

Infants proceed at their own rate and pattern of development. Some infants may stay in the crawling and cruising stage longer than others, whereas some spend no time at all in these stages, progressing rapidly from sitting to standing to walking. A characteristic feature of the infant's walk is standing on tiptoes and then lifting the legs high, reminiscent of the stepping reflex seen in the newborn.

Precautionary measures must be instituted to ensure a safe environment in which the child may explore. Furniture, dangling cords or cloths, open stairwells, and poisonous substances are but a few of the problem areas. (See Chapters 4 and 7, Safety.)

Although infants delight in cruising along holding onto furniture, even greater joy results from holding the hand of the caretaker and being able to walk across the room and down the halls.

That period of time when infants have learned to pull themselves to a standing position before learning to walk is often extremely frustrating to both infants and caretakers.

Infants learn to pull themselves to a stand before they learn how to let go and/or sit down again. Although the infant is delighted with the new skill of pulling to a stand, standing is tiring, and the infant soon cries for the caretaker to come to the rescue. Once rescued, the infant immediately practices the new skill again and again and again. Perhaps the most frustrating aspect of this new skill is that it is practiced most often at nap or nighttime sleep periods. Eventually the child does learn to release gently and sit down or lie down without help.

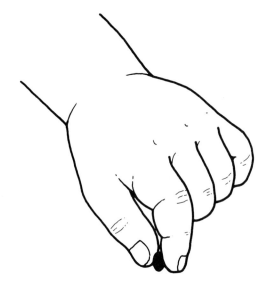

Fig. 3-1. Finger-thumb apposition. Finger-thumb apposition evident in late infancy period.

GROWTH AND DEVELOPMENTAL LANDMARKS	ANTICIPATORY GUIDANCE

Finger-thumb apposition occurs during this late infancy period and quickly becomes a refined act (Fig. 3-1).

Infants delight in learning how to pick up small objects using just the index finger and thumb. Once the infant has learned the trick, long periods of time will be spent in picking lint off blankets or small objects off the floor or ground.

Caution: Remember that infants continue to investigate the environment by putting things into their mouths.

To take advantage of the infant's newly refined skill, the caretaker should be encouraged to offer finger foods to the infant and encourage self-feeding. Examples of finger foods include non-sugared cereals, small pieces of toast, and crackers.

Safe and good eating habits can be developed by always having the infant eat only when in a high chair or at a table. (See Chapter 18, Feeding Techniques.)

Increased mobility strengthens muscle development of both arms and legs.

Infants should be provided with toys and equipment, such as pull toys, large blocks, big trucks or dolls, scooter chairs, and balls, that encourage muscle development.

Push toys, such as play vacuum cleaners and lawn mowers, will be more readily manipulated by the child in the next stage of development, toddlerhood.

Childproofing the rooms in which infants are permitted reduces the need to constantly negate an infant's exploratory behaviors. Removing nontouchable or breakable dishes, vases, or decorations during this period is recommended.

Children can be taught to respect objects of art used to decorate rooms at a later period of development.

Exploration of the outdoors is interesting to the infant who, through touch and taste, investigates new things such as grass, leaves, pebbles, dirt, cement, and insects.

Infants are challenged by uneven surfaces and coarse textures.

Caretakers can place a blanket on the ground so the infant can move from the familiar to the unfamiliar.

Psychological

DEPENDENCY

Although still dependent on others for physical needs, this age infant is entering the rudimentary period of decision making. This is evident in the infant's ability to change body position, select favorite objects, and discard items not wanted.

Caretakers are sometimes surprised to discover that decision making begins in infancy. Infants quickly determine the type and amounts of food they will eat. They try to determine their own nap and evening bedtime. Consistency of expectations and a sense of humor are valuable assets for caretakers during these battles of wills.

SELF-CENTEREDNESS

Self-centeredness appears more dominant at this stage as infants assert themselves more forcefully and more frequently than in the first 6 months of life.

Caretakers may have to begin setting limits for the infant at this stage because of their exploratory nature and lack of a sense of danger. (See Chapter 4, Discipline.)

Social

SOCIAL AWARENESS

Sociability in 7- to 12-month-old infants is more evident now because they desire to be in the company of other people.

The increased attentiveness and abilities of the infant enable them to participate in social exchanges with others such as simple games.

The infant wants to be in the presence of the caretaker and can be placed in a "teeter-chair," high chair, or playpen.

Participation games such as "peek-a-boo," "pat-a-cake," and "so-big" offer excellent opportunities for social interaction between the infant and others.

Further socialization with the caretaker or others can be provided by holding infants and reading to them. Books that will hold the infant's interest are those which have various textures, sounds, and bright colors. Infants should be permitted to examine and touch the various textures and assist in identifying the objects and colors.

27

GROWTH AND DEVELOPMENTAL LANDMARKS	ANTICIPATORY GUIDANCE

Social—cont'd

SOCIAL AWARENESS—cont'd

Infants may develop an attachment to a favorite toy or "security" blanket.

Infants often develop a fondness or attachment to a specific toy or blanket, requiring the object to be with them at night or naptime. The security object often becomes very dirty and quite ragged. Caretakers lament over the disreputable appearance of the object. The attachment frequently lasts well into toddlerhood and should not be discouraged because it provides comfort to the child during stressful situations such as illness, hospitalization, or separation from caretakers.

VOCALIZATION

Language development reveals a progression from meaningless babble to identifiable words. Initially, infants make sounds and later repetitively babble and coo sounds that are pleasurable to them. As early as 6 to 9 months of age infants begin to comprehend the meaning of words spoken to them, especially the word "no."

Infants usually imitate words or sounds that begin with consonants. At first the sounds have little meaning to the caretaker but gradually the sounds become more wordlike.

By the end of the first year, many infants will have a vocabulary of six to ten words. Some 1-year-olds exhibit no identifiable speech.

Remember, each infant develops at a unique rate. Learning is primarily through imitation and mimicry; it is important therefore to use correct terminology when teaching infants the names of objects and parts of their body.

The use of correct terminology provides a good role model for the development of proper speech patterns for the future.

Some infants develop a number of words by 1 year of age, although there are some who do not say any words at all.

TESTERS

The assertiveness and strong will of infants at this stage makes it possible for them to test caretakers to greater limits than in earlier periods of infancy. (See Chapter 4, Discipline.)

The battle of wills begins in infancy and frequently centers around eating and sleeping. If caretakers could be convinced that the negativistic behavior of the infant is not a deliberate act to annoy the caretaker, many problems would be substantially reduced.

Infants' desire to investigate and explore takes precedence over their pleasure with the eating process. Infants will eat enough to meet their needs, but perhaps less than the caretaker desires.

Infants' strong will is also demonstrated by their resistance to having their face and hands washed after meals or before bedtime. Caretakers should proceed firmly but kindly with the cleansing process, giving praise to the infant as it is being accomplished.

RELATIONSHIPS

Infants become more sociable, but relate differently to strangers than to caretakers or close relatives and friends.

Most infants, by 8 months, will have developed a strong attachment with a caretaker and become very anxious on separation. When reunited with the caretaker, the infant will cling with all four extremities as though fearful of another separation. (See Chapter 4, Hospitalization.)

Older infants enjoy being with people and delight in imitating adult behavior such as laughing, coughing, making faces, and gesturing.

Infants quickly learn that siblings might play with them, but adults will pick them up.

Although infants will fret over separation from caretakers, brief separations should be encouraged. As infants learn that caretakers will return, the sense of trust begun earlier in infancy becomes further established.

By the end of the first year, infants will initiate relationships with adults and siblings. They will try to go to the person and extend their arms to be picked up and held.

Infants likewise initiate play with siblings and adults by pointing at their nose or eyes and enjoy repeating this behavior.

CHAPTER 4

HEALTH MAINTENANCE FOR INFANTS

Health maintenance and the promotion of sound health practices started during the period of uterine development must continue once the infant is born. From birth through 1 year of age, the infant should be seen quite frequently by health care workers. Typically the visits begin at 4 to 6 weeks and are continued on a monthly basis through the fourth to sixth month. Health maintenance visits then usually decrease to every 3 months.

Patterns for eating, sleeping, and communicating will be unique for each infant. Adjusting to and anticipating routine needs of the infant the first few months are anxiety provoking for the caretaker.

As infants grow and develop, their new skills and abilities predispose them to accidents and injuries. Infants also have little natural resistance to disease. The antibodies that newborns received from their mothers disappear by 3 months of age. Most infants do not begin to develop antibodies of their own until they have been exposed to infectious organisms. During health care conferences, immunizations are given that enable the infant to develop these important antibodies.

The well-baby conferences provide the health care worker with opportunities to assess the progress of the infant and provide the caretakers with opportunities to discuss concerns they may have. Topics that frequently concern caretakers include diet, sleep, toys, and the progress of the infant. Caretakers (particularly first-time parents) need reassurance about the baby's progress and their own ability to care for this infant.

During this period of life, when infants are totally dependent on others for their care, the health professional's focus of attention for the teaching of sound health practices must be on the caretaker, since it is the caretaker who is responsible for the health care of the infant. If good health practices are established during infancy, this pattern of health care is likely to be followed in the future.

Areas of concern for the maintenance of a healthy infant plus helpful hints for the caretaker will be discussed in this chapter.

<table>
<tr><td>

AREAS FOR CONCERN

Health conference

The health care conference is one of the golden opportunities when health teaching and anticipatory guidance can be given for this stage of the child's life and to prepare the caretaker for expected future landmarks of development and achievement that warrant concern for safety, health protection, and additional health supervision.

Health care conferences during infancy are once a month up through 6 months of age, then at 9 months of age and at 1 year. (This schedule may vary with the needs of child.)

Health history

The health care conference begins with a health history, which provides the examiner with beginning baseline data in regard to health status.

At the first health care conference the examiner will review the pregnancy, labor, and delivery. Information will be gathered in regard to family members, particularly directed toward health problems that may exist.

During subsequent visits the examiner will continue to inquire about family members, although the major focus will be on the infant.

Information will be gathered on the habits and activities of the infant. Concerns the caretaker might have will be responded to by the health care workers.

Health assessment: physical examination

A physical examination will be performed, at which time the examiner will assess the infant's biological, psychological, and social development.

The unique pattern of growth and development for this infant will be revealed as an outcome of the examination and will provide a base for future health assessments.

Deviations from normal expectations of growth and development will be identified.

The health examiner might well identify health problems such as clubfoot (talipes equinovalgus or talipes equinovarus), a congenital dislocated hip, premature closure of the fontanels, cardiac murmurs, arrhythmias and/or developmental lags to name but a few.

A general examination will be performed by the examiner assessing the infant from head to toe. During the examination the infant will be undressed (although a diaper may cover the genitalia) and placed in a supine or prone position on an examining table. The caretaker is usually encouraged to stand at the head or side of the table.

Body measurements for height and weight will be obtained.

Vital signs of temperature, pulse, and respirations will be secured. Blood pressure readings are not usually secured during infancy.

Examination of the eyes, ears, nose, and throat will be performed.

Palpation and auscultation of the chest and abdomen will follow.

</td><td>

HELPFUL HINTS

The examiner will spend some time conversing with caretakers to make them feel comfortable and at ease.

Routine health visits are necessary to determine health progress, identify existing problems, and prevent future health problems.

The health history provides the health examiner with clues that may alert them to potential familial or congenital problems of the infant.

It is important at this time for the caretaker to provide any information regarding illness, high fever, injury (of any type), and stressful situations to which the infant has been exposed.

If for any reason the infant was seen by another health examiner since the last visit, this information should also be shared because a complete history is extremely helpful for the total picture of health assessment.

During the physical examination many of the areas listed for examination will be performed but not necessarily in the sequence presented here.

The examiner will gather data for many areas of assessment through only one or two procedures.

The presence of a caretaker during the physical examination provides the infant a sense of security.

If the infant wets or soils during the examination, caretakers should not be alarmed, since examiners expect this to happen.

As the mobility skills of the infant increase, it is essential that the caretaker or health personnel have a hand on the infant at all times.

The examiner may assess pulse, respiration, and chest sounds while the infant is being held by the caretaker.

Caretakers may be asked to assist during certain procedures such as holding the infant while the eyes, ears, nose, and throat are being examined or the temperature is being taken.

</td></tr>
</table>

AREAS FOR CONCERN

HELPFUL HINTS

Muscle tone and skeletal structure will be evaluated with the infant in both the supine (lying on back) and prone (lying on abdomen) positions. Throughout the first 12 months of life this portion of the examination will be directed to new abilities such as sitting, creeping, and standing.

Although the infant cries during the examination, caretakers should be assured that the procedures are not painful, and discomfort is quickly forgotten.

The presence or absence of landmark reflexes will be evaluated throughout the examination. (See growth and developmental landmarks for specific age.)

Permitting older infants to see and touch equipment, such as a stethoscope and/or tongue blade, may facilitate cooperation.

The infant will be given an opportunity to hold, reach for, grasp, and/or manipulate toys and other objects.

At times the examiner may speak softly, and at other times harsh or loud sounds will be deliberately made that cause the infant to startle or cry.

An external examination of the genitalia will also be included.

Permitting an infant to hold and manipulate toys or other objects provides evidence of increased motor skills and sensory development.

Health assessment: mental and social evaluation

The cognitive and affective abilities of the infant are assessed throughout the health care conference.

Health protection

Health protection in infancy focuses on immunization. Immunizations are available to prevent the occurrence of the following illnesses:

The initial series of immunizations (to protect the infant from certain diseases) is usually started about 2 months of age, provided there is no fever or illness.

1. Diphtheria (immunization begun before 1 year)
2. Pertussis (immunization begun before 1 year)
3. Tetanus (immunization begun before 1 year)
4. Poliomyelitis (immunization begun before 1 year)
5. Measles (immunization begun after 1 year)
6. Mumps (immunization begun after 1 year)
7. Rubella (immunization begun after 1 year)

Immunizations are contraindicated when the infant has an elevated temperature or illness.

At 2 months of age a diphtheria, pertussis, and tetanus (DPT) injection and trivalent oral poliovirus vaccine (TOPV) are given.

At 4 months of age, a second injection of DPT and TOPV are given.

At 6 months of age the third DPT injection is given. A third dose of TOPV might be given in some areas of the country.

Diphtheria, pertussis, and tetanus (DPT) vaccines are given by injection and protect the infant from diphtheria, pertussis (whooping cough), and tetanus (lockjaw). Caretakers may be asked to assist in holding the infant still when the injection is being given. Following injections the infant should be held and comforted by the caretaker. Three different forms of poliomyelitis vaccine (TOPV) are given orally to protect the infant from poliomyelitis (infantile paralysis or polio).

Infants might be irritable, have slight fever, and evidence a reddened area at the injection site within a few hours after immunization is given. These symptoms disappear within a few days.

If the caretaker reports an unusual reaction to the first DPT immunization, this may be sufficient reason to discontinue immunization. Unusual reactions include high fever, convulsions, or shock.

Some infants may exhibit more severe reactions to the immunization that will warrant alteration or postponement of the immunization series. If the infant reacted to an immunization, this information should be shared with the health professional.

Immunization records that are updated and kept at home are helpful reminders to caretakers of each child's series of protection.

At 12 months of age a tuberculin test (not an immunization) is given to determine the presence of tuberculin antibodies.

See Appendix A.

The tuberculin test is performed at this time to determine if the infant has been exposed to individuals who have tuberculosis. A positive test *does not* mean the child has the disease, but does indicate that the child has been exposed and has developed some resistance to the disease.

AREAS FOR CONCERN	**HELPFUL HINTS**

Health promotion

The health care conference includes discussion and review of the following topics, although not necessarily in the sequence presented:

1. Dentition: The number, position, condition, and pattern of tooth eruption. Recommend when to begin dental evaluation and periodic visits. Review measures of oral hygiene.
2. Nutrition: Discussion regarding changes in eating habits, dietary needs, and vitamin supplements.
3. Elimination: Review patterns of elimination.
4. Play and activity: Evaluation and discussion of a 24-hour period for play and activity.
5. Sleep and rest: Discussion will center on changing needs and patterns of sleep and rest.
6. Safety and accident prevention: Areas of concern will be discussed as they relate to the child's increasing sphere of activity.
7. Other areas to be included will be specific for each age period.

The health care conference is never complete without a period of clarification of the caretaker's questions in regard to the child's progress or additional concerns.

Many areas of concern will be discussed during the health care conference.

Caretakers can use the conference time most beneficially if they bring with them a written list of health problems and concerns that they have.

DENTITION

Tooth eruption begins between 5 and 7 months of age.

Each infant has a unique pattern and rate of tooth eruption. Tooth eruption typically follows this pattern: upper central incisors, lower central incisors, and upper lateral incisors.

Oral hygiene during infancy is best achieved by offering the infant a few mouthfuls of water after each feeding.

Tooth eruption (cutting teeth) usually begins by 5 to 7 months of age.

Excessive drooling, irritability, and desire to gum objects may be the first clues of tooth eruption.

By 1 year of age many infants will have six teeth. Some infants will have no teeth, whereas others have more than six at 1 year of age.

Zwieback, teething biscuits, or hard teething rings may provide comfort to the teething infant. Some teething rings can be refrigerated and prove to be very soothing when the cooled ring is gummed by the infant.

A mild fever may accompany teething. Providing cool clear liquids while the fever persists proves beneficial in meeting fluid needs and reducing fever.

Some teething infants may refuse nipple feedings and prefer drinking from a cup or being fed from a spoon.

NUTRITION

Fluid requirements

Daily fluid requirements for infants from birth to 1 year of age will increase in volume as the infant grows.

During the first few months of life, fluid needs are based on the infant's weight. The average fluid requirement is 2 to 3 ounces (60 to 90 ml) per pound of body weight or 150 ml* per kilogram of body weight. For example, if an infant weighs 7 pounds (3.1 kg):

7 pounds × 2 ounces = 14 ounces (420 ml)/day
7 pounds × 3 ounces = 21 ounces (630 ml)/day

This infant should receive 14 to 21 ounces (420 to 630 ml) of fluid every day.

This method of determining fluid needs ceases to be appropriate when the computation exceeds 1 quart (32 ounces; 1000 ml/day).

Every infant is unique. Infants usually drink the amount of fluid that their bodies need without much encouragement.

Some newborns might wish to be fed every 3 hours, whereas others might wish to be fed more often. The amount of milk (breast or formula) taken at each feeding varies, usually ranging from 2 to 3 ounces (60 to 90 ml). Water or glucose water (sugar water) can be offered between feedings. Newborns need a total of 14 to 21 ounces (420 to 630 ml) of liquid a day.

As the infant grows older, the amount of milk consumed at each feeding increases (3 to 4 ounces; 90 to 120 ml), and the number of feedings decreases. Often by 3 months, an infant fed at 9 or 10 PM will sleep through the night before waking for the next feeding. Water and clear liquids should continue to be offered between feedings. (Juices are added to the diet sometime after the first month).

*Milliliter (ml) is equivalent to cubic centimeter (cc).

AREAS FOR CONCERN

The amount of fluid taken at any one feeding will increase the first year:

1 to 2 months—3 to 4 ounces (90 to 120 ml) per feeding

4 to 6 months—5 to 6 ounces (150 to 180 ml) per feeding

8 to 12 months—7 to 8 ounces (210 to 240 ml) per feeding

The number of feeding times in 24 hours will also change from month to month as follows:

Birth to 3 months—six feedings per day

4 to 6 months—five feedings per day

7 to 12 months—four feedings per day

Fluids such as water or glucose water should be offered two or three times a day to the infant under 2 months of age. As the infant grows older, juices are added to the diet and may be substituted as one of the additional fluids.

Health professionals should caution caretakers that the amount of milk (breast, formula, or whole milk) consumed by the infant in any 24-hour period should not exceed 1 quart (1000 ml). If the child is thirsty, other liquids should be offered. If the child is hungry, solid foods should be increased.

One method to determine if fluid intake is sufficient is to test the infant's skin turgor. The skin should have a feeling of substance and solidity when grasped between the index finger and thumb. Skin turgor is normal if, when the skin is released, it quickly rebounds to normal position. If the skin does not rebound quickly, hydration or fluid volume may not be sufficient.

Caloric requirements

Daily caloric requirements for the first year of life range from 35 to 50 calories per pound (80 to 110 calories per kilogram) of body weight.

Neonatal period (first month)—35 calories per pound of body weight

1 to 12 months—50 calories per pound of body weight.

Caloric needs can be computed as follows:

Newborn weighing 7 pounds

7 pounds × 35 calories = 245 calories per day (3.1 kg × 80 calories = 248 calories per day)

5-month-old weighing 14 pounds

14 pounds × 50 calories = 700 calories per day (6.3 kg × 110 calories = 693 calories per day)

At 1 year of age the daily caloric requirement is 1000 calories per day.

There are 20 calories in each ounce of breast milk, cow's milk, and most prepared formulas. To determine the number of ounces of milk needed to supply the daily caloric requirement, the following formula can be used:

Newborn weighing 7 pounds

Formula (20 calories per ounce)

14 ounces (daily fluid requirement)

14 ounces × 20 = 280 calories

Most neonates will not consume the total amount of formula offered. There is no need for concern because caloric needs will be met. However, daily fluid requirements will have to be met by offering clear liquids between feedings.

HELPFUL HINTS

Infants 4 through 6 months of age average five feedings a day with amounts that range from 3 to 6 ounces (90 to 180 ml).

From 7 to 12 months the feedings decrease to four a day with amounts that range from 7 to 8 ounces (210 to 240 ml).

By the end of the first year, the infant usually drinks milk at each of the three meals, and another liquid feeding is taken at bedtime.

Avoid giving infants of any age more than 1 quart (1000 ml) of milk a day. More than 1 quart of milk per day can contribute to a health problem called *milk anemia*. Milk is a poor source of iron. (See Chapter 14, Iron Deficiency Anemia.)

Caretakers frequently are concerned that their infants are not receiving enough food. The newborn (through the first month of life) needs about 35 calories per pound of weight. Most newborns who are breast-fed or take prepared formulas receive many more calories than they need. Breast milk, cow's milk, and prepared formulas all average 20 calories per ounce.

If the infant weighs 7 pounds (3.15 kg) and drinks 13 ounces (390 ml) of formula then the calorie needs of the day are met.

7 pounds × 35 calories = 245 calories

13 ounces × 20 calories = 260 calories

Offering water between feedings provides the extra fluid the baby needs and prevents thirst.

As the infant grows older, it is still possible to meet caloric needs by increasing the amount of milk, but it is more important for good health that solid foods are added to the diet.

If the infant consistently requires feeding more often than every 3 to 4 hours, an alteration in formula or diet may be required.

Health promotion—cont'd

NUTRITION—cont'd

     5-month-old weighing 14 pounds

      Milk (20 calories per ounce)

      30 ounces (daily fluid requirement)

      30 ounces × 20 calories = 600 calories

      It is important at this time for the health professional to assess the total dietary intake, since solid foods added to the diet will increase the number of calories consumed.

Additional foods

   Solids are usually introduced during infancy when infants have hearty appetites and are willing and eager to try new foods.

   The involuntary forward motion of the tongue (extrusion reflex) that accompanies the sucking process will sometimes delay the infant's ability to ingest solid foods.

   During infancy the sense of taste is somewhat ill defined because taste buds are not yet fully developed.

Solid foods are introduced into the infant's diet somewhere between 1 and 3 months of age. Solids are not added earlier because the infant's digestive system is not mature enough to use the foods. (See Appendix B.)

Rice cereal is usually the first solid food given to an infant because it is easily digested and least likely to cause an allergic response. Introduction of whole wheat cereals is delayed because they are known to cause allergic responses. Cereal, when first introduced, should be prepared to a consistency much like the formula.

Infants will readily accept food placed in their mouths. Caretakers often mistakenly believe the baby does not like solid foods because the food is pushed back out of the mouth by an involuntary forward motion of the tongue. Remember, the baby is accustomed to sucking. The movement of the tongue for sucking purposes is directly opposite to the movement needed for eating solids. Infants quickly acquire the new skill if caretakers are patient and keep returning the food to the mouth. Successful introduction of solid food can be accomplished by supporting the infant in a sitting position, and, with a small spoon, place the food well onto the back of the tongue.

When infants are between 6 weeks and 3 months old, fruits, vegetables, egg yolk, and meats are introduced into the diet. Mashed ripe bananas and homemade applesauce are two foods that are most readily introduced into the infant's diet, since they are naturally sweetened and require little effort in preparation.

Neither solid foods (cereals, fruits, etc.) nor medicines should ever be added to the infant's bottle. Infant feeders that push food into the infant's mouth are also to be avoided.

Add only one new food at any given mealtime. A new food should be introduced several days in a row (4- to 7-day intervals) before the addition of another food. The purpose of this pattern is to note the child's tolerance as well as to identify any allergic response.

Some additional guidelines on feeding infants follow:

1. Not all infants will eat the same amount of food.
2. Prepare small portions (1 to 3 teaspoons) of food at a time.
3. Remove the quantity of food to be used from the baby food jar.
4. Place the baby food jar (with remainder of food) in the refrigerator between feedings.
5. Label each baby food jar with the date the jar was opened.
6. Discard the unused baby food within 48 hours after opening.

See Chapter 18, Feeding Techniques.

   Protein is necessary in the infant's diet, and the requirements are as follows:

     Birth to 6 months—2.2 g/kg of body weight

     6 to 12 months—2 g/kg of body weight

Protein is found in adequate amounts in milk for the young infant and in milk, cereal, and meats in the diet of the older infant.

AREAS FOR CONCERN	HELPFUL HINTS

Mineral and vitamin requirements

The rapid physical growth during infancy requires a number of minerals and vitamins that are necessary for cellular growth and organ function. Those minerals and vitamins of vital importance for the body metabolism and function will be briefly discussed.

Minerals

Calcium: For bone mineralization, tooth formation, and muscle and nerve function.

Daily requirement: 350 to 500 mg/day.

Iron: For formation of hemoglobin (the oxygen-carrying component of red blood cells.)

The fetal store of iron is depleted by the third to fourth month of life.

Daily requirement: 10 to 15 mg/day.

The best source of calcium is milk. However, caretakers should be cautioned about encouraging consumption of large quantities of milk because this may contribute to milk anemia. (See Chapter 14, Iron Deficiency Anemia.)

Breast milk or formula will not provide sufficient quantities of iron needed for the growth of the infant. Solid foods such as cereal, egg yolk, and meats provide the infant with adequate amounts. Egg yolks, a good source of iron, are added to an infant's diet between the third to fourth month of life. Egg whites are not usually introduced at this time because infants are not readily able to use the protein egg whites provide. The protein of egg whites has also been known to cause allergies.

Vitamins

Vitamin A: For tissue growth and resistance to infection. Vitamin A is especially important for development of the skin and eyes.

Daily requirement: 1400 to 2000 international units (IU) per day.

Vitamin C: For absorption of iron, tissue growth and healing, resistance to disease, and metabolic activities.

Daily requirement: 35 mg/day.

Vitamin D: For absorption of calcium and phosphorus necessary for bone growth.

Daily requirement: 400 IU/day.

Vitamin K: For blood clotting and the formation of prothrombin.

Vitamin E: For muscle and blood cell formation.

Daily requirement: 4 to 5 IU/day.

B-complex vitamins: Include thiamine, niacin, and riboflavin, all of which are important for enzyme activity, energy production, cellular oxidation, and metabolism.

B vitamins: For blood cell formation and muscle and nerve function. These vitamins include vitamin B_{12} (cobalamin), vitamin B_6 (pyridoxine), and folic acid (folacin).

Health professionals must assess nutritional intake of infants at each health conference. Caretakers will need to be counseled as to the necessity for meeting the daily mineral and vitamin needs of the infant as well as to not exceed the recommended daily amount.

Infants' diets usually provide them with an adequate amount of vitamins needed for growth. Liquid multivitamins are usually suggested as supplements and added to the diet in the first month of life.

Formulas and bottled milk are usually fortified with vitamins A and D.

Foods such as cereals, fruits, and vegetables contain sufficient quantities of the other needed vitamins.

ELIMINATION

Urination

Infants will urinate frequently within a 24-hour period.

Urine is often retained for several hours during sleep. Infants therefore have a wide range of normal frequency varying from five to thirty or more times every 24 hours. (Five to eight well-soaked diapers is quite typical.)

Infants urinate quite frequently each day, often on waking up and during or just after a feeding.

Cleansing of the genitalia and buttocks is necessary at each diaper change and more so when the ammonia odor prevails.

AREAS FOR CONCERN	HELPFUL HINTS

Health promotion—cont'd

ELIMINATION—cont'd

The urine normally is clear, pale yellow, and has a minimal ammonia odor. If the child is dehydrated, the color is darker, the odor stronger, and the amount eliminated is less.

A strong ammonia odor may be indicative of one or two things. The diaper has been wet for sometime and decomposition of urine is taking place, or the urine is highly concentrated because of poor hydration.

Diapers should be changed as soon as they are wet to prevent skin irritation and excoriation due to the decomposition of urine once it has been excreted. (See Chapter 5, Diaper rash; Chapter 18, Bathing an Infant.)

Urine that becomes cloudy or has noticeable changes in color may be indicative of a urinary tract infection (Chapter 8).

Bowel movements

Bowel movements will vary in frequency, consistency, and color due to dietary changes.

The neonate's stools are quite different from the stools of older infants.

Meconium (the first stools after birth or fecal waste) consists of thick sticky material that is dark green to black.

Transitional stools (stools that occur from the second through fifth day) consist of mucuslike material ranging from dark green to yellow green.

Infant stools (stools that occur after digestion of food such as formulas or breast milk) are indicative of the food ingested.

The breast-fed infant's stools are liquid or soft with small curds, have an almost pleasant odor, and are light yellow. Breast-fed infants have more stools a day than do formula-fed infants.

Formula-fed infant stools are soft to firm, with larger curds than breast-fed babies, have an inoffensive to strong odor, and are yellow to brown.

Infants receiving whole milk have stools that are firm to hard, have a strong odor, and are light to dark brown.

Older infants who eat solids have stools characterized by the foods eaten. Beets, peas, and green beans will change the color of the stool. An overabundance of fruits or foods high in sugar will contribute to loose stools. Diets high in cheese often lead to constipation. Diets high in fat lead to malodorous stools.

The number of bowel movements per day will vary depending on the food ingested and the infant's own pattern of elimination. Breast-fed infants will average two to four movements per day. Formula-fed infants and infants eating solids will average one or two bowel movements per day. The nature of the bowel movement is more important than the number.

Newborns will often have several bowel movements each day. The stools change in color, consistency, frequency, and odor as the baby grows older.

When the newborn first comes home from the hospital, the stool may be dark greenish to black and quite pasty or sticky. As the baby digests the milk obtained at each feeding, the stools change.

Breast-fed babies often have more frequent stools (2 to 4 a day) than formula-fed babies (1 or 2 a day). The breast-fed baby's stool is liquid or soft with small curds and is yellow.

The formula-fed baby has stools that are firm with large curds and are yellow-brown.

Infants receiving whole milk (4 months or older) have stools that are firm, formed, and brown.

Bowel movement consistency and color may be altered with the introduction of solid food. For example, beets will cause bowel movements to appear reddish, and green beans frequently will make the bowel movement green and softer.

As the solid food intake increases, the bowel movement becomes more formed or solid. Certain foods are known to cause constipation or diarrhea (Chapter 5).

PLAY AND ACTIVITY

Play in infancy refers to all forms of sensory stimulation that provide opportunities for development of physical, cognitive, and social skills.

Infants need to be exposed to different positions, materials, objects, sounds, and people.

Infants learn best through play.

Infants need time to play in and explore their environments from many different positions. Caretakers can change the infant's position during waking times to give the infants some time on their tummies, backs, and even propped on their sides. Different positions provide infants with opportunities to use different muscles, reach out, stretch, or even just view the world from different angles. As infants learn a new skill, they work to perfect it.

AREAS FOR CONCERN

Opportunities for infants to be alone with toys or safe objects that they can manipulate should also be provided.

Infants need to be held and cuddled. Talking, reading, and singing to infants provide additional pleasure.

Simple games such as "peek-a-boo," "pat-a-cake," "so-big," and identifying body parts should be introduced early in infancy. Infants quickly learn to mimic actions and sounds they see and hear.

Safety features must be considered when selecting toys for infants. Safety features to be included follow:
1. Smooth-edged objects
2. Sturdy and durable
3. Flame retardable or fire resistant
4. Parts that cannot be readily removed
5. Nontoxic paints (lead-base paints must be avoided)

SLEEP AND REST

The average sleeping time for infants may range between 14 and 18 hours a day. By the time the infant is 1 year of age, the amount of sleep required may be 12 hours.

Periods of sleep will be interrupted by periods of wakefulness.

The metabolic rate decreases when infants are asleep.

SAFETY AND ACCIDENT PREVENTION

The provision of a safe, secure environment is necessary to maintain health and promote the development of trust.

Through the third month of age muscular development is still immature and warrants support to the head and shoulder when lifting or holding the infant.

The motor ability is increasing rapidly. Infants learn to roll from the back to the abdomen in the second month, and in a few weeks will roll completely over.

Infants are able to push themselves forward with the knees and feet when on the abdomen at very young ages.

Hand-to-mouth coordination progresses rapidly after the third month.

HELPFUL HINTS

Infants must be provided with objects and toys that have different textures, sounds, and colors to enable them to learn more about their world. Avoid overstimulating the infant by providing too many things at one time.

Infants can entertain themselves for fairly long periods of time just looking at a mobile or moving their arms and legs.

Caretakers will notice that infants enjoy playing in water, feeling the wind against their faces, listening to new or sudden sounds, blinking at and staring at bright lights, and just plain enjoying new sensations.

Playing with and holding infants increase their social ability and desire to relate to others. Face-to-face contact is an excellent source of stimulation. Reading and singing to infants foster learning and intellectual abilities. Repetitive exposure to the same sounds encourage mimicry and lays the foundation for language development.

Beads and small toys are inappropriate for infants because they will put them in their mouths.

New stuffed toys should be inspected carefully to ensure that eyes cannot be removed easily.

When purchasing toys, inspect them carefully for safety features (flame resistance, smooth edges, nontoxic paint, and no small parts).

Infants need their own beds and preferably their own room. Ideally, the room is to be well ventilated and free from drafts. Opportunity for sleeping is provided after each feeding period during early infancy. (The amount of sleep needed decreases as the baby grows older.)

The safest position for sleep is on the side or abdomen after feeding. Pillows under the infant's head are not recommended because of the danger of suffocation. Lying on a flat firm surface is best for good posture.

A lightweight coverlet is desirable while the infant is sleeping to prevent chilling. Infants do not produce as much body heat when they sleep as when they are awake.

Sick infants may become fretful, often interrupting their own sleep at a time when additional rest is beneficial for the body to fight off the illness.

Selecting a crib must take into consideration the following points:
1. Siderails that can be adjusted to various levels and locked in place.
2. Bars on all four sides that are close enough to prevent the head from getting caught between them.
3. Free of lead-base paint.
4. Mattress firm and waterproof.

Infants suddenly develop the ability to turn over and roll anywhere after the sixth week. Keep a hand on the infant at all times when the infant is on a flat surface, such as a table, bed, or couch.

The use of plastic bags to protect surface areas from becoming soiled is a dangerous practice because infants can snuggle their faces into the plastic and suffocate.

AREAS FOR CONCERN	HELPFUL HINTS

Health promotion—cont'd

SAFETY AND ACCIDENT PREVENTION—cont'd

From 3 to 6 months of age the need for safety measures becomes more crucial. Gross motor skills are becoming more refined, curiosity is heightened, and mobility is increased. Infants will now readily place small objects into their mouths. It is not unusual by 6 months of age for the infant to be creeping about. Infants are now more stable in a sitting position and may even sit without support.

The ability of infants to place small objects into their mouths occurs about the fourth to sixth month. Caretakers must keep pins, beads, coins, and other small objects out of the crib and away from the reach of the baby.

Safety pins should always be closed and placed out of reach of the infant. (Avoid sticking pins into the mattress, since pinholes permit urine to enter the mattress.)

Infants often begin to creep by 6 months of age. When permitting the infant to creep about, "childproof" the area by placing all small objects out of reach. Infants by 6 months also enjoy scooter chairs in which they are able to place their feet on the floor and scoot themselves about.

By 1 year of age many infants will be walking, thus increasing the dangers to which they are exposed in the home.

Being able to travel, infants will be attracted to wall outlets and electric cords and fixtures. Place protective plates over wall sockets. Never leave extension cords plugged into a wall socket that is not being used. Infants will delight in pulling on lamp cords. Be extra vigilant in watching the infant when space heaters or fans are in service.

When using high chairs, secure the infant with a strap or safety belt. Even though infants appear secure in the high chair, never leave them alone because belts or straps do not totally inhibit the infant's ability to maneuver.

Safety of infants in a car cannot be overemphasized.

The caretakers should never permit the infant to sit on the lap while driving a car. Infants should be secured in an infant seat at all times when traveling in a car.

The use of an infant seat securely attached to the car safety belt (preferably in the back seat) can help minimize or prevent injury in case of an accident.

When moving about while carrying the infant, be aware of wet floors, toys, or other objects that may be underfoot.

A surprising number of injuries that do occur in this age are related to falls incurred by the caretaker while carrying the infant.

DISCIPLINE (LIMIT SETTING)

Discipline can be defined as the consistent guidance given to help children learn self-control and socially acceptable behaviors.

Children must be taught early in life that discipline by caretakers is necessary because they love them and want to protect them from the many dangers and pitfalls of life to which they will undoubtedly be exposed. Discipline has been likewise defined as those encompassing measures used by caretakers that are beneficial for children's physical, emotional, and social development.

The key to discipline is consistency, certainty, and authority, rendered with love.

Caretakers agree on behavioral expectations, rules to be followed, limits to be set, and methods of correction.

Inconsistency of limits will only cause confusion in the child, thus making difficult the differentiation of right from wrong as well as behavior that does or does not meet the caretaker's approval.

Hospitalization

Hospitalization may be necessary during infancy because of congenital defects, serious infection, diarrhea with dehydration, or for elective surgery such as a myringotomy or herniorrhaphy.

Adjustment for the infant to hospitalization will be less stressful if the infant has been accustomed to short absences from the caretaker and has been held by others for feeding or care in the presence of the caretakers. By 3 months of age the foundation of trust is becoming more firmly established.

If hospitalization is necessary for long periods of time, it is important that the caretaker stay with the infant. If the caretaker is not able to stay with the infant, consistency of care should be provided by only one or two health care workers.

If at all possible, the selection of a hospital in which the infant is to be confined should be one that permits and provides for the caretaker's presence at all times of the day or night.

AREAS FOR CONCERN

The strength of trust developed in the infant will be evident by the ease at which relationships are established with strange caretakers. Most 3-month-old infants will readily adapt to strangers. The 6- to 8-month-old infant will initially cling to the caretaker but quickly adapt to strangers. The 9- to 12-month-old infant finds this separation even more difficult. Separation anxiety increases in the later half of infancy because by this time the infant is well aware of caretakers and surroundings. Strangers and new surroundings increase the infant's anxiety.

The infant, prior to hospitalization, will likely need to have blood and urine tests performed.

For certain elective surgical procedures, preliminary laboratory tests are usually limited to a complete blood chemistry (CBC) test with a finger stick and urinalysis (preferably a clean-catch specimen). (See Chapter 18, Urine Specimen.)

When additional information is required, it may be necessary for more definitive laboratory tests to be performed.

The caretaker's cooperation and assistance are beneficial. Giving succinct, complete information about the tests and permitting the caretaker's participation will facilitate testing. (See Chapter 18, Immobilizing the Infant.)

Hospitalization and laboratory tests provoke anxiety in caretakers. Explanations and opportunities for the caretaker's expressions of concern and questions regarding procedures are encouraged.

Laboratory tests and a brief hospitalization are quickly forgotten by the infant who soon resumes typical behavior patterns. Infants at 3 months of age cannot readily localize the areas of pain or discomfort because receptors for pain are still immature. Therefore their response to discomfort or pain is a generalized response through irritability and crying.

Hospitalization may require the caretakers and health care workers to give extra love and sensory stimulation to the infant to maintain the basic sense of trust previously established. Providing periods of play is as important in the hospital as at home.

A golden opportunity exists during hospitalization for the health care workers to bring to the attention of caretakers those ways which nutritional patterns, needs for sensory stimulation, and safety of the infant will change.

Deprivation brought about by the absence of a loving caretaker can affect the growth and development of the infant. Following are some of the altered patterns of development:

1. Weight begins to fall below normal.
2. Motor development does not improve.
3. Infant evidences a decrease or lack of interest in surroundings and toys.
4. Sleep patterns are frequently altered.
5. The facial expression becomes passive, withdrawn, and shows little affect.

HELPFUL HINTS

Health care workers can more quickly relate to an infant if they develop a relationship with the caretakers. The initial approach to an infant should be while the infant is being held by the caretaker.

Caretakers are often encouraged to bring a familiar toy with the infant to ease the transition to the hospital setting. When selecting the familiar toy, it should be one that, if lost or broken, will not cause undue concern.

Raising questions about the care of the infant relieves the caretaker's anxieties. The caretaker's anxieties can be allayed by reducing fear of the unknown.

Once the infant has returned home, typical behavior patterns will be quickly resumed if the caretaker assumes the usual pattern of care. Infants soon begin to reflect the patterns of the caretaker; therefore if the caretaker is calm and relaxed, the infant will be calm. If the caretaker is tense and anxious, the infant will emulate this behavior.

CHAPTER 5

HEALTH PROBLEMS OF INFANTS

Infancy is generally a healthy period of life. Health problems that occur are often related to birth defects, the birth process, or adjustments infants must make to extrauterine life.

The infant must adapt to eating, retaining, digesting, and using nutrients and eliminating waste products in ways that are totally different from life in utero. Breathing on their own, regulating body temperature, and maintaining a physiological equilibrium in a new environment often predispose newborns to injury or illness. Whereas unborn babies were protected from many illnesses by their mothers' antibodies, infants must develop their own immunological defenses.

This chapter contains the most common health problems found during infancy. The problems, listed alphabetically, are approached from three points of view. First, each health problem is defined and described. Second, health care guidelines are included that assist health professionals in understanding the problem and managing the care. Third, helpful hints are provided to assist health professionals in increasing caretakers understanding and facilitating management at home of a child with a health problem.

HEALTH PROBLEM	HEALTH CARE GUIDELINES	HELPFUL HINTS
Brachial paralysis (Erb's palsy)		
Brachial paralysis: Paralysis of the arm caused by injury of nerve roots of the brachial plexus due to stretching of the neck during delivery (most frequently associated with breech delivery).	The affected arm is flaccid with the elbow extended and the hand rotated inward. The grasp reflex is usually intact. The Moro reflex is not present on the affected side. If the paralysis is caused by edema or hemorrhage, the condition will resolve itself within a few weeks. The prognosis is good. If the paralysis is caused by laceration of the nerves, healing may be prolonged, surgery may be required, and paralysis may be permanent. Initially, the affected arm is placed in a neutral position with the arm abducted, shoulder externally rotated, elbow flexed, and wrist supinated. Manipulation and range of motion are usually delayed for about 10 days.	Paralysis of a newborn's arm requires immediate treatment. Treatment is directed toward restoration of function and prevention of muscle deformity. Caretakers must be taught how to position the infant's arm. The arm may be immobilized by a splint, cast, or by pinning the infant's undershirt sleeve to the crib sheet. If a method other than the cast is used, the arm must be removed at intervals during the day for cleansing and gentle massage. Caretakers must be taught how to gently exercise the arm. *Caution:* During treatment the infant will always be placed on the back when in bed. Care must be taken to bubble thoroughly during and after feeding to prevent choking on food from involuntary vomiting.
Broken clavicle (broken collar bone)		
Broken clavicle: Fracture of the clavicle resulting usually from forcible efforts to deliver the shoulders during breech presentation.	A broken clavicle may be identified by the following: 1. Limitation of movement of the arm on the affected side 2. Unilateral Moro reflex 3. Muscle spasms 4. Crepitus (grating sound) at the site of the injury Although the signs listed are the most common for a broken clavicle, they are not always present. If a fracture has not been identified at birth, a callus will form, and a hard mass can be felt within 1 to 2 weeks at the site of the injury. Treatment usually consists of immobilization of the affected arm and shoulder. The arm is flexed at the elbow and wrapped securely against the chest.	A broken collarbone (clavicle) heals easily, quickly, and without deformity in about 1 to 2 weeks. The infant can be picked up and held, when the affected arm is secured in place, but must be handled carefully. Avoid putting pressure on the affected shoulder or putting the affected arm in sleeves because these maneuvers may cause further injury and/or pain. Skin care performed daily prevents irritation to those areas where the skin surfaces of the arm and chest come in contact. With the infant on the back, gently raise and support the affected arm (maintaining a flexed position) enough to permit cleansing and drying of skin surfaces. Replace and wrap securely the affected arm against the chest.

HEALTH PROBLEM	HEALTH CARE GUIDELINES	HELPFUL HINTS

Broken clavicle (broken collar bone)—cont'd

Positioning the infant for sleep and rest may pose problems. One method is to place the infant on the unaffected side and prop in position with firm support at the back. The other position is lying flat on the back. In either position, it is important to bubble the infant thoroughly before rest time to prevent choking from vomiting.

Caput succedaneum (swelling of scalp tissue)

Caput succedaneum: Edema of scalp tissue, usually at the presenting part, as a result of pressure on venous circulation during labor.

Caput succedaneum is effusion of serum in and under the scalp. The generalized edema is evident at birth and not limited by suture line demarcation.

Fig. 5-1 illustrates the bony structure and suture lines of the head with caput succedaneum and cephalhematoma.

Swelling of scalp tissue (caput succedaneum) is a self-limiting condition and requires no treatment.

The swelling will disappear within 7 to 10 days.

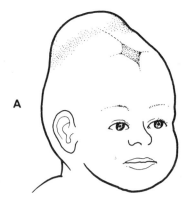
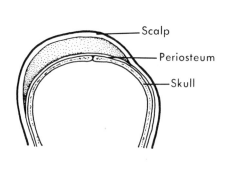

Scalp
Periosteum
Skull

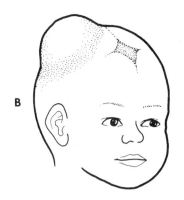
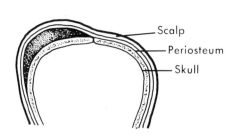

Scalp
Periosteum
Skull

Fig. 5-1. A, Caput succedaneum. Swelling is not limited to boundary of suture lines. **B,** Cephalhematoma. Bleeding under scalp tissue limited by margins of cranial bones.

HEALTH PROBLEM	HEALTH CARE GUIDELINES	HELPFUL HINTS
Cephalhematoma *Cephalhematoma:* Rupture of blood vessels between the skull bone and the periosteal covering because of pressure during delivery or application of forceps.	Cephalhematoma bleeding under scalp tissue is limited by the margins of the affected cranial bone, usually the parietal bone. Edema from bleeding appears within several hours to 1 day after birth. Initially, the swelling from caput succedaneum may conceal an existing cephalhematoma. Cephalhematoma is localized and never crosses cranial suture lines. Bleeding may continue for 3 days. Cephalhematomas are never aspirated because infection may develop. Jaundice of the area may occur as the hematoma is resolved.	Bleeding under scalp tissue (cephalhematoma) is a limiting condition and requires no treatment. Caretakers need to be reassured that this bleeding is not in the brain. Reassure caretakers that although the swelling may increase, it will disappear. It may take weeks or months for this to occur. As the swelling goes down, it is possible for the scalp skin to become discolored (yellow to yellow green). The discoloration will also fade without treatment.
Cleft lip (hare lip) *Cleft lip:* A unilateral or bilateral fissure of the lip that may be partial or complete. Cleft lip is more common in boys than girls.	Cleft lip is evident at birth and requires surgical correction. Surgical intervention may be planned within the first few days or weeks of life. The extent of the deformity and the neonate's ability to gain weight and be free of infection determine the timing for surgical correction. Cleft lip seems to appear in more than one family member. Cleft lip is frequently accompanied by other anomalies. The fissure(s) may be small, involving only the lip, or large, extending into the nostril. The extent of the deformity may influence the caretaker's reactions and ability to relate to the infant. The infant's ability to suck will be altered to various degrees by the extent of the deformity.	Hare lip (cleft lip) does not require immediate treatment but is correctable. Correcton is usually done in the second or third month or when the infant weighs 12 to 15 pounds (5.4 to 6.8 kg). Caretakers will need realistic support in accepting the child with this deformity. Assistance related to feeding and bubbling techniques will aid the caretaker in performing these tasks. The use of special nipples, a medicine dropper, or a syringe with a rubber tip may be necessary for feeding. The infant must be fed slowly and bubbled frequently. Babies with cleft lips swallow large amounts of air during a feeding. Bubbling them frequently permits them to get rid of the air. An easy position for bubbling the infant (with less interruption to feeding time) is to place the infant in a sitting position on the caretaker's lap, with one hand on the infant's back, and tilt the infant forward, supporting the infant's chest and head with the other hand. Formula feedings should be followed by a feeding of water to cleanse the mouth.

HEALTH PROBLEM	HEALTH CARE GUIDELINES	HELPFUL HINTS
Cleft lip (hare lip)—cont'd		After feedings, place the infant on the right side so that the food will pass more easily from the stomach to the small intestine.
		However, lying on the back will be used postoperatively for the infant after feedings to prevent injury to the repaired lip. Have infants lie in these positions (back and side) to have them accustomed to them prior to surgery.
	Postoperative care is directed primarily to prevention of trauma to the suture line either from feeding, positioning, or crying.	Caretakers are often quite involved in the immediate postoperative care.
		The primary emphasis after surgery is to prevent injury to the repaired lip. Crying causes tension on the stitches (suture line) and should be prevented.
		Caretakers are often permitted and encouraged to participate in the infant's care.
		It will probably be necessary to hold the infant more often than usual. Feeding slowly and bubbling well will eliminate discomfort from swallowed air.
		To prevent injury to stitches (suture line), infants are maintained on their backs when in bed. This position also warrants thorough bubbling after feeding and before placing the infant in bed.
	Methods of restraint, such as elbow restraints or pinning the sleeve to the diaper should be taught to the caretaker.	The infant's hands and arms may have to be restrained to keep fingers away from the mouth. This can be accomplished by the use of long-sleeve undershirts and pinning the arm down to the diaper.
	Restraints to the infant's arms should be removed at intervals to stimulate circulation and provide for passive range of motion exercises.	When removing restraints, remove one at a time so that the free arm is under control at all times.
		While restraints are used, the infant can be pacified by using mobiles or musical toys.
	Prevention of infection at the operative site is also important. Rinsing the infant's oral cavity and cleansing the suture line after feedings are measures that should be used.	Postoperative feedings for the infant will be followed by clear water to clean the mouth.
Cleft palate *Cleft palate:* A fissure in the roof of the mouth involving either the soft or hard palate or both, resulting in an opening between the oral and nasal cavities.	Cleft palate may occur as a separate anomaly or in conjunction with cleft lip. When one anomaly is identified, the infant should be examined carefully for other existing anomalies.	Cleft palate is an opening in the roof of the mouth. The opening may be small or large and involve the lip as well (cleft lip).
	There is a tendency for this condition to be found in more than one family member. Genetic counseling should be considered if familial tendencies are identified.	
	Cleft palate is evident at birth, but correction is delayed until anatomical structures of the mouth are more fully developed.	Surgical correction is at the discretion of the surgeon and is frequently performed after the infant is 18 months old.

HEALTH PROBLEM	HEALTH CARE GUIDELINES	HELPFUL HINTS
	The extent of the deformity may influence the caretaker's reactions and ability to relate to this infant.	Caretakers may need support in their acceptance of children with this deformity. They will need assistance in meeting the physical and emotional needs of these infants.
	Feeding and prevention of infection are chief concerns prior to surgical correction.	
	Children with cleft lip and palates are more prone to respiratory tract infections.	Children with cleft lips/palates pick up colds, sore throats, and ear infections easily. Avoid exposing these children to people with infections.
	Feeding is difficult because the opening in the palate prevents the infant from creating a vacuum when sucking.	Special nipples are available that cover the palatal opening and make sucking easier.
	Prosthetic devices that fit over the palate may be prescribed.	Because of the palatal opening, infants will swallow large amounts of air. Infants must be bubbled frequently.
	Introduction of solid foods, as with liquids, poses a problem because of the palatal opening, but must be encouraged.	Introduce solid foods into the infant's diet, even though feeding is quite messy and difficult, since this infant tends to expel food from the nose.
		Foods *should not* be placed in the bottle of formula because these infants, too, need to be introduced to different textures and tastes.
		Weaning from the bottle to a cup can be encouraged early. Cup feeding decreases the amount of air swallowed and is the recommended feeding technique after surgery.
	Surgical intervention is often delayed until the infant is 18 to 24 months old, but preferably before speech patterns are developed.	
	Palate repair may require more than one operation.	Caretakers are often involved in the post-operative care.
	Primary focus following surgical correction is directed toward the following: 1. Maintaining hydration and nutritional intake 2. Preventing trauma and/or infection to the operative site	
	The health professional will explain to caretakers alternative methods used for positioning feedings and reasons for the use of restraints. Some suggestions for caretakers are discussed in the helpful hint column.	Prior to corrective surgery, encourage sleeping on the abdomen because this is the position that will be used after surgery.
		Immediately after surgery, the initial feeding will be water, then formula and soft foods.
		Straws and nipples are never used during the healing period to prevent injury to the stitches in the mouth.
		Since nipples and straws cannot be used, liquids can be given with a spoon.
		Caution: Direct the liquid into the mouth from the side of the spoon. *Never* insert the entire spoon bowl.

HEALTH PROBLEM	HEALTH CARE GUIDELINES	HELPFUL HINTS
Cleft palate—cont'd		The quantity of food taken at any one time during the recovery period will probably be less than the child usually eats. Small amounts given at frequent intervals are helpful.
	Restraints that keep the child from flexing the elbow will be necessary to prevent the child from putting hands, toys, or other objects into the mouth.	It has been recommended that prior to hospitalization for surgery the infant have restraints, which keep the elbow from bending, applied for a few hours each day. This helps the infant become accustomed to being immobilized.
		Although the hands and arms are somewhat immobilized, infants and toddlers quickly adapt in amusing themselves with playthings.
	Restraints should be removed for short intervals during the day to stimulate circulation and provide for passive range of motion exercises.	Restraints should be removed one at a time, but care should be exercised to prevent the child from putting the hand in the mouth.
	The following sequelae may occur:	
	1. Dentition may be delayed.	Eruption of teeth may be delayed, and uneven placement of teeth may occur.
	2. Orthodontia may be necessary as determined by the extent of the defect.	Guidance for dental care and orthodontia should be secured during infancy.
	3. Speech may be delayed, as well as difficult to understand.	Encourage the child to talk. Do not ridicule the child for obvious speech impediments.
	4. Speech therapy may be needed.	Speech therapy is highly recommended so that parents can obtain reassurance, direction, and guidance in assisting their child in developing good speech habits.
		Socialization for this child during the first few years of life needs to be encouraged as much as for an infant without a structural deformity.
Clubfoot (talipes)		
Clubfoot: A foot that is turned to an abnormal angle and that cannot be readily moved to and beyond the normal position (frequently occurs bilaterally).	There are several recognized forms of clubfoot. The two most commonly seen are talipes equinovarus and talipes calcaneovalgus (Fig. 5-2).	Clubfoot (foot turned permanently in an abnormal direction) should be recognized and treated early.
	Talipes equinovarus: foot is extended and adducted.	An infant may have this condition in one or both feet. Clubbing is usually one of the two following types:
	Talipes calcaneovalgus: foot is flexed and abducted.	1. Foot points downward (as if infant were to walk on toes) and bent inward.
	Holding the foot in a clubfoot position is typical for the neonate, thus making a diagnosis difficult at birth. If true clubfoot exists, the examiner will have difficulty placing the affected foot in a normal position.	2. Foot is bent upward and turned outward.
	Treatment may consist of passive range of motion exercises to the affected foot or casting.	Medical supervision is required.

HEALTH PROBLEM	HEALTH CARE GUIDELINES	HELPFUL HINTS

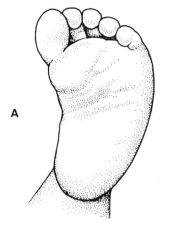

Fig. 5-2. A, Talipes equinovarus—foot extended and adducted. **B,** Talipes calcaneovalgus—foot flexed and abducted.

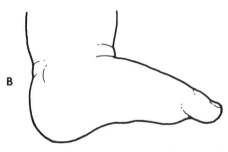

When a diagnosis of clubfoot is made and treatment is instituted early, correction is often quickly achieved. The infant will walk normally within the expected age period.

Caretakers may be requested to perform particular maneuvers of the affected foot (passive range of motion exercises). The frequency and extent of the maneuvers will be explained to the caretaker.

It is important that caretakers follow through on the exercise program if this form of treatment is to be of any value.

Casts might have to be applied to the affected foot to achieve full correction.

When casts are used, it may be necessary to change them to more fully correct the defect or because the infant grows so rapidly.

Infants rarely have any difficulty adjusting to a cast. Infants with clubfoot, like other infants, enjoy being held and cuddled.

The toes of the casted foot are exposed and should be checked daily to ensure that the cast is not too tight. (See the discussion of a dislocated hip for information on checking circulation. Also see Chapter 18, Cast Care.)

If clubfoot is diagnosed when the infant begins to stand or walk. Denis-Browne splints, casting, or even surgery may be required (Fig. 5-3).

The following are factors to consider when Denis-Browne splints are used:

1. Muscle cramps occur and can be relieved by changing the infant's position or removing the splint and gently massaging the calf.

2. Application of splints is easily accomplished when the infant is relaxed. This may be when the infant is sucking on a bottle or distracted by toys or a mobile.

3. Splints should be applied at night and at nap time only.

4. Splints will not impede the infant's ability to turn, roll over, or stand.

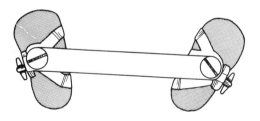

Fig. 5-3. Denis-Browne splint. Positioning device used for correction of clubfoot.

Colic

Colic: Paroxysmal abdominal pain usually associated with feeding and accompanied by crying.

Colic occurs in the first 3 months of life.

Infants with colic tend to be irritable, fretful, and cry more than other infants their age. The colicky infant often experiences painful abdominal distention with paroxysmal spasms or expulsion of large quantities of gas.

The exact etiology of colic is unknown, although environmental stress, maternal anxiety, or problems with feeding are all believed to contribute to this condition.

Abdominal pain may be attributed to the infant's inability to release tension.

Colic is one of the most trying problems of infancy for caretakers. Colic is characterized by unexplainable bouts of crying and abdominal cramps that do not respond to any comfort measures.

Feeding the infant slowly and bubbling frequently help prevent some of the discomfort.

Soothing music and a quiet calm atmosphere reduce tension.

HEALTH PROBLEM	HEALTH CARE GUIDELINES	HELPFUL HINTS
Colic—cont'd		Caretakers need to realize that their anxieties are transmitted to their infants and may trigger colic episodes.
	Treatment is symptomatic.	Holding the infant or the use of a pacifier may reduce some of the crying.
	Local application of heat to the abdomen has aided in reducing the frequency of paroxysms.	Placing the infant on the abdomen in a previously warmed bed may relieve the discomfort and possibly reduce the spasms or cramps and gas.
		The crib can be warmed by placing a hot water bottle under the top cover for 20 to 30 minutes. *Remove the hot water bottle before placing the infant in the crib.*
		Caution: Do not use electric heating pads, blankets, or hot water bottles under or over infants for warmth.
Conjunctivitis		
Conjunctivitis: An inflammation of the thin membrane (conjunctiva) that lines the eyelids and covers the eyeball.	Symptoms that are manifested in conjunctivitis can include redness, a clear discharge, and itching.	Eye infections (conjunctivitis) often occur in infants who have colds because they inadvertently rub nasal discharge into their eyes. The eyes become red (inflamed) and weep. Older infants may deliberately rub their eyes because they itch.
	Infectious forms of conjunctivitis are viral or bacterial. Other causative factors may be chemical or physical irritants and allergic responses.	The eye infection can occur in one eye or both. When it is detected in one eye, the caretaker should try to prevent the infant from rubbing the discharge into the other eye.
	Conjunctivitis can appear initially as a precursor to the common cold as well as a secondary infection following a cold.	Excessive drainage and direct secretions should be removed from the eye as they occur. Often on awakening, the infant's eyelid will be crusted shut. The crust can be removed by application of warm water. (See Chapter 18, Bathing an Infant.)
		Avoid the use of eyedrops or ointments unless ordered by the physician. (See Chapter 18, Instillation of Eyedrops.)
BLOCKED TEAR DUCT	Unilateral conjunctivitis persisting for several weeks may indicate the presence of a blocked tear duct. When this is suspected, pressure can be applied to the lacrimal sac to express contained fluid through the punctum or nasolacrimal duct. If this process is unsatisfactory, it may be necessary to probe the nasolacrimal duct.	Tear ducts may become blocked by drainage from eyes. Applying gentle pressure at the inner (against the nose) juncture of the eyelids will often assist the flow of tears and dislodge the plug.
	When seeking medical assistance include the following information: 1. Description of eye or eyes affected (redness, discharge, and itching) 2. Excessive tearing 3. Duration of existing condition 4. Presence of cold or other infection	Conjunctivitis that lasts several weeks or the presence of purulent discharge warrants medical advice.

HEALTH PROBLEM	HEALTH CARE GUIDELINES	HELPFUL HINTS
Constipation *Constipation:* A condition characterized by a decrease in the number of bowel movements with change in the consistency and color that eventually leads to increased difficulty of evacuation.	The best measure of constipation is the quality of the stool rather than the frequency of evacuation. The size and shape of the stool assist in determining constipation and the causative or contributing factors. Improper dietary habits, for example, can cause the stool to appear as small ball-shaped masses. If constipation persists even after review and change of the dietary pattern, a medical examination may be needed. When reporting constipation to the physician the following information should be included: 1. Usual pattern of evacuation 2. Size, color, and consistency of stool 3. Usual diet, any changes that have been made, and how long 4. Presence of abdominal distention 5. Signs of fever or infection	Some infants have very hard bowel movements (constipation) that may not pose any problem. Other infants with hard bowel movements may have difficulty in expelling them. It is not necessary that the infant have a bowel movement every day. Each infant will develop a consistent pattern of elimination. For some infants the bowel elimination will occur when awakening in the morning, and for others evacuation may occur immediately after a meal. The pattern will become important during the toddler period when toilet training begins. Should the infant have constipation, the following dietary changes may be considered: 1. Add fruits to the diet such as peaches, plums, or prunes 2. Add fruit juices such as pineapple juice and diluted prune juice 3. Add vegetables such as green beans and carrots 4. Increase fluid intake with fluids other than milk or formula Recommend that if the infant is receiving more than 1 quart (0.95 L) of milk a day, cut back on the amount of milk, and give water and juices. Adding sugar or honey to the formula or giving honey water to infants who have not yet been given solid foods will also aid in softening the stool.
Diarrhea *Diarrhea:* Excessive passage of stools that are loose and watery.	Diarrhea stools are frequently green, may contain mucus, and are occasionally tinged with blood. Mild diarrhea: 2 to 10 loose stools per day Severe diarrhea: 2 to 20 stools, liquid consistency and expelled with force	Some infants develop loose watery bowel movements (diarrhea). Note the number of stools expelled in a 24-hour period. Review the present dietary pattern for possible reasons for change in stool consistency. Foods that may contribute to diarrhea include the following: 1. Food with high sugar content 2. Excessive amounts of fruit (whether raw or cooked) 3. Some fruit juice such as orange juice, apple juice, pineapple juice, and Hawaiian punch

HEALTH PROBLEM	HEALTH CARE GUIDELINES	HELPFUL HINTS
Diarrhea—cont'd	Management of diarrhea is directed toward reduction of the number of stools and fluid replacement. An oral feeding of Pedialyte might be recommended for electrolyte replacement.	Larger amounts of fluid should be given to replace fluid loss. It may be advisable to discontinue formula feedings and other solids for a 24-hour period to permit the bowel to rest. During the 24-hour fasting substitute clear liquids. Do not give just water. Fluids such as gelatin water, diluted tea, and honey and water are usually available in the home and are recommended. After a 24-hour fast from formula and solids, if the frequency of diarrhea decreases, the older infant (9 to 12 months) may be given crackers, puffed rice, pretzels, gelatin, Popsicles, and fruit sherbets. Other solids, formula, and fruit juices may be added as bowel elimination becomes more normal.

Prolonged periods of diarrhea may lead to dehydration, coma, and death. Following are early signs of dehydration:

1. Dry skin, lips, and mucous membrane
2. Decreased skin turgor
3. Rapid and weak pulse
4. Depressed fontanel and sunken eyes; most evident in infants under 1 year old
5. Decreased urinary output
6. Weight loss

Diarrhea is frequently accompanied by vomiting and an elevated temperature.

Medical advice should be sought when dehydration is evidenced. The following information should be included when seeking medical assistance:

1. Duration of the diarrhea
2. Frequency, color, and consistency of stools
3. Presence or absence of vomiting
4. Presence or absence of elevated temperature
5. Behavior of infant
6. Number of wet diapers
7. Color and odor of urine

Extreme dehydration is characterized by the following:

1. Extreme prostration
2. Increased irritability and restlessness
3. Stupor
4. Pallor
5. Flaccidity

Monitor the urinary output. Scanty urine may indicate impending renal shutdown, and indicates that the child definitely needs medical attention.

Convulsions may occur as a result of loss of fluid and severe electrolyte imbalance.

If severe diarrhea persists for more than 24 hours, seek medical advice.

When large amounts of fluid are lost, the infant becomes dehydrated. Dehydration is characterized by dry lips and skin (older infants, 10 months and above, will be seen licking their lips), irritability, fewer wet diapers, urine darker in color, and visible weight loss.

The infant's lips may be moistened with a cotton applicator dipped in water, glycerin and lemon juice, or petroleum jelly.

Vomiting frequently accompanies diarrhea, which causes dehydration more rapidly.

Elevated temperatures are also common in infants with diarrhea and will cause fluid loss.

Keep a record of the number, color, and consistency of each bowel movement.

Determine if the diaper is wet from urine or from the stool or both.

Frequent loose stools will cause skin irritation (excoriation). The infant's buttocks can be protected by the application of baby oil, petroleum jelly, or A & D ointment. Exposure of the infant's excoriated buttocks to the air will aid in drying and healing.

Infants will often assume a knee-chest position for comfort. This position predisposes the infant to reddened chafed knees, elbows, chin, and cheeks.

Lotion or ointments applied to these skin surfaces offer some protection.

HEALTH PROBLEM	HEALTH CARE GUIDELINES	HELPFUL HINTS

Dislocated hip
 	
Dislocated hip: A congenital dislocation (partial or complete) of the head of the femur from the acetabulum.
Dislocation may be unilateral or bilateral (unilateral is more common).
This condition is found more frequently in girls than boys.
	Dislocated hips can be missed during the initial examination of the neonate because the infant's joints are very pliable. The condition becomes quite evident by 1 month.
	The shallow acetabulum permits the head of the femur to become dislocated. Therefore treatment is directed toward enlarging and deepening the socket. This is accomplished by maintaining constant pressure on the acetabulum, which is created by complete abduction of the affected leg.
	In the first examination of the neonate the dislocation is often partial rather than complete.
	Complete dislocation of the hip is identified by the following signs:
	  1. Asymmetry of gluteal skin folds.
	  2. Limited ability to abduct the affected leg (this is the first and most reliable sign).
	  3. The affected leg is shorter than the unaffected leg.
	  4. During the examination a "click" can be heard when the leg is manipulated.
	  5. If the infant walks, a limp or waddle will be observed.
	Treatment must be started immediately on diagnosis. Delayed treatment may cause a partial dislocation to become completely dislocated.
	
	Abduction of the affected leg may be maintained in a variety of ways, depending on the age of the child:
	  1. Pinning the diaper to the sheet with both legs abducted
	  2. Splinting
	    a. Use of a pillow or rolled diapers between the thighs with the leg in a froglike position (abduction)
	    b. Frejka pillow splint—a firm square pillow set firmly between the thighs against the diaper, and strapped in a position of abduction
	
	  3. For an older child, constant prolonged immobilization may be required. A body cast (hip spica) encircling the waist and extending to the toes is used to hold both legs in an abducted position.
		Dislocation of the hip (leg bone does not remain in hip socket) occurs in some infants and requires treatment immediately after detection. Medical supervision is required.
		If the condition is detected and treated early, the problem is usually resolved without difficulty.
		Health supervision and well-baby conferences within first month of life make it possible for early detection.
		It is important that the condition be detected and treated before the child learns to stand or begins to walk because additional damage could occur. When treated early, the infant will learn to walk on schedule and without a limp.
		
		Treatment for a dislocated hip depends on the degree of involvement, but in all instances, requires periods where infant is immobilized, and the legs are maintained in a specific position.
		Immobilization periods should be carried out with the infant lying on his back. The best times are during rest or sleep.
		Corrective positioning methods using pins or splints are the most effective for infants under 2 months old. Beyond this age, infants learn to roll over and will not stay on their backs.
		Many splinting devices are available. The physician will order an appropriate type.
		When applying and removing splinting devices, *never extend the affected leg.*
		Skin care and gentle massage to the buttocks and back should be given when infant is out of the splint to improve circulation and prevent skin irritation.
		If a cast is applied, an opening is left in the cast at the genital area for elimination.
		Inspection of the cast for chipped edges or impairment of circulation should be done daily.
		Check for impaired circulation as follows:
		  1. Note the skin temperature of the toes on both feet. Both should feel the same.
		  2. Inspect the color of the toes for bluish tint (cyanosis).

HEALTH PROBLEM	HEALTH CARE GUIDELINES	HELPFUL HINTS

Dislocated hip—cont'd

3. Test circulation to the toes by pressing on the nail bed. Initial blanching occurs with a pressure, changing to a normal pink color within moments after the pressure is released.
4. An older child will complain of pain or discomfort and point to the area involved.

See Chapter 18, Cast Care.

Epispadias

Epispadias: Congenital malformation of the urethra, in which the urinary meatus is on the dorsal surface of the penis (Fig. 5-4).

This condition is more common in boys than girls.

Occasionally epispadias occurs in girls, where the urethral opening is located in the separation of the labia minora.

Surgical intervention is required for epispadias for cosmetic purposes.

When the opening through which urine flows is on the upper surface of the penis, this condition is called *epispadias*. Epispadias is identified at birth, but treatment may be delayed beyond 1 year of age.

Correction of this condition may require more than one surgical procedure. The condition can usually be completely corrected.

Correction is recommended for appearance and to permit males to urinate in a standing position.

Plans for surgical intervention should be at the physician's discretion.

See Chapter 4, Hospitalization.

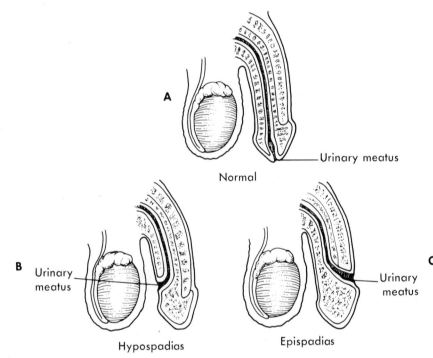

Normal

Urinary meatus

Urinary meatus

Hypospadias

Epispadias

Urinary meatus

Fig. 5-4. Congenital malformations of male urethra. **A,** Normal location of urinary meatus. **B,** Urinary meatus is located on undersurface of penis. **C,** Urinary meatus on dorsal surface of penis.

Facial paralysis

Facial paralysis: Paralysis of the facial nerve results from pressure of the forceps during delivery.

Facial paralysis is usually a transitory condition. Permanent paralysis is rare.

Paralysis will usually disappear within a few hours or days after birth.

The face on the affected side appears expressionless, the mouth may turn down, and the eye may remain open.

Corneal damage must be prevented.

Drooling may occur.

During the birth process, injury to the facial nerves can occur, resulting in a temporary *facial paralysis.*

Reassure caretakers that this condition will usually disappear within a few days after birth.

Assistance should be given to the caretaker with initial feeding of the newborn. Sucking is difficult, and some feeding may dribble from the newborn's mouth

HEALTH PROBLEM	HEALTH CARE GUIDELINES	HELPFUL HINTS
Hernia (rupture)		
Hernia: An abnormal protrusion of an organ or part of an organ through a weakened body wall that normally contains it.	Hernias can occur in many portions of the body, although the most common in children are inguinal and umbilical hernias. Hernias can be congenital or acquired. Congenital hernias are those which exist at birth because of failure of certain normal areas to close. Acquired hernias are those which develop after birth, usually as the result of excessive strain on the muscular wall.	A rupture (hernia) is a condition in which a weak spot in a body wall or muscle lining permits parts of underlying organs to bulge through. Hernias are commonly found in babies at the belly button (umbilical) area and at the groin (inguinal). Frequently these hernias are noticeable at birth.
INGUINAL HERNIA Inguinal hernias are more commonly seen in boys than girls. They may be unilateral or bilateral.	During embryonic life the testes descend (preceded by a sac of peritoneum) into the scrotum through an inguinal ring at the base of the abdominal cavity. Occasionally, the upper portion of this sac (which normally closes) remains open, permitting peritoneal fluid or the abdominal structure to herniate through. Peritoneal fluid enters the processes vaginalis, forming a hydrocele. The resultant swelling of the scrotum appears as a translucent, fluctuant oval sac. The fluid is usually absorbed within the first few months of life. Surgical correction is generally not necessary. A herniated loop of the intestine can become strangulated (incarcerated) from impaired vascular supply. In females, herniated sacs may contain an ovary. Hernias may be said to be reducible (disappear when pressure is applied by the caretaker's or physician's hand). When the hernial sac is empty, there are no symptoms. With increased intra-abdominal pressure, which occurs when the infant cries or strains, the intestine bulges through the inguinal ring. Pain, fretfulness, difficult defecation, and local pressure are the usual symptoms. Inguinal hernias that persist are usually treated surgically. Incarcerated hernias become surgical emergencies.	Inguinal hernias are more frequently found in boys than girls. Caretakers notice the "bulge" in the groin most often when changing a diaper while the baby is crying. The bulge often disappears or is less noticeable when the baby is quiet. When babies cry they increase the abdominal pressure, thus pushing part of the intestines through the weakened wall into the bulging sac. When the baby is quiet, the pressure is reduced, and the intestines can return to their normal position in the abdomen. Occasionally, the intestines get trapped and cannot return to their normal position. When this occurs the normal functions of elimination cannot occur. The baby becomes fretful, irritable, and has spasms or abdominal cramps. The stools may become diarrhea-like, be absent or passed with great difficulty. The hernia is then considered strangulated and requires immediate medical attention and surgery. Surgery is also the choice of treatment before strangulation occurs. (See Chapter 4, Hospitalization.)
UMBILICAL HERNIA Umbilical hernias are more commonly seen in girls than boys and in black children more than white children.	Umbilical hernias occur because the embryonic opening beneath the umbilicus does not close. The hernia becomes noticeable when the infant cries, coughs, or strains. The intestines bulge through the umbilical ring from the increased intra-abdominal pressure.	Umbilical hernias occur more frequently in girls than boys and more often in black children than white children. The caretaker will note a bulge at the belly button (umbilicus) particularly when the infant cries or is passing a stool. This type of hernia frequently closes in time without further intervention.

HEALTH PROBLEM	HEALTH CARE GUIDELINES	HELPFUL HINTS
Hernia (rupture)—cont'd UMBILICAL HERNIA—cont'd	Most umbilical hernias will disappear by the time infant is 1 year old. Surgery is contraindicated unless the hernia persists beyond 5 years or becomes strangulated.	In the past it was believed that taping a large coin over the bulge or strapping the area with an abdominal binder would relieve the condition. Neither method has proved to be helpful, and abdominal binders have proven to be dangerous. If the hernia does not disappear spontaneously by toddlerhood, surgical intervention may be necessary. (See Chapter 7, Hospitalization.)
Hypospadias *Hypospadias:* A congenital anomaly in which the urethral opening is located on the underside of the penis (Fig. 5-4). This condition is more common in boys than girls. Hypospadias may be found occasionally in girls; the urethral opening is located in the vagina.	Surgical intervention is required for hypospadias for cosmetic purposes. Circumcision may be delayed because of the location of urethral opening. A partial circumcision may be performed. Frequently, surgery is delayed until the child is 1 year old to permit maximum growth of the urethra.	When the opening through which urine flows is on the undersurface of the penis, the condition is called *hypospadias*. Hypospadias can be identified at birth. This condition does not interfere with normal urination. Correction is achieved in either one or more operations. The time when the surgical procedure should be done is at the discretion of the physician. Correction is recommended for appearance and to restore the ability of the male to urinate in a standing position. If surgery is performed during the early toddler period, the child will notice discomfort during voiding for a few days after surgery. Usually the toddler will not be able to localize the area of pain. Pain experienced by the infant is not remembered.
Nevus (birthmark) *Nevus:* A congenital discoloration of the skin.	Nevi range from a small circumscribed area of the skin to an extensive diffuse condition that includes subcutaneous tissue and blood vessels. Nevi are usually benign, although some can be malignant. Treatment, depending upon the extent of nevi, may range from no treatment to surgical excision for cosmetic reasons. If malignancy is suspected, therapy is more extensive.	Birthmarks (nevi) are small discolored areas commonly found on the face or neck. Birthmarks frequently fade and require no treatment. Surgical excision, if necessary, will be at the discretion of the physician and caretaker.
Otitis media (middle ear infection) *Otitis media:* Inflammation of the middle ear characterized by pain.	Acute otitis media is usually secondary to an upper respiratory tract infection such as nasal pharyngitis, which causes mucous membranes to swell, obstructing the eustachian tube. The most evident signs and symptoms are as follows: 1. Irritability 2. Rubbing the affected ear against bed surface	Ear infections (otitis media) in infants often follow respiratory tract infections because of the shortness of the eustachian tube (tube from the ear to throat). Otitis media can be readily identified in infants by their behavior. Infants with ear infections will be irritable, cry, and might rub the affected ear against the bed surface. Older children tug on the lobe of the infected ear.

HEALTH PROBLEM	HEALTH CARE GUIDELINES	HELPFUL HINTS
	3. Elevation of body temperature 4. Drainage from the ear 5. Nausea and vomiting 6. Meningeal irritation characterized by a high-pitched cry and twitching of the extremities	Because of the discomfort associated with this condition, the infant's eating patterns may change. In place of the usual milk or formula feedings the infant may more eagerly take warmed fluids such as apple juice, sweetened tea, gelatin water, or just plain water. If the infant has an elevated temperature, small amounts of clear fluid should be offered at frequent intervals to prevent dehydration. (See Diarrhea.) Perseverance and calmness are key factors to keep in mind while encouraging the infant to take fluids. Caretakers will quickly learn the infant's pattern of behavior during the infection: when to encourage fluids and methods that are most successful for hydration and comfort. If an ear infection is suspected, seek medical advice to avoid a ruptured eardrum (ruptured eardrum can cause hearing problems). A behavior change with less crying and irritability may be a clue to the fact that the eardrum has ruptured. On closer inspection the caretaker will notice light blood-tinged drainage from the ear or on the bed linen.
	Infants suspected of having otitis media must receive medical attention to treat the existing infection, prevent chronic otitis media, and prevent rupture of the eardrum. Serosanguinous (light blood-tinged) drainage from the ear and decreased irritability may indicate a spontaneous rupture of the eardrum. When notifying the physician, the following information should be provided: 1. Infant's temperature 2. Infant's behavior 3. Signs and symptoms of concomitant upper respiratory tract infection or prior infection 4. Evidence of drainage 5. Evidence of decreased appetite 6. Presence of nausea and vomiting 7. Onset and duration of these signs 8. Previous pattern of ear infection, if any The usual medical treatment for otitis media will include antibiotics, analgesics, nosedrops, and decongestants. For infants who have repeated bouts of acute otitis media or persistent chronic otitis media, a myringotomy is indicated. A myringotomy is a surgical incision of the tympanic membrane (eardrum) under anesthesia to permit drainage of the middle ear. Frequently small plastic tubes are inserted during the myringotomy to prevent closure of the eardrum and to facilitate continued drainage.	Medicines the physician will prescribe are primarily to resolve the infection, relieve pain, and decrease swelling of the ear membrane. Avoid treating ear infections without medical advice. Cotton pledgets, oil-base eardrops, or ear medicine bought over the counter may do more harm than good. Follow the physician's instructions for administration of medicines. (See Chapter 18, Administration of Medications.) When the physician orders medicines, caretakers should ask the physician and/or pharmacist about the purpose and potential side effects of these medicines. (See Chapter 18, Administration of Medications.)

HEALTH PROBLEM	HEALTH CARE GUIDELINES	HELPFUL HINTS
Otitis media (middle ear infection) —cont'd	If otitis media persists without treatment, the following complications can occur: 1. Repeated rupture of the membrane, resulting in scar tissue that can lead to impaired or complete loss of hearing 2. Mastoiditis—inflammation of air cells of the mastoid process 3. Meningitis—inflammation of membranes covering the brain and spinal cord 4. Septicemia—spread of an infectious organism to the bloodstream.	
Phimosis (tight foreskin) *Phimosis:* A condition in which the foreskin cannot be retracted (pushed back) over the penis because of a narrowed preputial opening.	The urinary stream will be small, requiring effort on the part of the infant to void. Treatment consists of circumcision. The circumcision site should be checked frequently during the first 24 hours for bleeding. Bleeding tendencies have been identified in some infants following circumcision.	Occasionally in males who are not circumcised, the foreskin will be so tight (phimosis) that it cannot be pushed back from the tip of the penis. Urinary flow is blocked. Treatment (circumcision) should be instituted once phimosis has been diagnosed. After circumcision, apply loose-fitting diapers for the infant's comfort. Change the diaper as soon as the infant soils or wets to prevent irritation and discomfort to the circumcision area. Healing takes place within a few days.
Regurgitation (wet burp) *Regurgitation:* Small amounts of swallowed food returned from the stomach during or shortly after feeding.	Regurgitation is a natural occurrence during the first 6 months of life. Regurgitation is less frequently seen in breast-fed infants probably because the curd of breast milk is more easily assimilated and digested. Regurgitation can be reduced as follows: 1. Bubbling the infant to release swallowed air ("eructation") 2. Gentle handling and holding during feeding 3. Placing the infant on the abdomen or right side immediately after feeding	Wet burps (regurgitation) occur shortly after feeding. Wet burps usually involve very small amounts of formula. The infant usually displays no stress or anxiety—the burp is merely formula pushed out due to the release of swallowed air (gas) from the stomach. To reduce the number of wet burps, bubble the infant at intervals during the feeding. Under 1 month of age—after each ½ to 1 ounce (15 to 30 ml) of fluid. 2 to 6 months of age—after every 2 to 3 ounces (60 to 90 ml) of feeding Fig. 18-9 shows the position for bubbling infants.
Rumination *Rumination:* Spitting out or reswallowing of regurgitated food.	Rumination is evident when solids are first introduced into the infant's diet, or when the diet has been changed.	Occasionally, infants reswallow regurgitated formula or food (rumination). To reduce rumination, small amounts of new formula or food should be given slowly to permit the infant to adapt to new tastes and textures.

HEALTH PROBLEM	HEALTH CARE GUIDELINES	HELPFUL HINTS

Rhinitis/pharyngitis/coryza (upper respiratory tract infection, common cold)

Rhinitis/pharyngitis/coryza: A condition characterized by sneezing, coughing, nasal congestion with clear nasal discharge, and a minimal elevated temperature.

Infants are highly susceptible to upper respiratory tract infections due to the immature mucosal lining of the air passages.

Rhinitis, pharyngitis, and coryza (upper respiratory tract infections) are usually the result of viral infections.

Rhinitis—inflammation of the nasal mucosa

Pharyngitis—inflammation of pharyngeal tissue

Coryza—acute catarrhal inflammation of the nasal mucous membrane

Functional activity of the cilia-fed mucous membranes becomes diminished after viral invasion, thus increasing the infant's susceptibility to bacterial complications.

Upper respiratory tract infections frequently lead to additional involvement of the respiratory system.

Frequent complications include conjunctivitis, otitis media, and tracheobronchitis.

Changes in respiratory rate and breath sounds are indicators of the extent and location of the infection.

Abnormal breath sounds might include rales, rhonchi, and wheezing.

Rales—a range of sound that varies with the patency and lumen of the bronchi.

Dry rales are sounds produced when air is being forced through narrowed bronchi caused by a thickened mucous membrane, viscid secretion, spasms of the bronchial wall, or external pressure.

Moist rales are sounds produced when air is forced through fluid in the bronchi.

Crepitations are small rubbing sounds produced when air is forced through the smaller collapsed bronchi.

Rales may be described in many ways by the sound that is heard or the location in which they are detected.

Rhonchi—loud rales heard over the trachea or bronchus.

Wheeze—a whistling sound as produced when forcing air through a narrowed passage.

Infants will frequently develop a runny nose followed by sneezing, coughing, and nasal discharge characteristic of a common cold or mild upper respiratory tract infection (Rhinitis/pharyngitis/coryza).

The immaturity of infants' breathing apparatus makes them vulnerable to respiratory tract infections.

When respiratory tract infections occur, the air passages become obstructed by mucus and swollen tissues (nasal congestion).

The infant may have difficulty with feeding because of nasal congestion. Clearing the nasal orifice of excess mucus will enable the infant to breathe and feed more easily. (See Chapter 18, Bathing an Infant.)

Milk tends to increase mucus production; therefore if nasal congestion is severe, milk feedings should be omitted. Offering clear liquids frequently is recommended as a substitute for milk feedings while the infant has the infection.

Cool moist air produced by a vaporizer helps decrease nasal congestion and moisten air passages, thus decreasing irritation to the mucosal lining.

For a common cold, cough syrups, expectorants and nosedrops are to be avoided unless ordered by the physician.

HEALTH PROBLEM	HEALTH CARE GUIDELINES	HELPFUL HINTS
Rhinitis/pharyngitis/coryza (upper respiratory tract infection, common cold)—cont'd		When the infant has a cold, reduce contact with others to prevent exposure to additional infection.
		Provide additional periods of rest to promote a more rapid recovery.
	When seeking medical advice the following information should be included:	If symptoms become prolonged, with an elevated temperature or if nasal discharge changes from clear to a yellow or green color, becomes thicker, and has a purulent odor, seek medical advice.
	1. Temperature: how it was obtained, when it was taken, and how long it was elevated.	
	2. Presence or absence of coughing, sneezing, or nasal discharge.	
	3. Type of cough and/or nasal discharge.	
	4. Amount and type of food and fluid ingested during the previous 24-hour period.	
	5. Last bowel movement and its consistency.	
Skin eruptions		
DIAPER RASH		
Diaper rash: A rash that will range from a papular erythematous appearance to extreme raw excoriation of the skin.	Diaper rash has been found more frequently in infants who are formula fed than infants who are breast-fed. This may be due to the difference in waste products.	Diaper rash (red raised areas on the buttocks and perineum) is caused by urine and feces irritating the tender skin of infants.
Diaper rash is caused by irritation of the skin of the buttocks and perineum by urine and feces.	Infants with sensitive skin may develop diaper rash more than one time.	Changing diapers as soon after soiling as possible may prevent diaper rash.
		The best remedy for healing diaper rash is through exposure of the irritated skin to air. Heat lamps may be prescribed but should be used with extreme caution.
	Reusable diapers are often the cause of diaper rash.	Reusable diapers must be washed and rinsed thoroughly and preferably dried in the sun. This care of diapers reduces the potential presence of decomposing urine and feces.
		Plastic panties should be avoided.
INTERTRIGO (CHAFING)		
Intertrigo: An inflammatory skin reaction due to accumulation of moisture where skin surfaces rub together, such as the folds of the neck, axillary areas, and groin.	Intertrigo occurs frequently in heavy infants or during hot weather.	Infants can develop raw, red, moist skin reactions (intertrigo) when two skin surfaces rub together. Folds of the neck, groin, and under the arms are the areas most frequently affected.
	A frequently overlooked site where intertrigo can occur is behind the ears, where the skin surface rubs the scalp.	Cleanse thoroughly those areas where skin surfaces come together. The infant's neck may require additional cleansing after feeding when formula dribbles down over the chin into neck folds.
	Skin is red, raw, and moist and can become infected. Infection is suspected when seepage is green or purulent.	Perspiration can also cause intertrigo. Avoid the use of plastic diapers and panties, plastic-lined overalls, or plastic bibs until the irritation is gone.
		Should intertrigo occur, avoid the use of powder or lotions; expose the area to air, and continue to keep the area clean and dry.

HEALTH PROBLEM	HEALTH CARE GUIDELINES	HELPFUL HINTS
MILIARIA (PRICKLY HEAT, HEAT RASH) *Miliaria:* A condition characterized by a dry, papular erythematous (bright red) rash.	Miliaria is associated with sweating that is brought about by excessive clothing, a viral illness, or summer heat. The rash may cover the entire body but is most prevalent in the skin folds and at the neck. Skin that is exposed to the air is not as likely to have this type of irritation.	Prickly heat (miliaria), a dry, bright red rash, can be found over the entire body, and is caused by overdressing or extreme heat. Recommend dressing the infant appropriately for the climate and avoid overdressing, particularly when the infant has an elevated temperature. Cotton clothing and polyester material will more readily permit evaporation of perspiration. Cleanliness and additional tepid sponge baths are recommended. Dry the irritated surfaces thoroughly by patting but avoid rubbing. Expose the irritated skin area to the air, but avoid direct sunlight or drafts.
Undescended testicle(s) *Undescended testicle(s):* Failure of the testicles (one or both) to descend into the scrotal sac before birth (frequently associated with inguinal hernias).	Because of the absence of the testicle(s) the scrotum will appear small. The testicle(s) may remain in the inguinal canal or descend normally without treatment. If the testicle(s) does not descend, surgical intervention is necessary. Surgical intervention should not be delayed after puberty because sterility may result.	At birth, in some boys, the sex glands (testicles) are not located in the scrotal sac, creating a condition called *undescended testicles.* This condition can be diagnosed at birth and may correct itself without any treatment. Undescended testicles do not interfere with urination. If the testicles do not descend into the scrotal sac by school age, surgery will be necessary. Delaying surgery beyond the school years may cause sterility (inability to father children).
Vomiting *Vomiting:* The forceful ejection of the stomach contents from the mouth shortly after feeding.	Vomiting may be due to overfeeding, feeding too rapidly, or introducing new foods. Vomiting frequently accompanies infection or illness. Projectile vomiting is the forceful ejection of stomach contents at a distance greater than 1 foot (30 cm). The presence of projectile vomiting indicates the need for medical supervision. Information for the physician should include the following: 1. Time vomiting occurs—before, during, or after feeding 2. Type of food being offered when vomiting occurs 3. Frequency of vomiting 4. Color, consistency, and amount of vomitus 5. Presence of discomfort at the time vomiting occurs	Vomiting is the forceful return of the stomach contents. The following guidelines can help reduce vomiting: 1. Allow the feeding time to last at least 20 to 30 minutes to provide satisfaction of sucking and to help the infant retain the feeding. 2. Feed the baby in a sitting position. Food is more likely to be retained if the baby is fed in a sitting position. Swallowed air will remain above the formula, thus diminishing regurgitation when the baby is bubbled.

HEALTH PROBLEM	HEALTH CARE GUIDELINES	HELPFUL HINTS
Vomiting—cont'd	Prolonged episodes of vomiting in addition to depleted nutritional intake will lead to an electrolyte imbalance.	
	Irritability is heightened as a result of electrolyte depletion.	
	Persistent vomiting of green material should be reported to the physician because it may indicate an intestinal obstruction. Other indications of an obstruction are a distended abdomen (rigid or firm to touch) and a decrease in the number or absence of stools.	If persistent vomiting occurs, seek medical advice.

UNIT TWO

TODDLERHOOD *seeking autonomy*

EVELYN N. BEHANNA

Children 1 through 3 years of age seem to have boundless energy, tremendous curiosity, and the desire to do things for themselves. Toddlers seek autonomy through their desire to be independent. This desire of the child to become independent and learn self-care skills frequently sets into motion four tug-of-war areas with caretakers that continue well into adolescence (although the behavior takes different forms). The tug-of-war is essentially a battle for control of situations or the ability to decide for oneself the actions to be taken. Nutrition, elimination, cleanliness, and discipline are four areas of concern that present frustration and consternation to toddlers and caretakers alike.

The nutritional needs of infants were, for the most part, decided on by the caretaker, offered to the infant, and usually accepted without too much stress. Toward the end of infancy, as the child started self-feeding, the battleground was established. In toddlerhood, the little ones assert their will and their desires to be self-sufficient by preferring to feed themselves and eat what they want, when they want it, and in the quantities they choose. The wise caretaker will realize that children will not starve and will eat sufficient amounts of food, although perhaps less than that desired by the caretaker. Mealtimes should be delightful periods because the entire family can eat together and engage in a mutual sharing of each member's activities.

Patterns of elimination identified during infancy by the caretaker now become irregular as toddlers become involved in other more desirable activities. Caretakers' insistence on strict toileting times and toilet-training procedures can establish this as a second battleground, which can be seen in later years as over-concern with constipation or the need for laxatives.

Cleanliness, too, becomes a battleground as caretakers insist on baths and clean hands, faces, and clothes at times when toddlers wish to continue their activities of play and exploration. Although patterns of cleanliness are essential, compromise should be established by the caretaker.

Discipline and limit setting begun in infancy now take on new parameters and meanings for both caretakers and toddlers. Caretakers need to be supported and reassured that limit setting is necessary, but that the typical toddler's behavior during this period is a natural expected outgrowth of development and the desire to be independent. Unfortunately, the toddler's negativism, temper tantrums, ritualism, and sibling rivalry often cause caretakers needless distress and anxiety.

The positive side of the development of autonomous behavior deals with the toddler's desire to interact with others. The development of language, social skills and graces, and the desire to please are characteristics common to most toddlers. They mimic, clown, and try to amuse caretakers and others. Play activities move from independent to parallel play with children in their own age range.

If toddlers are permitted the opportunity to assert themselves while learning self-care activities within limited parameters of love and security, a favorable self-concept becomes better established. The trusting relationship of the toddler with caretakers and others will be strengthened, autonomy established, and the stage set for the preschool period of development.

CHAPTER 6

TODDLERHOOD *1 through 3 years*

Toddlerhood, ages 1 through 3, is a period where the growth pattern of infancy begins to slow down, but the pattern of development gains speed. Toddlers become more independent in their abilities and activities, although they are still dependent on others to provide for basic needs.

Caretakers and toddlers are quite comfortable with each other, since they have developed daily routines together. Caretakers feel more secure in permitting these little ones more freedom to explore the environment. Toddlers need this freedom to develop new skills and to begin to assert their own personality and independence.

As children enter the second year, many new physical skills are learned. Toddlers have new worlds to explore, new abilities to develop, and limitless energy. Caretakers frequently find the period from 1½ to 2½ years very trying. The children are viewed as being in the "terrible twos." They are trying their wings.

By contrast, the 2½- to 3½-year-old is busy refining skills. This period, sometimes referred to as the "trusting threes," seems to give both the toddler and caretaker a chance to catch up with the changes and establish new bonds of closeness.

Suggestions for anticipatory guidance for caretakers are offered in conjunction with the expected biological, psychological, and social landmarks for this age.

GROWTH AND DEVELOPMENTAL LANDMARKS	ANTICIPATORY GUIDANCE

Biological

WEIGHT

The average weight gain for this period will range from 6 to 8 pounds (2.7 to 3.6 kg) per year.

By 2 years of age, the weight varies between 24 to 32 pounds (10.9 to 14.5 kg).

At 3, weight will vary from 30 to 40 pounds (13.6 to 18.2 kg).

By 2 years of age, children will likely be four times their birth weight, and by 3, they will be five times their birth weight.

No two children progress at the same rate, comparisons of different children's progress should be avoided.

HEIGHT

Toddlers grow approximately 3 to 5 inches (7.5 to 12.5 cm) per year.

By 2 years of age, toddlers will be approximately half their adult height.

The 3-year-old will be able to stand erect on an adult scale for both height and weight measurements.

HEART RATE

The average heart rate for this age ranges between 90 and 120 beats per minute. The pulse rate will increase when the child is upset or active.

Heart rates must be reviewed in relation to the child's emotional state and activity.

Palpation of the heart over the chest wall is less apparent by the end of third year than during previous periods.

Pulse rate is best obtained by the use of a stethoscope at the apex of the heart although it is palpable at the wrist (radial artery).

Heart rate, rhythm, and volume should be well established. Variations in cardiac rate and arrhythmias that persist should be evaluated by professional health care workers.

The circulatory system by this time is well established. Changes in skin color are noticeable with exertion or environmental changes, varying from flushing to blanching. Skin color returns to normal when circumstances are changed.

RESPIRATIONS

The respiratory rate may range to the midthirties but are more typically found in the low twenties.

Individuals' respiratory rates must be evaluated in relation to their circumstances and activities.

Abdominal breathing still predominates, although some children in this period will begin to use the thoracic muscles much more than in earlier periods of life.

Respiratory patterns are now established with more regular and predictable respiratory rates.

The toddler will breathe very rapidly when under exertion or stress.

BLOOD PRESSURE

Blood pressure for this age period can be both palpated and auscultated for systolic readings that range from 85 to 90 mm Hg.

The diastolic reading is present but often difficult to hear. The diastolic reading is usually about 60 mm Hg.

To obtain accurate blood pressure readings, an appropriate size cuff and correct placement are necessary.

Special ultrasonic equipment is available and should be used if accurate blood pressure readings are necessary.

Blood pressure readings for this age child are not usually taken during the health conference due to the difficulty in obtaining accurate readings.

Excitement, stress, and activity alter blood pressure readings and thus reduce their value in health assessment.

TEMPERATURE

Body temperature for this age period continues to range from 96.8° to 99.6° F (37° to 37.6° C).

The rectal thermometer technique provides accurate readings within 1 to 3 minutes. The axillary method requires 5 to 10 minutes. Invasive procedures such as taking rectal temperatures may be bitterly resented by this age child.

Body temperature fluctuates normally with the child's activity, hydration level, and environmental changes. Temperature elevations above normal range may be indicative of infection.

GROWTH AND DEVELOPMENTAL LANDMARKS	**ANTICIPATORY GUIDANCE**

HEAD

The head size in comparison to total body size is approaching more adult proportions. Chest circumference now exceeds head circumference.

The anterior fontanel will be completely closed by 18 to 20 months.

The contour of the head is becoming more oval. The bony prominence of the jaw and eye sockets make facial features more distinguishable.

The receding chin of infancy has disappeared now that the lower jaw is in proximity to the upper jaw.

HAIR

Hair color, texture, length, quantity, and type (curly or straight) will be unique for each child.

Hair will usually be shiny when the child is healthy and the scalp and hair are clean.

Some children may have coarse, dry hair, whereas others may have fine, oily hair.

Children's scalps are kept clean to remove oily secretions and reduce the incidence of dandruff. Shampooing children's hair is necessary only about one or two times a week. More frequent shampooing may be necessary because of excessive perspiration, activity, and climate.

Shampooing provides an opportunity for the caretaker to inspect the child's head for bumps, sores, or vermin. (See Chapter 8, Pediculosis).

Children are often introduced to their first haircut during this period. If this experience is treated as a normal occurrence without overemphasis and concern by the caretaker, the child will require little distraction while the hair is being cut.

If the toddler is permitted to sit in the barber chair and/or observe someone else having his/her hair cut, anxiety will be diminished.

NOSE

The obligatory mouth breathing phase of infancy has passed, and the child will now breathe through the nose.

Difficulty breathing through the nose with the mouth closed may indicate the presence of some pathological condition.

Drainage other than clear mucus from the nose may indicate the presence of a foreign object or respiratory tract infection. (See Chapter 8, Foreign objects, Respiratory Tract Infections.)

Children of this age can be taught how to blow their nose.

To teach the toddler how to expel air forcefully from the nostrils, the caretaker can demonstrate the desired action.

Place a feather or cotton ball on a flat surface and make it move by blowing it only with air expelled from the nose with the mouth open.

The toddler will copy the behavior. Once the behavior is learned, have the child transfer to blowing into a handkerchief.

Caution: The caretaker should perform the action first. Remember, the mouth should be open when the nose is blown, because additional force is not needed or desired.

MOUTH

The child will have a full set of twenty temporary (deciduous) teeth by 3 years.

Children 3 years old can be taught to brush their own teeth and should be encouraged and assisted in developing good dental care habits.

Carbohydrates or concentrated sweets predispose the child to dental caries and should be limited in the diet. (See Chapter 7, Dentition, Nutrition.)

The sucking pads of the cheeks decrease in size and are no longer evident by the end of this age period.

Once the child has learned to drink from a cup and to eat solid foods, drinking from a bottle will be less desirable. Eventually, the child will have great difficulty sucking from a bottle because the effectiveness of the sucking pads is reduced from lack of use.

Voluntary control of the tongue and lips are very well established.

New skills in the use of the tongue and lips enable the child to learn how to stick out the tongue and to spit.

On examination, the tongue should be freely movable and easily extended and retracted. Difficulty with maneuvering the tongue may be indicative of tongue-tie.

Children who have difficulty maneuvering their tongues may need a relatively simple surgical procedure.

GROWTH AND DEVELOPMENTAL LANDMARKS

Biological—cont'd

MOBILITY

Muscle development continues from head to toe with greater agility evident in the use of large and fine muscles.

The 2-year-old is able to stand erect and has good use of thoracic and shoulder muscles. Lordosis with a protruding abdomen exists due to underdeveloped muscles of the abdomen and lower back. Thus the 2-year-old's sense of balance is somewhat precarious. The toddler will stand with the feet wide apart to provide a broad base of support (Fig. 6-1).

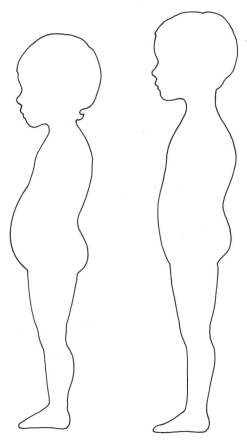

Toddlers walk, run, climb, and jump with boundless energy.

Two-year-olds can manipulate small objects. (See Chapter 7, Safety.)

Complete myelinization of the nerve tracts (enabling voluntary muscle control) is evidenced by the following two skills of toddlers:
1. Ability to sit, stand, and walk with ease
2. Ability to voluntarily pick up and let go of objects

Two-year-olds demonstrate the ability to work with the abstract, as well as concrete situations. They are now able to go from the simple peek-a-boo play of infancy to a hide-and-seek play to successfully locate the partner even though hiding place changes.

ANTICIPATORY GUIDANCE

Fig. 6-1. Posture of 2- and 3-year-old children. Two-year-old stature reveals pot belly with slight swayback as compared to three-year-old's erect position.

Two-year-olds will try out new skills at every opportunity. Because of the wide stance they assume for support, they will waddle and may have difficulty when attempting to walk quickly or run.

Because of the increased motor ability, caretakers should expect these children to enjoy activities such as running, rolling, beginning tumbling and somersaults, and climbing or crawling through and over objects. Supervision during play cannot be overemphasized.

Clues for the beginning of toilet training are evident at this age because children are able to stand erect and also demonstrate a "let-go" reflex. The "let-go" reflex is evidenced in the child's ability to play ball.

Playing hide-and-seek with the 2-year-old is valuable because it helps the toddler learn that people and objects return. Short periods of separation from the caretaker become easier.

GROWTH AND DEVELOPMENTAL LANDMARKS

The 3-year-old's posture is more erect than in earlier years and is much like that of the adult. The abdomen no longer protrudes, and the lordosis has been corrected. The sense of balance for 3-year-olds is more certain, and they will no longer need the wide stance for support (Fig. 6-1).

Toddlers continue to refine the motor skills learned earlier.

By 3 years of age, children are able to stand briefly on one foot, hop using both feet, and walk up or down stairs on alternating feet. They continue to use handrails for stability on stairs.

Psychological

DEPENDENCE-INDEPENDENCE

Toddlers continue to depend on others for physical, emotional, and social needs.

Toddlerhood initiates self-assertiveness as the child enters a rudimentary level of independence.

Two-year-olds are not aware of danger, nor do they realize just how dependent they are.

Three-year-olds have learned from experience that there are parameters of safety.

ANTICIPATORY GUIDANCE

The 3-year-old's limitless energy and eagerness to use new learned motor skills keep the caretaker very busy providing diversion and supervision.

Running ability is greater for toddlers than earlier in life, and they will run farther and longer. They derive great joy in attempting acrobatic skills of rolling and tumbling. They often attempt motor skills beyond their level of ability, such as leapfrog, and become upset when they are unable to complete the skill.

Placing toddlers in shopping carts eliminates losing a child and prevents the child from venturing into prohibited parameters. Shopping becomes pleasurable to both the child and caretaker when frustrating situations are minimal and excursions kept short.

Toddlers need opportunities to make choices, but choices should be limited to those which the 2- and 3-year-old can handle. When the toddler makes a choice, use that choice.

Do not offer a choice if there is no choice, since this will only frustrate and confuse the child. Toddlers who are continuously offered choices that are not granted may develop undesirable patterns of behavior, and autonomy may be delayed. Some patterns of divergent behavior have been noted: overt acting out (temper tantrums) or passive-resistant acts of thumbsucking or whining.

Examples of choices that could be offered a 2-year-old would include choosing between two different kinds of food, two different toys, or two different outfits.

Some 3-year-olds can make a selection from more than two items. On some occasions 3-year-olds can select an item entirely on their own.

Some 3-year-olds can be offered the opportunity to select a favorite cereal or snack food when accompanying the caretaker on food shopping trips.

Following are a few of the ways in which toddlers exhibit independent behavior:

1. Eating—they will decide how much they want and when they want it.
2. Dressing—they determine, often at inappropriate times, to remove their clothing.
3. Toileting—they find they can hold back or produce at will.
4. Sleeping—they are able to delay going to bed; have learned all kinds of tactics to postpone sleep time.
5. Stepping-out—when walking, they will let go of the caretaker's hand and take off on their own.

GROWTH AND DEVELOPMENTAL LANDMARKS	**ANTICIPATORY GUIDANCE**

Psychological—cont'd

DEPENDENCE-INDEPENDENCE—cont'd

Independence is demonstrated by the fact that toddlers will attempt more skills on their own.

Two-year-olds are curious and will perform thorough, although gross, investigation of objects, whereas the 3-year-old uses a more reflective technique. The 3-year-old wants to know the finer workings of an object and what makes it function.

> Toddlers need opportunities to develop their investigative skills. (See Investigative.)

Toddlers' behavior vacillates between that of older children and that of infants. They will revert to infantile behaviors when they are tired, fearful, angry, or uncomfortable.

> Toddlers often revert to infantile behaviors when they are tired, fretful, or upset.
> Toddlers want love, affection, and reassurance when frustrated. Quickly pacified, they will return to their endeavors.

SELF-ASSERTIVENESS

Toddlers are self-centered individuals with wills of their own who are beginning to assert themselves.

They quickly learn how to manipulate people within the environment through body language and vocabulary demonstrated by caretakers and others.

> Assertive vocabulary and body language are exhibited most often when the toddler's wishes are thwarted.

Toddlers have not learned the concept of sharing, although they are aware that others have possessions they frequently desire and claim for their own.

> Toddlers often play alone, choosing what they want to do. They think everything belongs to them so there may be times when playing with others causes problems.
> Although toddlers use the word *mine* in regard to their own possessions they are not able to understand the word *mine* when it relates to someone else's possessions.
> The caretaker's consistent firmness assists toddlers to learn the parameters of *mine, yours,* and *sharing.*

Social

SOCIAL AWARENESS

Children from 1 through 3 years of age progressively become more aware of others and more involved in the social scene. The parameters of their world are expanded.

> Opportunities for the toddler to be with other children and adults should be provided.

Exposure to others is increased through contact with baby-sitters, social gatherings, and nursery school.

Longer periods of wakefulness for this age permit more opportunities for socialization.

Toddlers learn to adapt to the different social expectations of caretakers and significant others.

One- through three-year-olds will learn social behavior if consistently exposed to the desired behavior.

> Social behavior such as using eating utensils are mimicked by toddlers as they watch others eat (at home, in restaurants, on television).
> Caretakers are the primary role models for the child.
> Many television shows provide good role models but some provide examples of undesirable behavior. Caretakers are responsible for monitoring the shows their children are permitted to watch.

INVESTIGATIVE

The increasing manipulative skills, mobility, and investigative curiosity of 2- and 3-year-olds keep them in constant motion.

Areas inside as well as outside the home that at one time were not available to the child now are easily accessible.

> The limitless energy of children between 1 and 3 years of age requires creativity and patience on the part of the caretaker.
> A child's curiosity makes many everyday experiences into new areas of exploration for the child. The neighborhood becomes a place of education from which they learn. Toddlers need opportunities to explore and investigate within parameters of safety. Pleasurable experiences excite children and further encourage them to try new things. Investigation of an object is not a one-time thing for the toddler but a behavior that is performed repeatedly (even watching an insect crawl).

GROWTH AND DEVELOPMENTAL LANDMARKS

ANTICIPATORY GUIDANCE

The toddler's curiosity prompts investigation of things that may be injurious. For example, toast in a pop-up toaster will intrigue the child to reach out to touch it, only to be burned.

Childproofing inside and outside the home is extremely important. (See Chapter 7, Safety.)

RELATIONSHIPS

Relationships of the toddler with people other than the caretakers continue to evolve. These evolving relationships are forming from different bases than those in the infancy stage.

The toddler initiates the relationship and develops close ties with people other than the caretaker. Toddlers will indicate their preference of those individuals they desire to be with.

Childrens' ability to relate now includes pets, inanimate objects, and, in later stages of development, even imaginary playmates.

Many toddlers become attached to a favorite object. Objects such as a blanket or toy will be very real to the toddler. Often, holding or fondling this favored object will be sufficient to pacify this age child when tired, hurt, or frustrated.

In infancy, relationships were developed and built on trust. Now the relationships evolve from curiosity.

Should a child relate only to inanimate objects and remain aloof from social contacts with individuals over an extended period of time, professional counseling should be sought.

A favorite toy or blanket gives security and comfort to the toddler and proves to be helpful when the toddler experiences stress.

This security object should not be taken away from the child, even when it appears so mutilated that it is ready for the trash. This object has a very special meaning for the child. Toddlers will give these objects up on their own, in their own good time, when autonomy is well developed.

VOCALIZATION

Vocabulary increases at a very rapid rate from 1 through 3 years of age. Language development progresses from the use of nouns, verbs, and simple sentences to the use of adjectives, adverbs, articles, and complex sentences. Word usage and sentence structure will fluctuate for each child.

Language development is an outcome of the exposure the child has to many people and things (radio, television, records, books).

Through language, the toddler expresses assertiveness and learns quickly which words to emphasize to get their meaning across. For example, the word "bread," spoken with emphasis does not have the impact on caretakers and others as the word "no."

One word expletives (swear words) used within hearing of the toddler will be mimicked immediately, not because the toddler knows the meaning of the word, but for the reaction it initiates from the caretaker.

At first expletives used by the toddler will be considered cute and bring positive responses from others in the environment. As the child becomes proficient in the use and timing of these words, alarm and overreaction become the typical responses of others in the environment.

Caretakers and others in the toddler's environment always seem to be surprised at the rapidity with which children learn new words.

To establish good language development, the use of correct terminology when speaking to the child cannot be overemphasized.

The association of words is limited within the child's ability to understand. A mental image of what children perceive is directly related to what *they* think they hear. An example of this is the child's version of the Pledge of Allegiance, ending with: ". . . one nation under God with liver, tea, and juice for all."

Early in the toddler period special one- or two-syllable words are taught to the child to encourage communication of needs, but by the end of the toddler period, children should be using words that are socially understandable and acceptable.

Crying continues to be a tool of communication. The toddler will cry when expressing anger, fear, uncertainty, pain, and fatigue.

Caretakers have learned the messages expressed in the cry of their toddler. Toddlers will still use crying as a tool to manipulate the environment.

If toddlers are totally permitted to control their own environment, problems with discipline will emerge.

CHAPTER 7

HEALTH MAINTENANCE FOR TODDLERS

The child from 1 through 3 years of age is usually a very healthy child. Routine visits to health care workers for health maintenance occur less frequently, usually at 6-month intervals. The major emphasis for this period is to keep the child healthy.

The child usually eats three meals a day and should certainly eat with the family. Most children prefer the foods that the adults enjoy.

Sleep time gradually becomes limited to the night hours with only occasional daytime naps for the average 3½-year-old.

Toilet training is well under way. By the end of this age period, most toddlers have complete bowel control and daytime bladder control. Some 3-year-olds will have day and night bladder control. Caretakers rejoice when they are no longer burdened with changing diapers and washing extra bed linens.

Accident prevention is a major concern for children in this age period. Providing safe environments in which the toddler can explore, investigate, and develop new skills is a primary responsibility of caretakers. Childproofing the home and the external environments to which the toddler will be most exposed is vital. Although many caretakers believe that they will teach their infants and toddlers to differentiate valuable objects and knickknacks from toys, this usually leads to frustration. To reduce frustration, provide safe environments, and permit toddlers new learning experiences, it is advisable for caretakers to remove knickknacks and valuable objects, provide safe play areas inside and outside the home, and be able to enjoy their child during a most delightful period of life. Although repetitious, "keeping the child safe" is the major health emphasis for the 1- through 3-year-old.

Areas of concern for health maintenance of the toddler with helpful hints for caretakers will be discussed in this chapter.

AREAS FOR CONCERN	HELPFUL HINTS

Health care conference

The frequency of routine health care conferences is reduced from that of infancy. Scheduled visits occur most often at 18 months, 2 years, and 3 years of age.

Before the health examination is performed, the examiner will usually take a health history. This gives the examiner an opportunity to have a social exchange with the toddler and caretaker and begin developing a rapport with the child.

The examiner usually spends some time conversing with the caretaker, providing opportunities for social contacts to be made with the child. If the caretaker holds the child or permits the child to stand close by, the child and examiner will get to know one another quickly.

Health history (reviewed and updated)

The examiner will ask about infections, illnesses, injuries, and other stressful situations that have occurred since the last visit.

Information will be requested regarding the possibility of the toddler having been exposed to any communicable disease.

The family history will be reviewed for health problems (congenital, familial) that may have significance for the health of this child.

When the health history is being taken, it is important for the caretaker to tell the examiner about illnesses, fevers, injuries (of any type), and stressful situations that have taken place since the child was last seen by health personnel.

The necessity for a review of family health history warrants cooperation by the caretaker because this provides clues that alert the examiner to assess for and rule out the presence of familial or hereditary problems.

Health assessment: physical examination

A physical examination will be performed, at which time the examiner will assess the child for continued progress in physical, mental, and social development.

Data gathered in this physical examination will be compared and contrasted to information from previous health care conferences and to expected normal standards established for the age.

Deviations from normal expectations of growth and development that may exist will be identified.

The presence of health problems requiring treatment or referral that were not identified in infancy may now be evident, such as a congenital dislocated hip.

A general examination will be performed by the examiner assessing the child from head to toe.

Body measurements for height and weight will be obtained.

Vital signs for temperature, pulse, and respiration will be obtained. Blood pressure readings may also be secured.

Most of the listed areas for examination will be performed but not necessarily in the sequence presented. Examiners gather data for many areas of health assessment through only one or two procedures.

Some of the physical examination can be performed with the child on the lap of or standing beside the caretaker.

The caretaker may be permitted to assist or actually perform some of the vital sign procedures. The intrusive procedure of taking a rectal temperature will be facilitated by permitting the caretaker to take the temperature.

Examination of the eyes, ears, nose, and throat will also be performed.

Auscultation and palpation of the chest and abdomen will follow.

The skeletal structure and musculature will be evaluated while child is in sitting, standing, and lying positions. Reflexes will be tested and evaluated.

The child will be requested to perform a few gross and fine motor skills.

An external examination of the genitalia will be included.

Giving the child opportunity to examine and handle some of the examining equipment prior to the examination will enhance the child's ability to cooperate and demonstrate motor skills. For example, the toddler may be permitted to shine the otoscope light or flashlight, hold the tongue blade, and manipulate the stethoscope.

The examination of the toddler can be facilitated by first performing portions of the examination on a doll or even on the caretaker.

External examination of the genitalia may seem unnecessary to the caretaker; however, the examination provides information on anatomical structure, the presence of infection (fungal, yeast, or other) and conditions such as hernias, which require monitoring or correction.

AREAS FOR CONCERN	HELPFUL HINTS

Health assessment: mental and social evaluation

Cognitive and affective abilities of the toddler will be assessed during the initial social exchange that takes place between the child and examiner.

A test for developmental progress such as the Denver Developmental Screening Test may be performed.

If the Denver Developmental Screening Test is performed, the caretaker will be requested to leave the room. The presence of the caretaker tends to alter results of the test.

Health protection

Health protection will continue. An immunization series will be continued. If, for any reason, the child has not had any immunizations, the series will be initiated. At 18 months, the following should be given:

1. Booster DPT (diphtheria, pertussis, tetanus)
2. Booster TOPV (trivalent oral poliomyelitis vaccine)
3. Measles-rubella (MR) or measles-mumps-rubella (MMR) (if not given at 15 months)

If the child has not had any immunizations up to this time, the initial series of immunization will be instituted. (See Chapter 4, Health Protection.)

Keep updating the personal immunization records of the toddler.

Maintaining adequate levels of immunity are contingent on the child receiving the initial series of immunizations and the necessary boosters at the recommended times.

Childrens' ability to benefit from measles immunizations given prior to 1 year of age has been questioned in recent research.

The recommended time for the child to receive measles-mumps-rubella vaccines is now in the toddler period (15 to 18 months).

Caretakers and health workers should review immunization records of older children for the age at which they received the measles vaccine. It may be necessary for some children to receive the vaccine again.

Tuberculin tests not performed in infancy will be included in early toddlerhood. If there is an increased incidence of tuberculosis or if the child has been exposed to the disease, it may be necessary that a tuberculin test be performed again during toddlerhood.

At health visits at 2 and 3 years of age immunization records will be reviewed and updated as necessary.

Health promotion

The health conference includes discussion and review of the following topics: dentition, nutrition, elimination, play, sleep and rest, safety, discipline, negativism, sibling rivalry, and hospitalization.

DENTITION

The pattern of tooth eruption is usually symmetrical.

At the beginning of the toddler period most children will have six teeth. These are usually the upper incisors (lateral and central) and the lower incisors (central).

The pattern of tooth eruption is unique for each child. Some children may not have any teeth at 1 year of age, whereas others may have six teeth.

Usually tooth eruption does not cause pain, but some children may experience discomfort that affects eating and sleeping patterns. Each toddler reacts differently to teething. Even toddlers who have no discomfort may chew on objects that should not be in their mouths.

Caretakers could offer toddlers hard biscuits, bread sticks, and Popsicles.

Some children may have a mild fever associated with the teething process and altered eating pattern. Fluids should be encouraged. Offer puddings, gelatin, sherbets, and ice cream, which are more appealing to the toddler than liquids.

Fevers that persist beyond the eruption of a particular tooth may be indicative of a condition requiring medical advice.

AREAS FOR CONCERN

From 12 to 18 months tooth eruption continues to be rapid. The typical progression of tooth eruption is as follows: lower lateral incisors, lower first molars, upper first molars, upper canines, and lower canines.

From 18 through 30 months, eruption of deciduous (temporary) teeth is completed (twenty teeth). The last teeth to appear are the second posterior molars (upper and lower).

Toddlers are capable of being taught oral hygiene practices such as eating foods helpful in reducing plaque formation, rinsing the mouth after eating, and brushing the teeth.

Brushing a toddler's teeth is best started after the fifteenth month because gingival tissue is tender and easily injured prior to that time.

Dental visits must be initiated in this age period. The number of visits will vary from one or two times each year.

NUTRITION

Dietary patterns for the toddler are now similar to adults, three meals a day plus a snack(s).

The daily caloric requirement for toddlers is 1300 to 1400 calories.

Minerals, vitamins, and protein requirements are as important as caloric needs, since this is the time of life when the body is developing muscle tissue and strengthening bones.

HELPFUL HINTS

The practice of following meals with a drink of water begun in infancy should be continued by the toddler.

To encourage the toddler to develop toothbrushing skill and later to assume responsibility for this practice the following suggestions may be followed:

1. Provide a toothbrush appropriate for the size of the child.
2. A soft-bristled toothbrush is initially recommended.
3. The place where the toothbrush is stored should be accessible to the toddler.
4. Color coding for identification of toothbrushes for each member of the household enables toddlers to easily locate their own.
5. Demonstration of toothbrushing by the caretaker will be imitated by the toddler.
6. Toothbrushing should be performed at least in the morning and evening, although other health professionals may recommend more frequent brushing.
7. Start when the toddler is about 15 months old (gum tissue is very tender).

Caretakers should not be overly concerned if the toddler swallows the toothpaste rather than spitting it out.

Raw vegetables such as celery and carrots and fruits such as apples are believed to be helpful in reducing plaque formation because of the coarse consistency that necessitates biting and chewing.

Caretakers will find that toddlers adjust easily to dental visits if the initial visit does not involve more than the examination of the teeth, but permits the child to become acquainted with the dentist and the office.

Subsequent visits may require inspection and some form of treatment.

Controversy exists in regard to filling or not filling primary teeth that have cavities (caries); most authorities seem to recommend the former.

The quantities of food consumed by the toddler at any one meal or on any particular day will vary.

Toddlers will usually select quantities sufficient for their energy needs, provided they are not overfilled by snack foods and liquids prior to mealtimes.

To stimulate appetites and enhance interest in mealtime, toddlers can be offered opportunities to select food items they would enjoy. Keep the choices simple, that is, offer a choice between two items for the 2-year-old and among three items for the 3-year-old as opposed to free choice from all available items.

The struggle for autonomy need not make mealtime a battleground. Eating and mealtimes can and will be pleasant experiences if they are viewed as a positive means for toddlers to express their growing needs for independence.

AREAS FOR CONCERN	HELPFUL HINTS

Health promotion—cont'd

NUTRITION—cont'd

Between meal snacks recommended for toddlers would include crackers, dry cereals, fruits, and raw vegetables. Snack foods high in carbohydrates and sugar in the form of candy should be discouraged.

Because some children of this age have difficulty chewing and digesting potato chips and have choked on nuts and popcorn, these snack foods should be discouraged.

The caretaker's concern with the decreased appetite of the toddler can be alleviated by the knowledge that the quantity of food is not nearly as important as the quality of food eaten. Ensuring meals high in protein, minerals, and vitamins needed to strengthen bones and build muscles requires caretakers to know the foods that contain these elements and how to prepare them.

The discussion that follows is not all inclusive regarding nutrition but should provide helpful hints for caretakers in planning and meeting the nutritional needs of the toddler.

Raw fruits and vegetables provide vitamins and minerals that may be destroyed if cooked.

Whole wheat bread and whole grain cereals may provide more vitamins and bulk than those prepared with refined flour.

Avoid foods containing additives, such as sugars, colorings, and preservatives, since they have been found to cause allergic responses, dental caries, and other health problems.

Toddlers may eat meats, cheese, eggs (hard boiled), fruits, and vegetables more willingly if permitted to eat them as finger foods.

Introduction of new foods into the diet always carries with it the possibility of an allergic response. (See Chapter 8, Allergy.)

Daily diets of toddlers should have representation from each of the four basic foods groups:
Milk and milk products
Meats
Vegetables and fruits
Breads and cereals

Caretakers should avoid reliance on milk for provision of all nutrients because milk contains very little iron. Iron is one of the substances necessary for bone and muscle growth in this stage of development. Two to three cups of milk per day is sufficient. More milk than this could satisfy the child's hunger, but decrease the appetite and contribute to milk anemia. (See Chapter 17, Iron Deficiency Anemia.)

Fluid requirements for a 24-hour period are as follows:
1-year-old: at least 1 quart (1000 ml)

A 1-year-old needs 1 quart of fluid a day and takes at least two thirds of that in the form of milk. Juice, water, and other liquids should be offered throughout the day. Caretakers should be reminded not to exceed 1 quart of milk per day.

2-year-old: at least four and a half 8-ounce (1100 ml) glasses

Two-year-olds need five glasses of fluid a day. Half the daily fluid requirement will be in the form of milk but they should be drinking other fluids as well (avoid highly sweetened beverages).

3-year-old: at least five 8-ounce (1200 ml) glasses

The 3-year-old will need six glasses of fluid a day. Half the daily fluid requirement can be in the form of milk.

A rule of thumb to remember for calculating normal daily fluid requirements: *The average 1-year-old requires 1000 ml. For each year thereafter, up to the age of 10 years, add an additional 100 ml.* Thus by 10 years of age the child will consume the average adult fluid requirement (1900 to 2000 ml per day).

The glass size should equal 8 ounces.

Fluid requirements for the toddler may be met not only through liquids but also with the following:
1. Gelatin
2. Junkets
3. Custards
4. Puddings
5. Sherbets and ices
6. Ice cream
7. Popsicles
8. Soups

AREAS FOR CONCERN

Health professionals should alert caretakers that alterations in hydration levels occur when children are teething, when the environmental temperature is hot, when children have fever from infection, or when children perspire because of increased activity. Daily fluid intake might be increased to one and a half times the usual 24-hour requirements when hydration levels are altered.

During the conference health professionals should discuss with caretakers methods that can be used to make mealtimes pleasurable. Methods that capitalize on the toddler's behavior of ritualism, imitation, and mimicry also provide refinement of developmental skills.

HELPFUL HINTS

When a child has an elevated temperature and increased fluids are recommended, avoid milk and milk products. Milk products are harder for the body to digest than clear liquids. When the child has a fever, the body needs extra rest not extra work.

Clear liquids such as tea, gelatin, gelatin water, and uncarbonated beverages are also better tolerated than milk products.

To encourage toddlers to drink more fluids offer small amounts frequently, use small receptacles, and use a straw cut in half (a shorter length of straw will require less effort on the part of the child and will reduce spilling when the child manipulates the glass).

Toddlers learn through ritualistic patterns where meals will be served, which utensils to use, and the behaviors that are expected.

Toddlers enjoy being a part of the household routine and derive pleasure from helping set the table. They enjoy eating meals with the other members of the family. Setting the table serves several purposes; it involves the child in socially acceptable activities, assists in the development and refinement of several motor skills, aids in teaching toddlers appropriate utensils, and reinforces the place where food is to be served.

Toddlers enjoy being actively involved in the eating process. Use of appropriate sized utensils for toddlers enables them to learn how to manipulate the utensils and feed themselves (small spoons are best). Mealtimes may become quite messy because toddlers use their fingers to place food on the utensil and tend to turn the utensil upside down to fit the contours of the mouth and tongue. Until this motor skill becomes more refined, food ends up on the floor, in the lap, on the face, and in the hair as the toddler becomes engrossed in developing these new skills. Caretakers often resent toddlers "messy eating habits," but should understand that toddlers do not deliberately try to spill their milk or drop their food on the floor. Caretakers can protect their floors by placing plastic or paper under the toddler's feeding chair or table area.

Toddlers will develop acceptable eating skills if (1) they are permitted opportunities to feed themselves, (2) they are provided with utensils and plates they can manage, (3) finger foods are incorporated into meals, and (4) caretakers stay calm during this period of learning.

The social graces of eating are learned with each additional opportunity that the toddler has to eat meals with others. Therefore for children to learn expected behaviors when eating with others, they must be included at family mealtimes:

1. Toddlers can be taught to eat at the table.
2. Toddlers can be expected to stay at the table throughout the mealtime.
3. Toddlers, as well as other members of the household, should be discouraged from eating in front of the television.

When caretakers consider taking toddlers to restaurants, they should remember that toddlers have short attention spans and cannot be expected to sit in one place for extended periods of time. Mealtime in restaurants is much longer than eating at home. Preparation of food, meal service time, as well as length of eating time must be considered.

AREAS FOR CONCERN	HELPFUL HINTS

Health promotion—cont'd

NUTRITION—cont'd

Many foods are often omitted from diets because of the food likes and dislikes of the one preparing the meals.

ELIMINATION

Patterns of elimination are more established for both the bowel and bladder.

Most children have one bowel movement per day, although it is not unusual for a child to occasionally have more than one movement per day. Some children's bowel elimination pattern may be less than one bowel movement per day.

Characteristics of the bowel movement (color, consistency, and odor) as well as frequency and amount can be altered by foods, medicines, other ingested substances, infections, illnesses, and stressful situations.

Urinary elimination is also becoming more predictable. The toddler's bladder now holds greater quantities of urine than in infancy. The infantile involuntary reflex is being replaced by voluntary control.

The amount, color, and odor of the toddler's urine can be altered by substances ingested or by infection, illness, and stress.

Bladder and bowel control (toilet training)

Bowel control is usually achieved by the time child is 18 months of age.

Toilet training (bowel) can begin when the child is about 1 year of age.

Myelinization of nerve tracts usually occurs about the end of the first year.

If the calculated time span exceeds 1 hour, the likelihood exists that the toddler will become restless and irritable, thus disrupting the meal not only for the family but for other people eating at the same place.

Caretakers' likes and dislikes should not influence toddlers' introduction to and reception of new foods.

During this period of life, toddlers develop strong likes and dislikes in regard to food.

Rejection of certain foods by toddlers may be related to texture and consistency as much as to taste and odor; for example, melons such as cantaloupe and honeydew will frequently be rejected because of their texture and consistency.

Children develop their own unique patterns of elimination.

Caretakers should be aware that the consistency of the bowel movement is as important as frequency in determining constipation or diarrhea. Before laxatives or enemas are considered, caretakers should review both the food and fluid intake of the child for the past 48 hours.

When caretakers are concerned about the toddler who has not had a bowel movement, increasing fluids and foods high in roughage, such as fruits, vegetables, and cereals, may be beneficial. Foods such as cheese products, because of their binding effect, could be withheld for a couple of days.

Laxatives and/or enemas should never be used routinely because these practices may become a habit.

If constipation occurs frequently, even after following the previously suggested nutritional recommendations, seek advice from a health professional.

Caretakers should be alerted to the fact that foods such as beets and string beans may change the color of the bowel movement.

The odor and consistency of bowel movements will change as the child's dietary pattern changes

Caretakers may frequently become annoyed or exasperated with this stage of their child's development. It seems that children should have control of the urinary flow because the amount of urine released at any one time is so much greater than it was in infancy, but this is not the case.

Caretakers have stated, "My child just stood there, stared into space, grinned from ear to ear, and piddled through diaper, pants, and socks, and made a puddle on the floor."

Just as with every other skill for the toddler, learning the appropriate time and place for emptying the bowel and bladder come as a result of development.

Children can learn bowel control before bladder control. Training for bowel control is best started when the toddler's nervous system and muscle control have been established. This is evidenced by the child's ability to stand and walk and to engage in activities that demonstrate control of the "let-go" reflex such as deliberately throwing a ball. These abilities are usually developed at about 1 year of age.

AREAS FOR CONCERN	HELPFUL HINTS

AREAS FOR CONCERN

Voluntary muscle control of anal sphincters becomes possible. Evidence of readiness is observed when the child stands and walks alone and can deliberately throw a ball.

HELPFUL HINTS

Potty equipment for the child should be small and rest securely on the floor or on the adult toilet seat. If the child's feet can be placed firmly on a step or floor it will make the child feel more secure as well as provide a more natural position (hips and knees flexed) for elimination.

Attempts to train the child to use a potty-chair prior to 1 year of age may meet with limited success. The child does not actually learn this behavior, but rather the caretaker anticipates the need for toileting based on knowledge of the child's typical elimination pattern. Attempts to toilet train a child before 1 year of age tend to cause frustration and anxiety in both the caretaker and child.

Toddlers learn from ritualistic and repetitive experiences. Toilet training patterns, to be successful, *must be consistent.*

Observe bowel patterns of the child over a 72-hour period to establish approximate times for taking the child to the toilet.

If the child's pattern of bowel elimination is in the morning, place the child on the potty-chair immediately after breakfast. Stay with the child and help with evacuation through grunting sounds. (When demonstrating grunting sounds, place the child's hand on your abdomen so that tightening of the abdominal muscles will be associated with grunting. Reverse the procedure, placing the child's or the caretaker's hand on the child's abdomen, and the child will mimic the behavior of grunting with abdominal straining.)

The amount of time on the potty-chair should not exceed 5 minutes. Do not be surprised, however, if on removing the child from the potty-chair or shortly thereafter, the child has the movement (defecates) in the diaper.

Several attempts may be necessary before the child will have success in having a bowel movement when placed on a potty-chair.

After several successful occurrences, the toddler will associate straining and defecating as being appropriate only when on a toilet or potty-chair.

Toddlers will usually have established bowel control well before bladder control.

Bladder control does not usually occur until after 18 months of age.

Daytime bladder control is achieved before night control. On the average, by 3 to 3½ years of age, children will have achieved both daytime and nighttime bladder control.

The inability of the child to achieve daytime bladder control beyond 3½ or 4 years of age warrants the need for medical advice.

Some children may have difficulty achieving nighttime bladder control. (See Chapter 10, Elimination.)

Caretakers may find the following clues and suggestions helpful during the period of bladder training:

1. When the child awakens in the morning, immediately place on the potty-chair. A wet diaper does not always indicate that the bladder is empty. Anticipate a full bladder, particularly if the diaper is dry.
2. Automatically place the child on the potty-chair after each meal, before and after nap time, and before going to bed.
3. Identify clues in the child's behavior that announce the need to empty the bladder, such as grasping the genitalia and/or dancing on one foot.
4. Establish a socially acceptable term to be used by the child to communicate the need to urinate. Use this term each time the child is taken to potty.
5. Provide different clothing as the child's pattern of elimination becomes regular. Training pants and trousers that can be easily pulled up and down will enable toddlers to independently take care of toileting needs.
6. Wiping and cleansing the toddler's genitalia following urination and defecation must be performed by the caretaker.

AREAS FOR CONCERN	HELPFUL HINTS

Health promotion—cont'd

ELIMINATION—cont'd

By this age, children have learned many skills and are able to follow simple directions. The toddler quickly associates the behavior with the appropriate time and place as approval and pleasure are elicited by the caretaker. (See Discipline.)

Most little boys will begin learning bladder training by sitting on potty-chairs, since this is a natural follow-up from the method used for bowel training. By the end of the toddler period, boys will have observed and imitated the male behavior of standing when urinating.

When standing to urinate, the toddler may miss the mark because of distractions in the environment. Toddlers enjoy this new skill and find it interesting to be able to aim the stream of urine in whichever direction they wish.

Following are overall suggestions for toilet training:

1. Praise the child when successful.
2. Avoid scolding when the child is unsuccessful.
3. Permit the child to flush the toilet when finished. Although this may seem unimportant to the caretaker, the toddler has produced as requested and cannot understand why it should be flushed away. Receiving praise and being a part of the flushing process makes the entire experience pleasurable for the child.
4. Washing hands after toileting fosters good habits of personal hygiene.
5. Terms taught to children to communicate toileting needs should be those which are familiar to adults. Once learned, language is difficult to unlearn; therefore it is recommended that terms such as "toilet," "bathroom," "bowel movement" ("defecate"), and "urinate" ("void") be used.
6. By the end of the toddler period, children have learned to wipe themselves after toileting. This skill can be taught after bowel and bladder control have been established. Because of incomplete muscular coordination and manual dexterity, the toddler's skills may not be fully developed until well into the preschool years. It is important that girls be taught to wipe from the front of the genitalia back toward the rectum, thus decreasing the possibility of infection to the urinary opening (urethra) from contamination with the stool (feces).
7. Capitalize on the child's imitative behavior and use a "diaper-wetting" ("Betsy-Wetsy") doll to show the child the expected behavior. Children learn many skills through play and will imitate the caretakers demonstration and terminology when playing with the doll.

Accidents in controlling both bowel and bladder elimination will occur during the toddler stage, since these children become very preoccupied in exploration and play activities. Likewise, moments of excitement and stress may cause the toddler to have a lapse of bowel and/or bladder control.

PLAY

Play has been described as the essential work of children. It provides opportunities for the development of new skills and abilities.

Children's play can reveal their capabilities in all realms of development, as well as portray areas in which they are having difficulties.

AREAS FOR CONCERN	HELPFUL HINTS

Solitary play permits time for the child to refine previous skills, try out new skills, and be creative. Playing alone frees the child from the criticism of others, as well as the need to compete.

Parallel play is typified by two or three children each doing a similar task but not performing it together or with give and take between them. Each child is playing separately but physically in the same area. Toddlers (and some preschoolers), when in the company of other children their own age, will engage in parallel play.

Biological development through play is evidenced by the refinement of both gross and fine motor skills.

Toddlers need time to play alone. At these times children are uninhibited in their expression of feelings. Children reveal in play their concept of the roles of others in the environment, as well as how they perceive others' attitudes or feelings toward them.

Toddlers need time to play with others their own age. When playing with other children their own age, it is helpful if there are similar toys available for use by each child. For example, if playing in sand, each toddler needs a pail and shovel or a pot and large spoon, so that they can perform similar play activities.

Gross motor skills are those abilities children learn in using the large muscles of arms, legs, and the body. Pounding, pedaling, climbing, jumping, reaching, and stretching are a few of the many activities that enhance gross motor skills.

Other forms of play and play materials include wooden beads, sewing cards, puzzles, blocks, crayons, and paints. These types of activities reinforce eye-hand coordination and contribute to the refinement of fine motor skills.

Toddlers need opportunities to express themselves through a variety of media, playing in water, playing with clay or Playdough, and playing in sand.

Provide the place and proper clothing and permit the child to get wet or dirty when involved in these kinds of play activities. Different media provide opportunities for creative expression and release of tension.

Provide experiences with items of different forms and textures such as cotton balls, sandpaper, yarn, wood, pieces of cloth, nylon stocking, mirror, plastic cup, etc.

Permit the toddler to assist in household tasks such as stirring pudding, kneading dough, rolling cookie dough, hammering nails into a block of wood, and using a screwdriver.

Toddlers who are permitted to assist in tasks that are being performed by the caretaker learn the skill of performing a task and how to follow directions.

Play activities influence the psychological development of children. Through play, children are able to ventilate feelings as well as begin to learn measures of self-control.

The attitudes of others and situations to which toddlers are exposed for long periods of time will influence the internal feelings they eventually develop.

Play can be a mode through which children can be assisted in ventilating their feelings.

Negative behaviors are expressions of the toddler's feelings of frustration experienced in attempting to develop more complex skills and to meet the expectations of others.

Toddlers will mimic and imitate in play the roles of mother, father, and others. In their play activities toddlers can be seen practicing voice intonations, body gestures, and methods of awarding approval and discipline as perceived in the parenting role models. Patterns of behavior practiced by the toddler while playing, become the foundation for the patterns that will be used by them as they assume these roles later in life.

Objects or materials such as dolls, teddy bears, and pounding boards should be provided for the toddler to express feelings of love and affection, as well as anger and frustration.

When a toddler is inflicting injury on another child, the toddler's attention should be diverted to toys and inanimate objects.

Many toddlers bite other children and adults. Biting the child in return (not breaking the skin) is often the best solution so the child learns that this is painful.

When toddlers play together, differences of opinion will occur. If given the opportuniity, they will frequently be able to work out their differences on their own.

Social development through play is evidenced by the way children learn how to get along with others, how to lead, follow, cooperate, and compromise.

Provide times when the toddler can have socializing experiences with children of the same age. They also need time with older children, siblings, parents, grandparents, and other adults.

AREAS FOR CONCERN	HELPFUL HINTS

Health promotion—cont'd

PLAY—cont'd

Those social behaviors demonstrated by others will be the behaviors eventually mimicked by the toddler. Since the toddler's social contacts are primarily in the home, *it is important that caretakers practice what they preach.*

Television should not be used as the major form of entertainment. Television *is not* an adequate substitute for solitary play, parallel play, or group play.

Although some television programs are educational, the method of presentation may distort the child's impression of the real world. Toddlers are impressionable; they lack the ability to differentiate between the real and the unreal. A large percentage of television programs and commercials distort the child's impression of the real world by their method of presentation. Constant exposure to speaking letters, dancing numbers, talking animals, and costumed adults suggests to the toddler that these things exist in the real world.

Just as toddlers imitate and model themselves after caretakers and other individuals in their environment, so too will they imitate and pattern their behavior from the antics and roles portrayed on television. The violence and slapstick that are frequently portrayed cannot help but influence the toddler's behavior patterns now and in the future.

SLEEP AND REST

A child 1 to 2 years of age requires approximately 12 to 14 hours of sleep and rest for each 24-hour period.

The 2- to 3-year-old child requires approximately 10 to 12 hours of sleep and rest for each 24-hour period.

Consistency in preparing the toddler for bed becomes the ritual with which the toddler will associate sleep. A nighttime ritual could consist of bathing, reading a story, placing the child in bed, saying good night, and turning on a night-light.

Rest periods should be provided for each day.

The younger toddler may need both a morning and afternoon rest period. The older toddler may require only one rest period per day. Rest periods may fluctuate in length from day to day and are usually based on the amount and type of activity and health status of the child.

Although all toddlers should have rest periods each day, it is not essential that these periods include sleep.

Rest periods can include quiet time while the child listens to music, "reads" a book, or plays with puzzles.

Sleeping and awakening patterns are unique for each child.

Children, when being prepared for bed, use delaying tactics. Some common delaying tactics include asking for another drink of water, kissing caretakers goodnight, rearranging toys, needing to go to the bathroom, saying more prayers and needing one specific object that cannot be found.

Set and maintain the limits of acceptable nighttime ritualism.

Once the nighttime ritual has been completed and the child settled for sleep, caretakers should not acquiesce to new demands made by the child. Tears may result, but if consistency is maintained by the caretaker, the toddler will conform to the expected behaviors.

Uninterrupted periods of sleep and scheduled times for rest are essential to permit restoration and conservation of energy necessary for the toddler's growth.

Some children awaken cheerful, playful, and content to be alone in their crib for varying periods of time. They can be heard talking to themselves, to their toys, or other objects in the room.

Other children will awaken from sleep fretful, irritable, and anxious for immediate attention from the caretaker.

The consistency with which the caretaker meets the needs of the awakening child will determine the ease with which the child conforms to expected behaviors.

Situations that might contribute to interrupted sleep patterns could include strange surroundings, an environmental temperature change, an illness, or a family crisis.

If a child's sleep is interrupted, it is quite likely that the child will be irritable and have difficulty in falling asleep again.

Clues to the need for rest periods can be evidenced in the child's behavior. For example, some children will rub their eyes, become irritable, whiny, or more easily frustrated than usual.

AREAS FOR CONCERN	HELPFUL HINTS

By the end of the toddler period, most children will have advanced from a crib to a small bed. The mattress for every bed should be firm to provide adequate support to the skeletal structure. Ideally, the mattress should also be waterproofed, since toddlers may not yet have achieved full bladder control.

The toddler's bedtime apparel should be loose fitting and appropriate to the climate. It may be necessary for caretakers to add a cover after toddlers fall asleep because body temperature decreases during sleep.

SAFETY

Accident prevention should be of primary concern to everyone who works with or around the toddler. Their ability to move with ease, innate curiosity, desire to investigate everything and anything, and lack of a sense of danger makes toddlers prone to a host of accidents.

Beginning skills of problem solving through tasting, manipulating, pulling, and climbing make toddlers highly vulnerable to situations both inside and outside the home that could be injurious.

Accidents will occur in toddlerhood despite the most vigilant efforts of the caretaker. Efforts should be geared to reduce the incidence of occurrence.

Childproofing the home is essential when the child gains mobility and is given access to investigate the environment.

Childproofing the home should be an organized procedure. Keep in mind the eye level from which children perceive their environment.

One way to begin childproofing the home would be to examine the environment for things that could be classified as "not-to's" for the child. Childproofing is necessary until the child can understand the following:

1. Cords that can be pulled are usually attached to lamps, radios, or other appliances *and are not* meant to *be used to pull* themselves erect.
2. Unattached cords hanging from electrical sockets are *not to be chewed.*
3. Rickety furniture will *not support body weight.*
4. Medicines are *not meant to be eaten* like candy.
5. Gasoline is *not to drink.*
6. Valuable objects of art are *not* playthings.

Once caretakers have carefully examined the environment for hazard areas, then safety measures should be established and adhered to.

A few of the safety measures that should be used when childproofing the environment are listed here:

1. Place gates at stairways.

Remember that children in late infancy, as well as in the toddler period, enjoy climbing and pulling. These children can climb up onto furniture and stairs but do not learn to reverse this process for quite sometime.

Suggestion: Place the gate at the second or third step from the bottom to permit the child the opportunity to develop this new, desirable skill with some degree of safety.

Caution: Remember that ladders and the stairs to sliding boards will attract the child to try out new skills.

2. Store all medications in cabinets (with doors) out of the reach of the child.

Most bathroom medicine cabinets are highly accessible to toddlers who will climb from one piece of bathroom equipment to the other (i.e., toilet seat to sink to medicine cabinet or bathtub to sink to medicine cabinet). Realize also that the toddler may be attracted to the mirror front to see "the baby," but once there discovers new thrills.

Frequently caretakers store their daily medicines on the kitchen table or in kitchen cupboards, which are also easily accessible to the toddler.

Caution: There is no such thing as a harmless medication when it is accessible to children.

AREAS FOR CONCERN	HELPFUL HINTS

Health promotion—cont'd

SAFETY—cont'd

3. Store all household cleansers, polishes, and detergents in cabinets or cupboards out of the child's reach. Always store cleansers and detergents in appropriate, well-labeled containers. *Do not place these substances in bottles, cans, or boxes formerly used to store foodstuffs. Toddlers learn by association and will assume that food is in the container. They do not test by smelling and/or tasting before they swallow.*

Should the child eat or drink medications, seek medical advice. (See Chapter 8, Poisoning.)

In most households supplies such as cleansers, polishes, and detergents are kept under the sink, on the floor of closets, and in floor-level cabinets, all of which are easily accessible and arouse the curiosity of the child to investigate.

Remember that caretakers spend a great percentage of their time in the kitchen and laundry areas; therefore it is likely that the toddler will also be there to socialize.

Suggestion: It would be helpful to provide the toddler with a low cupboard or large container or box for playthings in the kitchen or laundry area.

Caution: Be sure to check every area for injurious substances. The toddler will not differentiate dangerous substances by the area in which it is found.

Should the child eat or drink any of these substances, seek medical advice. (See Chapter 8, Poisoning.)

4. Check all electrical cords for condition and location.

   Cover all unused electrical wall sockets.

   Remove any extension cords that are connected to the wall socket, but are not attached to an appliance.

   Prevent dangling of cords attached to appliances such as toasters, coffee pots, frying pans, or hot plates.

Be sure that electrical cords are intact, not frayed, attached to an appliance, and in place in the wall socket.

Reduce the likelihood of the older infant and young toddler from poking fingers or other objects into a live electrical socket by covering it when not in use.

Older infants and toddlers will pick up the free end of dangling electrical cords and place them in their mouths, with disastrous results.

The older infant's and toddler's skills of reaching, cruising, and standing on tiptoes enable them to pull the cord to see what will happen. Serious burns, scalds, and other injuries frequently are the result of pulling down irons, coffee pots, or lamps.

5. Be alert to the position of pot handles on the stove, sink, counter, and table or places above the toddler's line of vision but within reach.

Toddlers reach and pull at items that attract their attention and trigger their curiosity.

Caution: Caretakers may have to change meal preparation habits, deliberately and consistently remembering to turn pot handles inward.

6. Stoves, ovens, broilers, microwave ovens, and toasters have the potential to inflict severe burns when in operation.

Caretakers will find it necessary to use firm words such as "no" or "hot" consistently and emphatically. Only use those words in reference to things that do get hot. (See Chapter 8, Burns.)

7. Tablecloths, hanging plants, dangling curtains, towels, and items of clothing also must be viewed as potential items of investigation for toddlers.

To investigate objects on the table, the toddler will pull the tablecloth, bringing everything with it.

Caution: Tablecloths may be decorative, but very dangerous to toddlers.

8. Household furnishings such as end tables, lamps, and bookcases may be potential causes of injury.

Toddlers will use any lamp table, coffee table, lamp pole, magazine rack, or other available piece of furniture to climb upon and to pull erect. Remove rickety furniture or items that can be easily broken.

9. Check the location and accessibility of dangerous yard and garden equipment.

Toddlers will wish to imitate lawn mowing efforts of the caretaker.

Caution: Power lawn mowers can throw stones and other debris with great force and distance. *Keep toddlers out of the range of mower debris!*

Since toddlers like to mimic and imitate the adult, provide safe imitation equipment.

Sharp instruments such as hoes, scissors, saws, knives, and other cutting devices should be stored in areas that are not accessible to toddlers.

AREAS FOR CONCERN	HELPFUL HINTS

Electric hedge clippers, trimmers, weeders, and other electrical equipment are also potentially dangerous items.

10. Storage of liquid fuels, pesticides, motor oils, and polishing and cleansing substances must be in containers in cupboards or cabinets well out of the toddler's range. *Do not place any of these substances in bottles, cans, or boxes formerly used to store foodstuffs. Toddlers learn by association and will assume that food is still in the container. They do not test by smelling and/or tasting before swallowing.*
Caution: Harmful substances such as these are also stored in garages, outdoor cabinets, basements, automobile trunks, camper vans, and boats to name but a few places.

11. Clear the play area or yard of all rusty or inoperable equipment such as old swings, slide boards, lumber with rusty nails, trash, etc.

12. Safety measures must be consistently adhered to whenever toddlers are in or near water (bathtubs, pools, rivers, ponds, lakes, oceans, or quarries).

Items that make sounds or move intrigue toddlers. Never leave electrical tools plugged in and unattended because the toddler will investigate.

Toddlers by nature will investigate and try everything that is new and available to them. *Limits must be set and adhered to for play areas and safe areas of exploration.*

Because of increased mobility, although still unstable, toddlers will run, climb, jump, and fall. To prevent serious injury, provide safe areas for play.

Toddlers must have responsible supervision when in the water, whether they are being bathed or playing in a pool.

Caution: Children can drown in as little as 1 inch (2.54 cm) of water if they should fall and bump their heads and end up face down in the water.

Children in later infancy usually have no fear of water. They can drown in a small child's pool because of their limited ability to pick themselves up after a fall.

The fearless exploratory nature of toddlers spurs them to run head on into situations they are not able to handle, such as the impact of an ocean wave or the depth of an unknown body of water.

If toddlers are on a boat, they must have a floating vest or jacket on at all times.

Children can be taught to swim, even in infancy. It is highly recommended that children be taught to swim at an early age, particularly if the child is exposed to water frequently.

Caution: Flotation devices should never be substituted for responsible supervision. These devices are merely an additional safety feature for the exuberant unpredictable toddler.

All above-ground pools or built-in pools should be enclosed by fencing with lockable gates.

Inflatable backyard pools should be emptied after each use. Too often these small pools are not emptied for a few days and then become a medium for bacterial growth.

Set ground rules of safety at pools that are clear, concise, and enforced. Although the following list is far from complete, a few suggested rules are provided:

1. When children are in the pool, adult supervision must be provided.
2. Running around the pool should not be permitted.
3. Food and beverages should not be permitted in the pool area.
4. Children who do not know how to swim must wear flotation devices and stay at the shallow end.
5. Diving and jumping into the pool are to be done only in areas where it is safe.
6. Roughhousing should be prohibited.
7. The pool is not to be used as a bathroom.
8. If dirt and grass surround the pool, rinse the feet before entering the water.

AREAS FOR CONCERN	HELPFUL HINTS

Health promotion—cont'd

SAFETY—cont'd

13. Yard safety measures are essential. Supervision of the toddler at play must be provided because the toddler lacks the knowledge and experience to differentiate pleasure from danger.

When childproofing the yard, caretakers must keep in mind the toddler's limited motor skills and inability to perceive danger. For example, toddlers like to swing and when approaching the swings will be unaware of the potential danger of being hit by another child already swinging.

Caution: Potential dangerous equipment in backyards includes swings, gliders, sliding boards, or seesaws.

Scrutinize the toddler's play area inside and outside the home for trees, shrubs, and plants that may be poisonous.

The curious toddler will be attracted to and investigate gardens, trees, shrubs, and flowering plants. Many of these have poisonous components. For example, sumac, poison ivy, and poison oak are dangerous to touch, as well as to eat. The berries of some plants and blossoms and leaves of others can also be poisonous.

Caution: Avoid burning poison ivy in a trash or leaf fire because inhalation of the smoke fumes can cause a severe generalized allergic response.

14. Fires and burns. The flickering flame of a fire and billowing smoke will attract curious toddlers. Clothing becomes ignited when toddlers are too close to the flame.

Vigilance is necessary on the part of caretakers in keeping the toddler from being burned.

Areas of play once perceived to be free of danger may become a hazardous playground. For example, equipment used on a part-time basis such as space heaters, open gas heaters, Franklin stoves, and fireplaces become potential hazards.

Burning leaves or trash can also become a source of danger for the exploring toddler. Burning cigarettes, pipes, cigars, and candles also attract curious toddlers.

Out of doors, the toddler can be attracted to fireplaces, barbecue grills, camp fires, and trash fires.

15. Electrical fans of all types lure the toddler into close investigation of the blades and possible injury.

Toddlers will examine with their fingers and poke pencils or toys into the blades of fans, thus resulting in injury. To provide safeguards, caretakers should place fans in areas or at levels to which toddlers do not have access. In addition, some fans on the market have a safety feature in which the fan will stop if any object comes in contact with the rotating blade.

16. Windows offer toddlers avenues to the outside world and must be viewed as potential sources of danger.

Every window must be assessed for features of danger such as the manner in which it opens, how it is secured, placement, and depth of the sill.

Toddlers should never be permitted to stand or sit on window ledges as vantage points for viewing activities outside. Although the window is closed or a screen is in place, these measures will not ensure the toddler's safety.

17. Other objects of danger in the toddler's environment include scissors, knives, lollipop and Popsicle sticks, pencils, and pens.

Insist that toddlers sit down when eating a Popsicle or when sucking a lollipop. New motor skills along with imperfect balance cause tumbles and falls.

Sharp cutting objects such as knives and scissors must be kept in safe places out of reach of the toddler. If scissors are to be moved from one area to another, teach toddlers to carry the scissors holding the points down.

AREAS FOR CONCERN	HELPFUL HINTS

DISCIPLINE

Areas of discipline to consider during toddlerhood include setting limits, punishment, control (expectations of others), and self-control.

Discipline must be consistent and agreed on by caretakers and revised at each period of life.

Toddlers quickly learn to play one caretaker against another to gain their own way and assert their autonomy.

Limit setting

Toddlers must have limits set that are consistently maintained. Physical parameters—places permitted for exploration.

Caretakers must set limits for toddlers. Toddlers need to know what they can do and where they can play.

Limit setting for toddlers should not be beyond their ability to meet or constructively use.

In the home, a low cupboard in the kitchen area may be set aside for toddler's toys. Only this cupboard may be used by the toddler.

Toddlers are unable to identify safe from unsafe areas, thus limit setting helps provide safety and security.

In the yard introduce toddlers to the fenced area. They can then be outside alone but cannot leave the fenced area.

Danger areas such as hot stoves and fireplaces have already been discussed. Impress on the toddler that these *are not* areas for investigation.

Avoid overprotection. Permit toddlers to explore and investigate and expect that bruises and bumps will occur.

Behavioral expectations—with family members and with others. Limit setting in regard to behaviors with others enables toddlers to learn basic patterns of socialization.

Toddlers can be taught that different behaviors are expected with different activities. For example, although mealtime is a period of socialization, it is not playtime. Children should be expected to eat food, not throw it.

A few simple basic rules or guidelines must be established and enforced to assist toddlers in learning new social behaviors. Rules must be simple and directed to only one situation.

Toddlers need rules for security, but too many rules will confuse them.

On a shopping trip the toddler is expected to stay in the cart or walk holding onto the cart. Punishment for infraction *should be* meted out immediately.

Words such as "stop" and "no" spoken firmly have a definite place in the area of discipline. These words should be used to enforce rules, clarify meanings of directions, and gain immediate attention.

The word "no" is a powerful word and should be used *only when absolutely necessary*. Frequent use of the word "no" weakens its impact and clouds its effectiveness.

Punishment

Methods of inflicting penalties for nonacceptable behavior, infractions of rules, and/or violations of limits may include pain, loss of freedom, and/or forfeiture of privileges.

Points for the caretaker to consider when child's misbehavior merits punishment include the following:

1. Control the *self* before attempting to control the situation, do not react or overreact.
2. Clarify whether the incident was an accident or a misbehavior.
3. Punish the child immediately. Do not threaten with delayed punishment such as "wait until your father comes home."
4. Keep punishment realistic for the age of child and the offense committed.

   Spanking the child (two to three swats on the bottom)
   Having the child sit still (5 to 10 minutes)
   Taking away a favorite toy (1 day)
   No television (1 day)

Punishment, although at times necessary, should not cause physical injury or humiliation.

Control

Controls are the external measures used by others to guide and direct the activities and behaviors of people to conform to family and/or societal norms.

External controls for directing and guiding others in acceptable activities and behaviors will change in scope and expectation as children progress from one stage of development to another.

Behavioral expectations and methods of control differ with each individual. If toddlers are to be exposed to many caretakers it will be most difficult to maintain consistency of discipline.

When toddlers are engaged in unacceptable behavior, distract them by providing an acceptable activity.

Distraction works well with toddlers because they have such heights of curiosity and short attention spans.

AREAS FOR CONCERN	HELPFUL HINTS

Health promotion—cont'd

DISCIPLINE—cont'd

Caretakers react immediately when misbehavior or accidents occur. Avoid *reacting negatively* to situations that occur normally with children during toddlerhood.

Incident	*Reaction*
The toddler, reaching out for one item of food, accidently knocks over cup of milk.	The caretaker responds, "Ooops, everybody grab a napkin." Everybody, including the toddler, is involved in cleaning up the spilled milk.
	The caretaker, speaking pleasantly to toddler, "We'll fill your cup half full this time and put it farther back on the table."
The 3-year-old is pulling the 1-year-old sibling by the seat of the pants (diaper) across the kitchen floor.	The caretaker immediately verbally reprimands and spanks the 3-year-old.
	When the 3-year-old stops crying she informs the caretaker that she was saving her sister from falling down the cellar steps by pulling her away from the open cellar door. The caretaker then apologizes for having punished the child when the child actually was *not* misbehaving.

Caretakers *must* admit when they are in error, not only at times of punishment, but at all times. The result will be that children learn that all people *will* make mistakes.

It must be made clear that punishment is not an outcome of the caretaker's displeasure with the child, but displeasure with the unacceptable behavior.

When reacting to misbehavior, caretakers should describe what they see, feel, and expect. Avoid lowering the child's self-esteem by humiliation with expressions such as "You're so stupid!" "Why are you so dumb?" Instead, state, "I am angry, I am hurt, and/or I am very disappointed with your behavior."

Self-control

Self-control: The internalization of expected norms of behavior, among which are decision-making methods, choosing right from wrong, viewing circumstances from many sides, expecting and accepting punishment, and delaying gratification.

Toddlers learn the basic concepts of self-control through the examples of the behaviors of others and through the external controls imposed on their behavior by others.

Self-control is an ongoing lifetime process.

As in every other realm of development, several opportunities for learning the expected behaviors and norms must be provided.

If caretakers react in anger or prejudge situations, the toddler will mimic that same behavior in future play periods. For example, a toddler may be seen hitting and shaking a teddy bear, screaming, "Dumb, stupid teddy, why you do that?"

If caretakers consistently take the time to gain information before reacting, then the toddler also mimics that behavior. For example, a toddler with two stuffed animals will ask, "Bear—what you do to Teddy? Teddy—who hit first?"

Viewing circumstances from many sides and learning control measures help children develop insight into their own behaviors.

It is our belief that children want to please. Toddlers derive great pleasure and satisfaction from moments when they know that behaviors or activities of theirs have brought pleasure and satisfaction to the caretaker.

Children are very sociable and will seek attention and approval. If attention and approval are not provided for the toddler's good behavior, it is not unusual for the toddler to revert to bad behavior. *Some attention, even in the form of painful discipline, is better than no attention at all.*

NEGATIVISM

Patterns of speech and behavior of a negative nature displayed by toddlers may be labeled as *negativism*.

Toddlers often display negativism through speech and behavior. Toddlers learn that certain words such as "no" have much more impact than words like "bread" or "dolly." They enjoy the power of the word.

86

AREAS FOR CONCERN	HELPFUL HINTS
Negative speech includes such words as "no," "shut up," "bad," "naughty," swear words, or any other word that has a meaning of power to the toddler.	The caretaker and toddler may use the same "power word." The "power word" has different meanings for caretakers than it does for toddlers. Toddlers will frequently use "power words" at appropriate times and places without understanding the full ramifications of these words. This use of "power words" may cause consternation on the part of the caretaker. The use of "bad words" by the toddler should be ignored, and caretakers should avoid using these words in their own vocabulary. Remember, toddlers learn through mimicry.
Negative behavior may range from facial expressions, spitting, hand gestures, slapping, and kicking to full-blown temper tantrums. Circumstances that frequently precipitate negativistic behavior include the following:	Toddlers remain self-centered beings who are trying to assert themselves and gain autonomy. Their negative speech and behaviors are attempts to gain their own way by mimicking the external controls set by others.
1. Denial of a desired object or activity.	Toddlers must know the limits for acceptable behavior and can only learn through consistent guidelines that have been established by the caretaker. One- through three-year-old's live in the "immediate present" and lack the ability to conceptualize the "future." Thus denial of an object or activity with promise of it at some future date is incomprehensible to the toddler. If it is necessary that an object or activity be denied, give a simple explanation and expect compliance.
2. Interruption of activity.	When it is necessary for the caretaker to interrupt the toddler's activity, precede the interruption with a warning. A timer set to go off in a period of 5 to 10 minutes will be the signal to end play. Toddlers will learn a concept of time as well as to cease play activity when a time set is used by the caretaker.
3. Ignoring a request.	Children learn that requests made will not always be pleasurable to them. As caretakers' expectations of children's behavior remain consistent, children will learn to meet those expectations. Refrain from unnecessary requests.
4. Overtired.	Toddlers seem to have boundless energy; however, caretakers learn to identify those behaviors unique for each child that signify the need for rest. Some of these behaviors are sucking fingers or the thumb; rubbing the eyes; whining voice; irritability; desire to be picked up, then put down; clinging; and even short spurts of increased activity.
5. Fear of separation from the caretaker. Toddlers become very attached to the caretaker with whom they spend long periods of time and will react negatively when the caretaker leaves them.	To accustom the child to separation and assist in teaching the concept of "future time," brief periods of separation should be planned with someone familiar to the toddler. The caretaker informs the toddler when and where they are going and when they will return. It is important that the caretaker uses phrases the toddler knows, such as "I am going shopping now," "Aunt Ruth will stay with you," "I will be back after you have had lunch." Be truthful because a deceived toddler begins to doubt the caretaker's honesty and dependability. If caretakers are honest and dependable, toddlers will respond to brief separations with trust and confidence. Thus toddlers become more secure in their quest for autonomy.

AREAS FOR CONCERN	HELPFUL HINTS

Health promotion—cont'd

NEGATIVISM—cont'd

Temper tantrums

Temper tantrum: A lack of emotional and physical control by the toddler characterized by a variety of actions. Some of these actions could include the following:

1. Holding breath
2. Screaming
3. Throwing self on floor
4. Kicking
5. Pounding hands and arms
6. Stamping feet
7. Attacking caretaker or younger sibling
8. Banging head

Temper tantrums are means by which toddlers seek attention and attempt to get their own way.

Immediate retaliation on the part of the caretaker to the tantrum permits the toddler to succeed in accomplishing the first goal—getting attention. Further compliance of the caretaker to the toddler's tantrum opens the way for them to accomplish the second goal—having their own way.

The toddler soon learns that a tantrum is an effective tool to control the environment and to manipulate other people.

Preventing temper tantrums is the *best* practice. Keep at a minimum those circumstances which frequently precipitate negative behavior.

The time and place toddlers choose for having a temper tantrum is frequently frustrating and embarrassing to the caretaker. Ignoring the tantrum is probably the best response to be taken by caretakers, yet is difficult to do, particularly when the tantrum occurs outside the home.

When temper tantrums occur in the home, the caretaker should acknowledge that the child is upset and invite the child to another room.

If the toddler has a temper tantrum in a store, acknowledge that the child is upset, tell the child you are leaving, proceed to the next aisle, and invite the child to come along.

Although the caretaker has left the toddler, demonstrating disapproval of the temper tantrum behavior, the fact that the toddler was invited to join the caretaker in another area helps the toddler learn to develop self-control and differentiate acceptable from nonacceptable behavior.

Toddlers rarely inflict injury on themselves although their tantrums look violent and may cause damage to inanimate objects or hurt the person on whom they are venting their feelings.

Caretakers become alarmed when toddlers hold their breath, turn blue, and faint. The body reacts spontaneously to a lack of oxygen and the child *will* take a breath, the skin will return to normal color, and the child will awaken. Caretakers become so alarmed that in attempting to thwart the behavior, they accede to the child's wishes.

During the health conference, information should be gathered about the pattern of temper tantrums to assist health professionals in determining whether this behavior is indeed a tantrum or perhaps is a neurological problem that requires additional investigation and follow-up.

Tantrums must be differentiated from seizures because both can be triggered by frustrating or stressful situations. (See Chapter 8, Convulsive Disorders.)

Additional suggestions for the management of temper tantrums include the following:

1. Avoid restraining the child during a tantrum unless the child is injuring another person.
2. Avoid bribery as a method of stopping the tantrum because this acknowledges that tantrums do work.
3. Avoid threatening with punishment during the tantrum because child is too out of control to be able to attend to this knowledge.
4. Avoid spanking after the tantrum because child has finally gained self-control.
5. Avoid offering either food or liquid during or immediately after a tantrum; this may trigger vomiting. When the child is calm, offer comfort. After a calming period, offer food and drink, since a great deal of energy was expended during the tantrum.

AREAS FOR CONCERN	HELPFUL HINTS

When toddlers are calm, suggest that in the future they work out their feelings of anger and frustration on a pounding board, punching bag, pillow, or even a doll. Be sure that the objects are available to them.

SIBLING RIVALRY

Sibling rivalry can be defined as that behavior exhibited by an individual who feels threatened by the existence of a brother or sister.

Children should be prepared for the arrival of a new baby.

Preparation of the toddler for a new brother or sister (sibling) should not be started too early in the mother's pregnancy, but in the sixth or seventh month. Keep explanations simple and concise.

Make changes in the home environment prior to the new baby's arrival to provide time for the toddler to adjust to the new situation.

Moving a toddler from a crib to a bed should be based on the toddler's new abilities rather than an explanation that the crib is needed for the baby.

Praising the toddler's new abilities helps develop the understanding that toddlers have progressed beyond infancy, thus reducing the feelings of being deprived by the presence of new siblings.

A few of the behaviors toddlers may demonstrate when seeing a new baby include the desire to touch, pick up, and carry the baby, play with the baby's toys, and drink from the baby's bottles. Permitting and encouraging toddlers to assist the caretaker in caring for the new baby fosters independence in the toddler. Toddlers then see that babies are dependent on others.

Toddlers need to feel loved and wanted, not replaced by the new baby.

The existence of a sibling may generate within the toddler feelings of jealousy, envy, anger, and resentment.

In attempting to cope with these negative feelings the toddler might be openly hostile or regress in behavior. If the coping mechanism used by the toddler is successful, this same mechanism will likely be used in the future life experiences whenever that individual feels threatened.

Open hostility is a behavior that may be manifested directly or indirectly.

Direct hostility may be evidenced by the toddler hitting the baby or calling the baby "bad names."

The toddler's feelings of anger may be directed to caretakers as well as to the new sibling. Providing love, affection and attention to the toddler as well as diversions prove beneficial.

Divert the toddler's attention to an activity that is socially acceptable such as pounding a pegboard or punching a punching bag. (Hitting the toddler merely reinforces the idea that hitting is an acceptable behavior.) Simple explanations of desirable behavior expected by caretaker should accompany the diversional tactics. Avoid long-winded explanations.

Indirect hostility is manifested in the toddler's obvious clumsiness in bumping the baby or dropping a toy on the baby.

Regression is when the individual reverts to a former or more infantile level of behavior.

Toddlers who tend to internalize feelings may revert to infantile behaviors such as sucking thumbs, wetting themselves, clinging to the caretaker, or wanting to revert to bottle- or breast-feeding (regression).

These infantile behaviors are the toddler's way of saying "I want your attention too." If caretakers respond with love in meeting the toddler's desires for attention, the regressive behaviors will usually disappear quickly.

AREAS FOR CONCERN	HELPFUL HINTS

Health promotion—cont'd

SIBLING RIVALRY—cont'd

If one caretaker is involved with the care of the new baby the other caretaker should find time to provide individualized attention for the toddler.

If only one caretaker is present, an opportune time to provide attention to both the toddler and the new baby is at feeding time. While holding the infant in one arm, the caretaker could encircle the toddler with the other arm, permitting the toddler to nestle against her as the baby nurses or is fed.

Sibling rivalry is expected. The outcome can be positive or negative depending on how the situation is handled.

Help toddlers ventilate their feelings and assist them in developing positive coping mechanisms.

Hospitalization

Toddlers may need hospitalization because of accidents, infections, elective surgery, or corrective surgery.

The toddler period is a more difficult time for hospitalization than infancy because of an increased attachment to the caretaker.

Toddlers have difficulty understanding abstract concepts and may be unable to understand the need for absence of or separation from the caretaker.

Toddlers fear separation from caretakers. They may have difficulty relating to new people and strange places.

Toddlers are beginning to develop a sense of autonomy and to have some control over the environment in which they live. Placed in a strange building with strange people would be most threatening to toddlers and will frequently cause them to regress to previous infantile behaviors.

To assist toddlers' adjustment to strange new places it frequently proves helpful to bring their favorite object(s) from home. These familiar objects provide a sense of security. Labeling the object with the child's name is desirable to prevent loss during the period of hospitalization.

It might be necessary for preadmission laboratory tests to be performed. To facilitate the ease with which some of these tests can be performed, it will be necessary to immobilize or secure the cooperation of the toddler. If the caretakers are willing to assist, they should be encouraged to do so.

Due to toddlers' difficulty in adjusting to a hospital environment, it is helpful if caretakers can stay with them.

Explanations of the procedures and their purpose should be given to the caretaker. Toddlers should be given simple explanations and directives to assist them in cooperating so that the procedure can be performed quickly.

Although hospitalization of toddlers is traumatic to caretakers, their presence and assistance are beneficial. At times it may be beyond the caretaker's ability to handle the toddler during these stressful procedures.

It is extremely important that toddlers be told that the procedures will hurt, they will be helped in holding their position, and they can cry. Following the procedure it is equally important to commend and praise toddlers for their cooperation, although they may have cried, kicked, and otherwise rebelled throughout the entire period.

There may be some procedures performed during which the caretaker's presence is not permitted; however, the caretaker can stay nearby to be present when the procedure has been completed.

When it is necessary for the caretaker to leave (for long or short periods of time) it should be expected that the toddler will become upset, cry, and even cling to the caretaker. This behavior is usually of short duration.

Toddlers will cry and fuss when the caretaker leaves. This period of protest is usually of short duration because toddlers are easily distracted. Once good-byes have been said, leave and do not come back and start the entire separation process over again.

It is essential that caretakers be truthful in their explanations to toddlers about their leaving. After a truthful explanation, caretakers should leave quickly without a prolonged exit. A sense of trust can be further established or reinforced by the honesty of the caretakers and health professionals at times such as these.

Some toddlers may reject the caretakers on their return but within minutes they are receptive to the love and attention being given.

AREAS FOR CONCERN

During hospitalization, health professionals should capitalize on the toddler's accomplished skills by the following:
1. Providing eating utensils that the toddler can manipulate.
2. Providing foods appropriate in quantity and appeal for the toddler.
3. Expecting and encouraging toddlers to feed themselves.
4. Providing appropriate toileting equipment for the toddler's use if toilet training has been started.
5. Providing appropriate play areas and materials.
6. Maintaining appropriate safety measures.

HELPFUL HINTS

Although attempts may have been made to facilitate the toddler's previously developed skills, it should come as no surprise that following hospitalization the toddler's behavior will have regressed. This regression is quickly overcome as the caretaker's expectations and typical patterns of behavior for this child are reestablished.

Safety measures within hospital settings are instituted for the safety of children and others.

Hospital cribs are higher than cribs usually found in the home; therefore crib rails should be up all the way when the toddler is in bed.

Areas such as kitchens and utility and treatment rooms are off limits because of the various types of solutions and equipment contained there. Inquire as to the areas where children are permitted to roam and play.

CHAPTER 8

HEALTH PROBLEMS OF TODDLERS

Although the toddler is usually very healthy, this is the time of life that tries the caretaker's soul. Toddlers are extremely accident prone because of their insatiable curiosity and their ability to travel and investigate.

Accident prevention becomes a major family concern. First aid kits should be available in the home and in the automobile. In addition, first aid supplies should accompany the family on all trips and outings, such as picnics, family gatherings, and boating and camping expeditions.

In everyday activities, the toddler acquires bruises, abrasions, cuts, and lacerations. Because of a limited sense of danger, the toddler often oversteps the bounds of safety, and more serious injuries occur.

Many of the illnesses of infancy, such as earaches and common colds, are typical health problems of this period of life and will not be discussed again. Accidents, bites, stings, allergies, urinary tract infections, and respiratory tract infections will be discussed, with health care guidelines and helpful hints provided for each problem area.

HEALTH PROBLEM	HEALTH CARE GUIDELINES	HELPFUL HINTS
Accidents *Accident:* The occurrence of a sudden, unexpected event with a resulting unfortunate outcome.	*Prevention* is the *key factor* in protecting toddlers from accidents.	Major concepts in prevention of accidents are supervision, safe internal and external environments, and limit setting.
ABRASIONS (BRUSH BURNS, SCRAPES) Abrasions result from a fall where skin is brushed across a rough surface, such as pavement or cinders. The most common sites of injury for the toddler are knees and elbows.	The skin surface exhibits small, multiple nicks accompanied by small drops of blood. The skin may also be completely brushed away and foreign material embedded in it. The area should be cleansed and treated with an antiseptic. The preferred treatment is to expose the site to air. Conditions such as the age of the child, extent of the injury, or activity of the child may dictate the need for the application of a sterile dressing.	Scrapes and brush burns (abrasions) occur when the child falls. Very little bleeding occurs. Rinse the dirt from the skin wound with a cool water spray. The injured area should be washed with mild soap and water before applying the antiseptic. If a covering is necessary, apply a sterile dressing. Some dressings on the market are sterile, do not stick to the scraped (abraded) area, and are therefore easier and less painful to remove. *If soil is in the abraded site check with the physician as to the need for tetanus toxoid or antitoxin injections.*
BRUISES (BUMPS) Bruises usually result from a blow or fall. They may be combined with an abrasion and/or laceration.	Bruised skin is not usually broken but appears red and swollen. Within 24 hours the area changes color to "black and blue" because of broken blood vessels under the skin.	Bruises appear as swollen reddened lumps, can accompany scrapes, and turn black and blue while healing. If there is no break in the skin, immediately apply a cold pack or cold compress to the injured area. If there is broken skin, cleanse it with an antiseptic and cover it before applying cold to the bruised area. *Caution:* The application of cold to skin surfaces can cause pain. Always cover the cold pack with a cloth (towel) before applying it to the injured area. Limit the cold application to less than 20 minutes at one time.
BURNS A burn is trauma to tissues caused by heat, radiation, chemical, or corrosive substances. *External burns:* Trauma to external tissues that varies in extent and depth of severity; classified as first, second, or third degree. 1. Superficial (first-degree) burns: Red, painful, and swollen, involving epidermal layer of skin and/or mucous membranes. 2. Partial thickness (second-degree) burns: Redness, blisters, and extreme pain, involving epidermal and dermal tissue.	Burns on toddlers are usually because of accidents that could be prevented. (See Chapter 7, Safety.) The immediate treatment of first- and second-degree burns covering less than 20% of the body is immersion of the body part into ice cold water or running ice cold water over the affected part of the body until pain subsides. If pain returns after removal from ice water, resume the treatment. After the cold water treatment, pat the area dry and avoid friction.	Preventing burns and other accidents cannot be overemphasized with caretakers. Burns that only redden the skin are considered *superficial,* or *first degree.* If the skin blisters or the burn involves more than just the outer skin, it is considered a *second-degree burn.* Icy cold water or ice cubes applied immediately provide the best home care for first- and second-degree burns. The initial application of cold will be extremely painful. It may be necessary to insist on and maintain treatment against the child's wishes.

93

HEALTH PROBLEM	HEALTH CARE GUIDELINES	HELPFUL HINTS
Accidents—cont'd BURNS—cont'd 3. Total thickness (third-degree) burns: Destruction of the epidermal and dermal layers, including nerve endings, sebaceous glands, and hair follicles. Can also involve muscle and bone tissue.	Analgesic ointments or first aid creams may be applied to first- or second-degree burns. Light bandaging may also be used. All burns that cover more than 10% of the body should receive immediate medical attention. When seeking medical advice give the following information: 1. Cause of burn 2. Extent of burn 3. Description of burn areas 4. Level of consciousness The rule of nines (Appendix F) can be used to estimate the amount of surface area that is burned.	First aid creams or ointments can be applied judiciously to first- and some second-degree burns. *Avoid applying thick, greasy substances such as butter, lard, or petroleum jelly to burned areas.* If second-degree burns are excessive, seek medical advice. *Third-degree burns* destroy the top layers of the skin and can involve muscle tissue and bones. Third-degree burns should always be treated by health professionals.
Internal burns: Trauma and/or destruction of internal tissues and organs.	Swallowing of caustic substances is the most common type of internal burns seen in toddlers. When drinking, toddlers tend to swallow without testing, thus the mucous membranes of the mouth, oral pharynx, and esophagus are all involved. These burns require immediate medical attention. When seeking medical advice, give the following information: 1. Substance swallowed 2. Presence or absence of vomiting 3. Level of consciousness Signs and symptoms will include pain, swelling, and the inability to swallow. Tissue that comes in contact with the corrosive substances will be affected. Tissue ulceration and perforation of the esophagus are common results. The child's pulse becomes rapid, weak, and thready. Prostration follows quickly. *Vomiting is to be discouraged because it increases the severity and extent of the trauma.* Management is directed toward neutralizing the ingested substance and maintaining a patent airway. Damage to the esophagus may warrant the need for a gastrostomy. If trauma to the oral pharynx is sufficient to obstruct the child's airway, a tracheostomy will be necessary. With healing, scar tissue forms that can cause strictures within the esophagus. In this case, dilation of the esophagus will have to be done.	Toddlers can burn themselves internally by swallowing corrosive substances like lye. When it is suspected that a toddler has swallowed a corrosive substance, *never induce vomiting or offer fluids.* *Swallowing lye, caustic soda, or other corrosives is an immediate medical emergency.* Swallowing caustic substances can lead to problems with eating and breathing. Lifesaving and life-sustaining operations may have to be performed. Recovery is long and often painful. Many follow-up operations may be needed.

HEALTH PROBLEM	HEALTH CARE GUIDELINES	HELPFUL HINTS
CONCUSSION A concussion is an injury to the head that may cause temporary or permanent damage to brain tissue. Falls from heights or blows inflicted with objects such as a shovel or toys are the usual causes of concussions.	Concussion symptoms will vary depending on the location of the impact to the head and the degree of injury. Symptoms can be as minor as transient dizziness or a headache to more serious changes, such as partial or total paralysis or unconsciousness. If injury is accompanied by vomiting and/or bleeding that cannot be stopped, medical assistance should immediately be obtained. If vomiting occurs, note the content, color, and amount. Seek medical assistance. Transport the child, if necessary, in a lying-down position. Give the following information: 1. Time of accident 2. Cause of injury 3. Extent of injury 4. Presence or absence of bleeding 5. Level of consciousness 6. Presence or absence of vomiting 7. Type of vomiting and amount	Injuries to the head are referred to as *concussions.* Apply cold compresses to the injured area. Have the toddler rest in a lying-down position with shoulders slightly elevated. *Do not give medication of any kind.* Observe the toddler for the ability to be awakened from sleep for 12 to 24 hours. If the toddler is difficult to wake, seek medical care. Bleeding from the injured area can usually be stopped by use of pressure to the site. If bleeding persists or the child begins to vomit, seek medical advice.
FRACTURES (BROKEN BONES) A fracture is a discontinuity of the bone that can be described as a complete or incomplete break. *Incomplete break:* Those fractures which involve one side of the bone but do not traverse the diameter of the bone.	Common sites of fractures in toddlers are arms and legs with a high incidence of fractured femurs. Incomplete fractures are more common in young children than are complete fractures because of the soft bone structure. As children grow older, the bones become harder and more brittle as full mineralization takes place. Incomplete fractures may produce pain, swelling, and a reluctance to use the limb, although in some cases there are no signs or symptoms at all. The management of incomplete fractures (if diagnosed) is directed toward symptomatic relief. This may include closed manipulation and/or casting.	A broken bone (fracture) can be either a complete or an incomplete break. An incomplete break (partial fracture) involves only a portion of the bone, but the child will be reluctant to move that bone. A complete break (complete fracture) crosses the entire diameter of the bone. Complete fractures may be visible because the bone may actually penetrate the skin. Toddlers' ability to climb and investigate predisposes them to falls and fractures. Toddlers frequently break arms or legs (upper leg bone [femur] is a very common site). Caretakers should be alerted to the fact that the initial management of toddlers with fractured femurs is hospitalization. Toddlers whose fractures (arms or legs) require traction will also be hospitalized. Toddlers whose fractures require casts are usually cared for at home. (See Chapter 18, Cast Care.)
Complete break: Fractures revealing a break across the total diameter of the bone. The pattern of the break will vary; the break may be spiral, transverse, or shattered.	Complete fractures are evidenced by pain, swelling, and contusions of the tissue at the fracture site. There may be perforation of the skin with some bleeding. In addition, there may be limited motion of the extremity or the inability to move it at all.	Complete fractures usually cause pain and swelling at the site of injury. Bleeding will be present if the bone punctures the skin. Medical advice must be sought.

HEALTH PROBLEM	HEALTH CARE GUIDELINES	HELPFUL HINTS
Accidents—cont'd FRACTURES (BROKEN BONES)—cont'd	Management of complete fractures is directed toward relieving muscle spasm, maintaining bone alignment, and preventing wound infection. Open or closed manipulation, traction, and/or casting may be used to maintain correct bone alignment. Analgesics and antibodies may be included in the medical regimen. Medical advice should be sought whenever a fracture is suspected.	Treatment may include surgery, traction, and/or casting. (See Chapter 18, Cast Care.)
LACERATIONS (CUTS) A laceration is an injury to a body part where a sharp instrument has cut or torn an area of tissue.	The injured area gives the appearance of two bleeding edges of the skin with oozing or spurting of blood from the afflicted area. The edges of the injured skin may appear jagged and irregular. Debris and/or dirt may be embedded in the injured tissue. If blood is spurting it must be controlled by pressure points and a compressed dressing. Bleeding will cleanse the wound; however, great blood loss will induce shock. Emergency treatment at a local hospital or by a physician may be required if bleeding cannot be stopped within 3 to 5 minutes or if the edges of the injured site need suturing.	A cut (laceration) is a wound caused by a sharp instrument. There may be bleeding (either oozing or spurting). The bleeding should be controlled. Pressure immediately applied over the wound will control oozing blood. Pressure applied at pressure points as well as directly over the wound will temporarily control spurting blood. If spurting of blood continues, seek medical advice. If dirt is in the wound, remove it with cool water, moistened gauze, or a soft spray of cool water. Be careful that bleeding has been stopped. The injured area may be cleansed with mild soap and water followed by an antiseptic and covered with sterile gauze or a no-stick dressing. Ragged edges of the wound may need to be united prior to application of dressings. Commercially prepared adhesive strips can be used for this purpose. If the edges of the wound pull apart with the use of adhesive strips, then medical treatment will be needed to suture the wound. *The need for tetanus toxoid or antitoxin injections may be required because of the nature of the foreign material in the wound.*
POISONING Poisoning is ingestion of any substance that may be injurious to body tissue or function. See Allergy for discussion on contact poison.	Toddlers will eat and drink substances that they believe to be edible. Toddlers often mistake medicine for candy because of the size and color. Poisonous liquids stored in bottles and cans may appear to be soda, juice, or milk to the toddler.	Children often swallow medicines or substances that cause poisoning. Childproofing the toddler's environment cannot be overemphasized. Be alert to the fact that baby aspirin resembles candy. If it is necessary to store leftover detergents, petroleum liquids, and other substances that are injurious to the body, it should be done with extreme caution.

HEALTH PROBLEM	HEALTH CARE GUIDELINES	HELPFUL HINTS
		Never store poisonous substances in bottles or containers that originally held food. (See Chapter 7, Safety.)

Toddlers are unable to differentiate those substances which are edible from those which are nonedible.

Substances commonly ingested by toddlers include the following:

1. Medications such as aspirin (salicylates), tranquilizers, amphetamines, and sedatives.
2. Insecticides such as ant traps and rat poisons, powders, or liquids.
3. Household products such as cleansers; detergents; polishes (shoe, silver, furniture); flush products containing lye, potash, or other caustic substances (See Burns); dry cleaning agents; and moth crystals or balls.
4. Flammables such as kerosene and gasoline. (Vomiting should never be induced when kerosene, gasoline, or similar products are ingested because there is danger of aspiration with injury to the respiratory system.)

This is not an all-inclusive list of substances that are toxic or harmful to toddlers.

When seeking medical advice, the following information is essential:

1. What substance has been ingested?
2. How much of the substance was taken?
3. When was the substance ingested?
4. Is there any nausea, vomiting, diarrhea, sleepiness, twitching, convulsions, or any other noticeable change in behavior.

If it is necessary to take the child to an emergency room, the caretaker should bring the container in which the substance was stored and a sample of the substance. If a sample of ingested substance is not available and the child vomits, bring a sample of the vomitus.

Medical management is directed toward neutralizing the toxic substance and/or removing the substance.

Vomiting may be induced if the substance is noncorrosive or not injurious to tissue. (See Burns.)

Gastric lavage may be performed. Antidotal medications, if administered, are administered with caution because detoxification and excretion of the poison have activated and increased liver and kidney function.

Antidotal medicines may prove to be ineffective and even dangerous because they are not absorbed and excreted in appropriate amounts.

Over-the-counter medications such as aspirin, cold medications, and sleeping remedies can be as dangerous to toddlers as those medicines prescribed by physicians. *All medicines should be locked in cabinets out of the sight and reach of the toddler.*

Medical advice should be sought as soon as poisoning is suspected. The telephone number for the local Poison Control Center should be kept at the telephone.

Do not induce vomiting if the swallowed substance is a corrosive or petroleum product or the child is unconscious.

After seeking medical advice by phone, the caretaker may be requested to assist (induce) the child to vomit. At home, vomiting may be induced by the caretaker inserting a finger in the back of the child's throat to stimulate the gag reflex or give the child syrup of ipecac. (One tablespoon is usually sufficient. A second dose may be given within 30 minutes).

97

HEALTH PROBLEM	HEALTH CARE GUIDELINES	HELPFUL HINTS

Accidents—cont'd

LEAD POISONING

Lead poisoning is the ingestion, inhalation, or absorption of lead or lead products leading to brain damage.

Lead poisoning in the toddler is insidious. Signs and symptoms usually become manifested long after the initial exposure to lead.

Toddlers frequently develop the practice of *pica*—ingesting nonedible substances such as dirt, wood, clay, or plaster. They are likely to chew on chips of paint (which may be lead based) either inside or outside the home.

Toddlers can continue to do this for long periods of time before any deleterious effects are noticed.

Symptoms of insidious onset (the more common type of lead poisoning) include irritability, muscle twitching, behavioral changes, decreased appetite, and decreased learning ability. Lead poisoning may also lead to convulsions, coma, and death.

Toddlers can be exposed to lead products or fumes if they live close to garages or stations where lead batteries and other lead-based substances are used and stored.

Inhalation of lead fumes may produce immediate symptoms. Immediate symptoms associated with inhalant lead poisoning includes abdominal pain, nausea, vomiting, irritability, convulsions, coma, and death.

Medical advice must be sought if lead poisoning is suspected because brain tissue is the body tissue most frequently affected, and brain damage is irreversible. Lead can be found in other body tissues and bone as well.

Medical management is directed toward reducing the concentration of lead found in the blood and soft tissues and encouraging excretion of lead by the kidneys.

PUNCTURE WOUND (STAB OR STABBING)

A puncture wound is when the body tissue is pierced by a pointed object, such as scissors, a nail, or a knife.

Puncture wounds usually occur by falling, being pushed on a pointed object, or being stabbed.

A sharp object puncturing body tissues leaves a small opening in the tissue. The site of the puncture generally has little or no bleeding.

Puncture wounds can cause trauma to deeper tissue. If the object is not easily withdrawn, leave it in place. Cushion the site to prevent movement of the object and transport the client to a medical facility for treatment.

HELPFUL HINTS (Lead poisoning)

Lead poisoning occurs in toddlers because they have either eaten lead-base substances or inhaled lead fumes. Lead is very harmful to the body and can cause permanent brain damage.

Toddlers tend to pick at loose plaster, wood, or paint chips and end up eating them. Eating nonedible substances should be discouraged.

Old homes are likely to have vestiges of lead-based paint on window sills and walls.

Avoid having toddlers play in areas where lead batteries or fumes exist.

Early detection, followed by treatment, may reduce the severity of the problem.

HELPFUL HINTS (Puncture wound)

A stab (puncture wound) occurs when the skin is pierced by a sharp object.

If the object can be easily removed, flush the wound with cold water and use a mild antiseptic to cleanse the site. Cover the area with a sterile gauze or nonstick dressing.

Caution: If the object is not easily removed, cushion the exact site to prevent movement of the object while transporting the child to the medical facility for treatment.

HEALTH PROBLEM	HEALTH CARE GUIDELINES	HELPFUL HINTS
	A puncture wound of the chest may enter the thoracic cavity and cause immediate respiratory distress (pneumothorax). The puncture site should be covered with a compressed dressing to prevent entrance of air. Probing the wound should be done only by medical personnel. It is important that the physician be informed of the type of object causing the puncture wound to ascertain the need for medical follow-up.	If the injury is a chest wound, do not use water or antiseptic; place a dry dressing over the wound and seek medical advice. *Tetanus toxoid or antitoxin injections may be necessary, depending on the object that inflicted the puncture wound.*

Allergy
Allergy: A hypersensitivity of the body to substances that are usually harmless. They are most commonly manifested by skin and/or respiratory disturbances.
	Allergens can enter the body through ingestion, inhalation, inoculation, or direct contact (touch).
	Any substance can be an allergen and produce a hypersensitive reaction in or on the body. These reactions usually do not occur on the first exposure to the substance because it takes time for the body to develop antibodies that attack the foreign substances producing the allergic reaction.
	All individuals can develop an allergy but they do not all react or become sensitive in the same way to the same substance(s). All too often individuals known to have one allergy are prone to be hypersensitive to other substances.
	Some individuals will manifest allergic responses early in life (e.g., babies to milk products, fruits, or eggs), whereas others may develop allergies after repeated exposures later in life to the substances (e.g., pollens, dust, animal hair, and some foods).
	The following list includes some of the more common identified allergens.
	Foods:
	  Orange juice
	  Milk and milk products
	  Eggs, particularly the albumin (whites of eggs)
	  Chocolate
	  Pork products
	  Spices
	Plants and trees:
	  Poison ivy, oak, and sumac
	  Pollens
	
	Animals:
	  Fur
	  Hair
	  Feathers
		Some toddlers have a hypersensitive reaction to common substances (allergies).
		Allergies are usually a response to substances that are eaten, inhaled, or touched.
		Allergic responses can occur with contact to almost any substance but rarely occur during the first exposure to the substance.
		
		Some children are more prone to develop allergies than others. The type of allergic response will be unique for each child.
		Children who have demonstrated an allergic response to one substance are usually hypersensitive to other substances as well.
		As the variety of foods in the child's diet increases, allergic responses may occur.
		Foods that caused no problem in infancy may now, with repeated exposure, precipitate an allergic response.
		
		Foods to which the child is allergic or is suspected to be allergic should be removed from the diet for a long period of time. When these foods are reintroduced into the diet, they should be added in very small portions and one at a time.
		
		Outdoor play areas should be cleared of poison ivy, oak, and sumac, since these plants are known to be injurious to most humans.
		Seasonal changes increase the pollen count in the air, which in turn triggers allergies.
		When the child is known to be hypersensitive to animal hair it is inadvisable to have a fur-bearing pet. It may be necessary to give away family pets when the allergen identified is animal hair or fur.

HEALTH PROBLEM	HEALTH CARE GUIDELINES	HELPFUL HINTS
Allergy—cont'd		Children may visit other homes or places where there are animals. Animal hair and fur dander are everywhere in the environment. The dander will cause the toddler's eyes to become inflamed, itchy, and swollen. Try to keep the child from aggravating situations.
		Pillows are frequently introduced at bedtime during the toddler period. Select pillows made of hypoallergenic material.

	Household substances:
	  Dusts and molds
	  Dyes
	  Soaps and detergents
	  Cosmetics
	  Medicines
	This list is by no means all inclusive, but merely representative of some of the more common allergy-producing substances.
		Soaps selected for the toddler's baths and laundry should be mild and nonperfurmed. Mild soaps cause fewer allergies.

		Cosmetics should be inaccessible to the child because some cosmetics cause severe allergic reactions. Remember, toddlers love to play with cosmetics.
		The danger of medicines lies not only in the immediate effect of the drug, but the possibility of stimulating production of antibodies. On future exposures to that same drug, the child could become violently ill.
	Emotional factors such as stress and/or anxiety are known to precipitate as well as prolong an allergic response.	Allaying fears and reducing stress will often alleviate allergic responses. Caretakers should try to remain calm during a child's allergic attack because this behavior helps relieve the child's fears.
	Skin reactions are a common manifestation of an allergic response. *Urticaria (hives):* Slightly raised reddened patches associated with itching. Hives can be either localized or generalized across the body. *Eczema:* Reddened rash associated with itching and frequently accompanied by oozing and scaling. Eczema usually develops from foods or substances that are inhaled, such as dust or pollens.	The appearance of a skin rash (eruption) is usually sudden and may be alarming to the caretaker as well as irritating to the child. Skin rashes usually occur on the face, neck, and extremities followed by the chest, abdomen, and back.
		Skin rashes are usually reddened spots appearing singly or in clusters. The rash may be raised red spots or flush with the skin. Itching may accompany a rash (hives). Some rashes may seep fluid, which dries. Crusts form but eventually peal off (eczema).
	Contact dermatitis: Rash that resembles eczema but occurs when the allergen comes in direct contact with the skin.	Itchy rashes cause children to scratch. When itching is intense, the child scratches repeatedly and intensely to the point of breaking the skin. Bleeding and oozing of tissue fluid occurs, which can become unsightly, as well as predispose the child to more infections.
		Damage caused by scratching can be minimized by keeping the child's nails cut short. Mitts over the child's hands may be used but have not always proved to be helpful.
		Eczematous rashes may or may not persist for long periods of time.

HEALTH PROBLEM	HEALTH CARE GUIDELINES	HELPFUL HINTS
		Caretakers may find it difficult to show affection by holding and cuddling the child covered with weeping, oozing lesions, but should be encouraged to try. An apron worn by the caretaker will prevent soiling or staining of clothing when in close contact with child.
	Inflammation of the body cells in response to allergens can be both external and internal, affecting any or all body systems (respiratory, gastrointestinal, cardiovascular, central nervous).	As the lesions disappear, the skin becomes dry and scaly. This in turn may cause additional itching, which precipitates another acute episode of eczema.
	Skin eruptions can occur as a result of stings or bites or contact with poisonous plants (such as poison ivy, poison oak, or poison sumac).	
	Reactions to bee or wasp stings can be extremely severe, affecting not only the skin surface, but underlying tissue and internal body systems as well. These responses may lead to an anaphylactic shock or even death.	
	Treatment for skin reactions is directed toward relief of symptoms, prevention of secondary infections, and alleviation of prolonged stress on major body systems.	Children with severe skin reactions need medical supervision.
	To alleviate allergic skin reactions, the following measures might be used: 1. Antihistamines 2. Lotions or creams 3. Baths 4. Soaks	Medications are frequently ordered to relieve distress and prevent infection. Caretakers should know the type of medications being used, expected effects, and side effects of these drugs. Caretakers must also be informed as to the frequency and extent to which ointments, creams, or lotions are to be applied on the child's body. Creams, lotions, or ointments seem to be more beneficial if applied immediately following a bath. When baths are being used for their soothing effect, avoid prolonged soaking (beyond 20 minutes) because this causes softening, puckering, and wrinkling, making the skin easily injured.

	Allergies also affect the respiratory system.
	Allergic rhinitis (hay fever)
	  Sneezing
	  Runny eyes
	  Itchy eyes
	Asthma
	  Wheezing
	  Shortness of breath
	  Coughs that can be productive or nonproductive
		Children in respiratory distress will automatically assume the positions of greatest comfort to them (upright or sitting). The child's body can be supported by placing one pillow at the back and one pillow at the front at chest level. To create greater air exchange, have the child raise the arms to shoulder level, and place them on top of the pillow used to support the chest.
		Wheezing and shortness of breath cause anxiety for both caretaker and child. Give the child quiet, calm reassurance. Reducing anxiety slows the rate of breathing and increases the depth of each breath. Breathing slowly and deeply should decrease wheezing and shortness of breath.

101

HEALTH PROBLEM	HEALTH CARE GUIDELINES	HELPFUL HINTS
Allergy—cont'd		It cannot be denied that children soon learn that their allergic reactions will gain the attention of the caretaker and other people in the environment. Children with asthma can control families through their periods of difficult breathing. Although the child is sick, caretakers should not permit the illness to control the family.
	Management of respiratory reactions to allergens might include the following: Antihistamines Bronchodilators Expectorants Anti-inflammatory drugs Mist therapies Bed rest	Medications are frequently ordered to relieve breathing difficulties.
	The initial acute allergic attack usually stimulates the caretakers to seek immediate medical advice. For caretakers whose children have a history of allergy, medical advice should be sought in the following situations:	Caretakers should know the type of medications being used, the expected effects, the side effects of these drugs, and how often they are to be given.
	1. Skin eruptions that are generalized, prolonged, and involve internal systems, or when secondary infections are suspected.	Mist therapy is often ordered. Cool mist is more beneficial than warm in relieving spasms associated with this type of breathing difficulty.
	2. Respiratory distress that becomes severe, is prolonged (status asthmaticus), or symptoms that are not relieved.	
	Medical management is directed toward the identification of the allergen(s). When allergens have been identified, sometimes they can be eliminated or avoided (such as foods, medicines, animals, or plants).	
	In some instances, a costly and time-consuming process known as *desensitization* can be undertaken. This is a process whereby the individual is exposed to the allergen in increasing doses until an immunity is established.	
Convulsive disorders (convulsions, seizures)		
Convulsive disorder: A problem of unknown etiology, resulting in involuntary spasmodic contraction and relaxation of the musculature.	Seizures are characterized by specific muscular movements. Tonic movement: Tightening of muscles, producing rigidity. Clonic movement: Opposing muscles contract and relax in an alternating rhythmic pattern.	Fits (convulsions or seizures) are sudden episodes of uncontrolled muscle activity often characterized by rhythmic jerking of the arms and legs.

102

HEALTH PROBLEM	HEALTH CARE GUIDELINES	HELPFUL HINTS
FEBRILE SEIZURES Febrile, or fever-induced, seizures are the most common form found in children 6 to 18 months of age.	Febrile seizures are triggered by a rapid rise in body temperature (102° to 104° F; 38.9° to 40° C). Febrile seizures may be familial. The seizure is characterized by a generalized reaction, including tonic and clonic movements. Children with febrile seizures may develop an idiopathic epilepsy.	Some seizures occur when a child's (typically 6 to 18 months old) temperature rises quickly to levels above 102° F (38.9° C). This trait often occurs in more than one family member. Caretakers are often alarmed because of the rapidity with which this occurs. The child's entire body is involved. This is called a *grand mal seizure*. Every muscle in the body is involved. The muscles contract and relax, giving a jerking appearance to the arms, legs, head, face, tongue, and trunk. (Often children are thought to be frothing at the mouth. This is not true, but saliva is pushed out of the mouth by the movement of the tongue and the inability of the child to swallow during a seizure.) The child seems to be thrashing about uncontrollably. Lack of consciousness may occur, thus the child cannot respond to direction. Soiling or wetting of the diaper or panties may occur. Shortly after the jerking movements stop, the child will awaken but appear drowsy and desirous of sleep.
	Management is directed toward reduction of body temperature through the use of antipyretics or tepid sponging. Anticonvulsant therapy may be used.	Reducing the body temperature helps avoid seizures. This can be achieved by bathing the child in cool water before a seizure occurs or after a seizure to avoid further seizures. Medications can assist—seek medical advice. The major emphasis of care during a seizure is to prevent injury and promote breathing. Turning the head to the side prevents the tongue from blocking the air passage. Forcing tongue blades, spoons, or any object between the gums (teeth) is not necessary, if the child is already having a seizure. Forcing an object into the mouth can cause greater damage than good. Be sure that the child is protected from injuries that could result from the jerking movements of arms, legs, or the head against objects in the environment (such as bedrails).
FOCAL (JACKSONIAN) SEIZURES Focal (jacksonian) seizures reflect a dysfunction in a localized area of the brain (sensory or motor).	Focal seizures are characterized by clonic movements, usually limited to one side of the body. Focal seizures are not usually accompanied by a loss of consciousness or tonic contractions. Brain lesions are suspected when focal seizures occur. Extensive diagnostic procedures may be necessary.	A seizure that affects only one side or a limited area of the body and is not usually accompanied by a loss of consciousness is called a *focal*, or *Jacksonian, seizure*. Medical advice is recommended.

HEALTH PROBLEM	HEALTH CARE GUIDELINES	HELPFUL HINTS

Convulsive disorders—cont'd

GRAND MAL SEIZURES

Grand mal seizures are also categorized as generalized seizures featuring both tonic and clonic major motor movements.

Typically, a grand mal seizure is preceded by an *aura*. An aura is a warning symptom that a seizure may occur (older children and adults report auras). The aura is subjective, such as feeling funny, a tingling sensation, a strange odor, visual disturbances, or dizziness.

The seizure consists of a sudden loss of consciousness followed by tonic contraction of the body muscles. (A child who is standing or sitting will fall down.) This phase lasts approximately 60 to 90 seconds.

Following the tonic phase, the body muscles will rhythmically contract and relax (clonic phase) giving a jerking motion to the body parts. The child may salivate, become cyanotic, and incontinent. This phase can last 5 minutes or more.

Following the convulsive activity, the muscles will ache, and the child may appear confused and want to sleep. Older children may also complain of a headache.

Management is directed toward prevention of injury, maintenance of respiration, and prevention of additional seizures.

Medical management is required. Anticonvulsant drugs are prescribed.

Children who have grand mal seizures (described under febrile seizures) that are not triggered by fever, are thought to have epilepsy. Epilepsy, however, is not a disease, but a term used to describe a variety of recurring seizures, including the grand mal type.

Children with recurring grand mal seizures need medical management and usually some form of drug therapy.

If drug therapy is recommended, it must be followed precisely and consistently to prevent further seizures. In addition, it is helpful if the child wears a Medic Alert bracelet to provide information to others should the seizure occur away from home.

PETIT MAL SEIZURES

A petit mal seizure is a brief loss of awareness without tonic or clonic muscular component.

These seizures are more frequently seen in girls than boys.

Petit mal seizures are characterized by brief lapses of awareness (stare).

A staring expression may last for a few seconds and be accompanied by slight twitching of the face, blinking, and nodding of the head.

This seizure is not usually accompanied by a loss of consciousness or change in body position. Children are rarely aware that a seizure has occurred.

Some children have brief staring spells, short blinking episodes, or twitching of facial muscles that occur with some frequency. These can be *petit mal seizures.*

This type of seizure is frequently identified in the school years by teachers, school nurses, or caretakers who note periods of inattentiveness or staring that the child is unaware of.

Medical evaluation is desirable.

PSYCHOMOTOR (TEMPORAL LOBE) SEIZURES

Psychomotor, or temporal lobe, seizures are characterized by periods of confusion often accompanied by awkward or poorly coordinated muscle movement.

Psychomotor seizures are often episodes of bizarre or purposeless behavior, such as running in circles or laughing inappropriately.

Psychomotor seizures may be preceded by an aura.

Clouding of consciousness or confusion may exist but rarely does a total loss of consciousness occur.

Following the seizure there may be continued confusion or drowsiness. Often, there is no memory of the affair.

Another type of seizure that can occur in children is a *psychomotor seizure.* The typical seizure consists of behavior that does not make sense. Child may cry, laugh, or run around for no reason at all. Following the activity, the child may seem confused or sleepy. The child usually has no memory of the event.

HEALTH PROBLEM	HEALTH CARE GUIDELINES	HELPFUL HINTS
Foreign objects *Foreign object:* The presence of an object within the body that is not normally found there. Foreign objects can lead to obstruction, perforation, or infection.	In the toddler, foreign objects are most frequently found in the nostrils or ears, but can be found in the respiratory or gastrointestinal tracts. Toddlers and older infants enjoy handling or picking up tiny objects such as beads, gravel, peas, beans, pins, buttons, and even insects. While investigating the object, they will not hesitate to place them in the ears, nose, or mouth.	Toddlers and older infants require constant and close surveillance because they enjoy placing small objects in their noses and ears (foreign objects). If the object is in the ear and is visible, it may be possible to remove it at home using tweezers. Warm water or oil irrigations may prove beneficial in removing some objects. *Caution:* Irrigation should not be used if the object is or is thought to be an organic object such as a pea or bean, since it will absorb fluid and swell. In all events, avoid pushing the foreign object farther into the ear. Objects in nostrils may be forcefully ejected if the child blows the nose. *Caution:* If the child has not learned to blow the nose, object may be inhaled further into the nostril. Medical attention would be needed.
	Foul or purulent drainage from the nose or ears or coughing may be the first clue to a hidden foreign object. Medical advice should be sought. The presence of a foreign object may be evidenced by pain or discomfort in the associated body part.	If there is reason to believe an object was inhaled, seek medical advice immediately. A hidden foreign object is suspected if the toddler has foul drainage from the ear or nose that is not related to an existing infection. If the caretaker knows the child has swallowed a foreign object that has sharp corners or points (pins, needles, nails), contact a physician immediately because these objects can puncture tissue. Some swallowed objects might pass through the intestinal tract and be found later in bowel movements.
	Medical management is always directed toward removal of the foreign object.	Hospitalization may be necessary for removal of foreign objects.
Parasites *Parasites:* Organisms that live in, on, or at the expense of the host and may reduce the energy potential of the host and produce uncomfortable signs or symptoms. *Helminths (worms):* Small, elongated, limbless invertebrates. *Ascaris lumbricoides:* A roundworm that resembles an earthworm and may range from 6 to 14 inches (15 to 35 cm) in length.	Roundworms are found in human feces used as fertilizer. They are usually ingested as larvae attached to foods that have not been thoroughly cleansed or cooked. Larvae then grow in the intestinal tract, pass into the bloodstream, and are transported to the lungs, only to be coughed up, swallowed, and returned to the intestinal tract, where they will grow to maturity. Signs and symptoms may include colic, abdominal symptoms, lack of appetite, and loss of weight.	Worms (parasites) are organisms that are found in the toddler's bowel movement or around the rectal area. Eggs (larvae) of the worm are usually found in the soil. Toddlers become infected from eating dirt, eating foods contaminated from soil, and individuals who have worms. Washing foods well and cooking them thoroughly reduce the chances of worms being eaten. Some worms resembling earthworms (roundworms) show up in bowel movements and/or vomitus.

HEALTH PROBLEM	HEALTH CARE GUIDELINES	HELPFUL HINTS
Parasites—cont'd	It is not unusual for the infection to pass unnoticed until the child either coughs, vomits, or passes a mature worm. Medical advice should be sought if worms are found or suspected.	Children with roundworms lose their appetites, have stomach cramps, and lose weight.
Enterobius vermicularis (pinworms): A small spindle-shaped roundworm less than ½ inch (1.3 cm) in size.	Pinworms can be acquired by direct contact with food, clothing, toilet seats, or other objects contaminated by the eggs and larvae of the organism. After ingestion, the eggs/larvae travel to the large intestine. Adult worms migrate to the rectum, usually at night, where they deposit eggs around the anal ring, which in turn cause irritation, itching, and disturbed sleep. The toddler tends to scratch the area, thus getting eggs under fingernails, which in turn reinfects the child when the fingers are placed in the mouth. Pinworms are diagnosed by microscopic examination of an anal swab.	Toddlers with pinworms (small round, spindle-shaped worms) often scratch around their rectums. The worms are rarely ever found except early in the morning. Cleanliness cannot be overemphasized. Washing the hands before bed, on rising, after toileting, and before eating is absolutely essential at all times. Take extra precautions with toilet seats, clothing, bed linens, and other laundry when pinworms have been identified in a family. Caretaker may be asked to obtain a specimen to assist in the diagnosis of pinworms. (See Chapter 18, Specimen Collection.)
Pediculosis (lice): Lice are living parasitic insects that can infest and multiply on mammals in a variety of ways.	Medical management of parasitic infections is aimed at eradication of the organism. The louse lives and multiplies on human blood obtained by biting the skin. The bitten area becomes red, sore, and itchy. This area may become infected from scratching.	Lice (pediculi) are parasites usually found in hair on the child's head, body, or genitalia. Lice live by biting the skin. They multiply by laying eggs (nits) that cling to the hair shaft.
Three common types of lice have been identified on humans:	Treatment of pediculosis of all types requires medical supervision and medication.	Lice infestations are highly infectious, traveling with ease from one individual to another through close contact (clothing of infested individual).
1. Body lice *(Pediculus humanus corporis).* Usually found in or on clothing. Bites are frequently found where clothing comes into close proximity with the body (at wrist or cuffs).	When infestation occurs, clothes and linens of all types must be boiled, autoclaved, or dry cleaned. Bed clothing, mattresses, and other inanimate objects will also need treatment.	If body lice are discovered, seek medical advice. The clothing and bed linen of the infested child must be kept separate from the family laundry and washed and boiled. Check the entire household environment, such as carpets and furniture, for further presence of body lice.
2. Crab lice *(Phthirus pubis).* Usually found in the pubic hair, although they are also found in eyebrows and eyelashes (and even in beards) of older individuals.	Crab lice are spread through body contact. They are seen more frequently in adolescents and the adult.	
3. Head lice *(Pediculus humanus capitus).* Found in the hair of the head.	The head louse is readily identified by examination of the head for oval seedlike eggs, called *nits,* that are attached to the hair shafts.	The treatment of head lice is usually carried out at home. Nits (eggs) can be removed by using a mild vinegar solution and combing the hair with a fine-tooth comb.

HEALTH PROBLEM	HEALTH CARE GUIDELINES	HELPFUL HINTS
		Lice are destroyed through applications of creams and shampoos that contain 1% benzene hexachloride. To purchase this substance, a physician's prescription may be necessary.
		Prevention of lice is the best defense. Cleanliness, frequent bathing, and daily changing to clean clothes are deterrents to all three types of lice infestation.

Respiratory tract infections

EPIGLOTTITIS

Epiglottitis: Inflammation of the epiglottis characterized by redness and swelling, resulting in severe respiratory tract obstruction.	Inflammation of the epiglottis is evidenced by redness and extreme swelling. Swelling may increase to the extent that complete obstruction of the airway occurs.	Few toddlers ever have a sore throat so severe that it obstructs breathing. When this occurs, it is called *epiglottitis*.
	The child will evidence extreme apprehension, assume an upright position, tug for breath, swallow infrequently and with great difficulty, and tend to drool rather than swallow saliva.	Symptoms arise quickly and include sudden difficult breathing and swallowing, drooling, and tremendous anxiety. This disease is a medical emergency, and medical advice should be sought immediately.
	Examination of the oropharyngeal cavity must be done with extreme caution and only one time by an experienced examiner, since muscle contractions of the epiglottis can occur and close off the respiratory passage.	Hospitalization will be required. The presence of a caretaker during this acute stage is advisable to reduce the child's apprehension.
	Management of epiglottitis is directed at reducing obstruction and fighting infection.	
	Vomiting is not to be induced, since this will force epiglottic movement that can obstruct the child's airway.	

LARYNGITIS (CROUP)

Laryngitis: A mild inflammation of the larynx characterized by spasms of laryngeal muscles and evidenced by a hoarse barking cough with crowing-type respirations.	Croup is a mild form of laryngitis. Spasms of the laryngeal muscles obstruct airflow, making breathing noisy and difficult. Stridulous breathing is accompanied by retractions, restlessness, and extreme apprehension on the part of the toddler.	Croup (laryngitis) is a swelling of the vocal cords that makes breathing noisy and difficult.
	The body temperature usually is not elevated.	The child frequently wakes up at night with a barking cough that upsets both the child and caretaker. This is an unexpected occurrence because the child usually has no other signs of illness.
	Signs and symptoms seen in mild upper respiratory tract infections, such as colds, are not usually present.	
	Laryngeal spasms will usually occur at night. The intensity of the laryngeal spasms is short lived and can be relieved through the use of a warm or cool mist or induced vomiting.	Harsh breathing is usually relieved quickly by placing the child in a warm moist environment. (See Laryngotracheobronchitis.)
		Moving the child from a warm moist environment to a cold room can trigger another croup spasm. Additional moisture should be provided by a vaporizer in the child's room.
		The child may be thirsty following the croupy spasm. Clear liquids are recommended at this time (avoid milk).

HEALTH PROBLEM	HEALTH CARE GUIDELINES	HELPFUL HINTS
Respiratory tract infections—cont'd LARYNGITIS (CROUP)—cont'd	Vomiting may be induced by the child's own anxiety or mechanically induced through the use of an emetic such as syrup of ipecac. Vomiting relieves the laryngeal muscle spasm, thus providing relief from respiratory distress.	Holding the child in an upright position during the spasm aids breathing. The child is usually anxious. The anxiety may induce vomiting, which is good, because the spasms of the laryngeal muscles will be relieved. *Caution:* Should the child vomit, place the head lower than the hips to prevent choking on the vomitus.
LARYNGOTRACHEOBRONCHITIS *Laryngotracheobronchitis:* Inflammation of the larynx, trachea, and bronchi, leading to obstruction of the air passages, making breathing difficult and noisy.	The inflammation may involve only the larynx, which is referred to as *laryngitis;* the trachea, *tracheitis;* or the bronchi, *bronchitis.* Young children tend to develop laryngotracheobronchitis because of the shortness of their air passages.	Infections involving the breathing passages (larynx, trachea, bronchi) are referred to as *laryngotracheobronchitis.* Infections that involve only the larynx are called *laryngitis* and are characterized by loss of voice. If the infection is in the passage leading to the lungs (bronchi), it is referred to as *bronchitis.* The severity of the infection will determine the extent of breathing difficulty. For disorders believed to be an allergic response, see Allergies.
	This inflammatory process of the respiratory system can be elicited by a number of agents such as foreign objects, viral or bacterial infections, or an allergic response.	Avoid exposing toddlers to individuals with colds, sore throats, or other respiratory tract infections. If members of the family have a respiratory tract infection, take the following precautions: 1. Use separate eating and drinking utensils (consider using paper cups during this period). 2. Shield the mouth and nose when coughing or sneezing. 3. Use disposable handkerchiefs. 4. Avoid kissing or close facial contact with others.
	The inflammatory process produces swelling of the mucous membranes, thus decreasing the diameter of the air passage. In some cases an exudate may be present, which further obstructs airflow and gas exchange. The exudate can range from thin to thick and become crusty. The color may vary from colorless to yellow or green with flecks of blood. There may be a foul purulent odor or no odor at all. Airflow becomes impaired, and the child must force respirations to maintain an adequate gas exchange. Compensation by the child becomes evident by the stridulous breathing during the inspiratory and/or expiratory phases of respiration.	Toddlers are prone to smear the discharge from the nose to the mouth (mucous exudate), across their cheeks, and even into their eyes. Mucus is irritating to the skin. The face and hands should be washed and dried frequently. As much as possible, prevent toddlers from spreading this discharge into their eyes, since it could cause a secondary infection, conjunctivitis. Noisy breathing (stridor) may cause caretakers to become overly concerned. The swelling of the throat (larynx and vocal cords) obstructs the airflow and is the reason that breath sounds can be heard.

108

HEALTH PROBLEM	**HEALTH CARE GUIDELINES**	**HELPFUL HINTS**

Accessory muscles are used to assist in respiration, resulting in suprasternal, substernal, intercostal, and/or diaphragmatic retractions. The nares of the nose will tend to flare to facilitate air intake.

Dyspnea and restlessness occur as a result of the hampered gas exchange. The child becomes anxious and cries, thus adding to the severity of the problem.

Upright sitting positions are assumed by the child with impaired respiratory function to facilitate respiration and alleviate discomfort.

Caretakers can assist children to breathe more easily by the following:
1. Propping pillows under the mattress at the head of the crib to provide a semi-lying position.
2. Sitting can be achieved by having the child lean forward over a folded pillow.
3. Holding the child in an upright position on the caretaker's lap or over the shoulder.

In some instances there may be an elevation in body temperature, particularly when infectious agents are the cause of the problem. The temperature may range from normal 98.6° to 104° F (37° to 40° C). As body temperature rises, there is usually a concomitant rise in the respiratory and cardiac rate.

If the toddler's temperature is elevated, avoid overdressing, keep the environment cool, and encourage clear liquids.

The respiratory rate becomes more rapid, and labored respiration can be noted on inspiration and expiration, depending on the portion of the respiratory tree that is affected. The respiratory rate may be as rapid as 40 to 60 breaths per minute.

The breathing rate increases because the child has difficulty getting air in and out.

Medical advice should be sought in the following circumstances:
1. Breathing that is very rapid (40 or more breaths per minute).
2. Nostrils spread wide.
3. Breathing becomes more noisy.
4. Temperature goes above 101° F (38.3° C).

When seeking medical advice the following information should be given:
1. Temperature: how obtained, when taken, and duration of elevation.
2. Respirations: rate per minute and character (noisy, grunting, difficult, painful).
3. Presence of cough and/or nasal discharge (exudate). Include description of exudate, consistency, odor, and color.
4. Duration of existing condition.
5. Previous exposure to someone who is/was ill.

Management is directed toward reducing the inflammation and obstruction of the air passages.

HEALTH PROBLEM	HEALTH CARE GUIDELINES	HELPFUL HINTS
Respiratory tract infections—cont'd LARYNGOTRACHEOBRONCHITIS—cont'd	Warm moist air reduces spasms of laryngeal muscles and aids in liquefying secretions from the inflamed mucous membranes.	Warm moist air can be provided quickly at home by turning on the hot water in the shower. The caretaker sits in the bathroom (not the shower stall), holding the child on the lap. If a warm moist mist is needed over a long period, it may be necessary to use a vaporizer. *Caution:* Hot steam vaporizers can cause burns—place them out of the child's reach. Cool moist air is provided by a cool mist vaporizer that is placed next to the crib, with the mist directed toward the child's head.
	Cool moist air decreases the swelling of the mucous membranes and liquefies secretions, facilitating better gas exchange. Both warm and cold mist therapies alleviate respiratory distress, thus reducing the child's anxiety and restlessness. Depending on the severity of the disease and the causative factors, drugs such as bronchodilators, antipyretics, anti-inflammatory antibiotics, antitussives, expectorants, and antihistamines are likely to be part of the medical management.	Medication is often ordered to aid breathing and/or decrease fevers. See Chapter 18, Administration of Medications.
	Bedrest during the acute phase of the illness decreases the need for greater cardiac output and gas exchange. Activity is gradually increased as the child's respiratory function and body temperature return to within normal ranges.	During the acute stage of the illness, caretakers will have little difficulty in keeping children in bed. Children will be more active as the severity of the disease decreases.
	Fluid loss occurs as a result of the increased respirations and elevation of body temperature. Fluids in excess of normal daily requirements should be encouraged. Increased fluid intake replaces fluid loss, liquefies secretions in the respiratory passage, and rids the body of toxic substances.	Children with respiratory tract infections lose fluid, which must be replaced. Encourage clear liquids. (See Chapter 7, Nutrition.)
	Milk and milk products tend to increase secretion of mucus and therefore should be eliminated from the diet. If there is reason to believe that the respiratory problem is an allergenic one, milk and milk products should not be included in the diet at all.	For the child who is having difficulty breathing, milk, puddings, ice cream, or foods made with milk such as French toast should be eliminated because milk tends to increase and thicken mucous secretions.
	Clear liquids are given during the acute phase of the illness because they are easily assimilated and will cause less irritation to the mucous membrane if the child should choke and inhale the fluid. Water, diluted tea, ice tea, ginger ale, cola, Kool-Aid, gelatin, and broths are some clear liquids to consider.	Clear liquids such as Popsicles and/or slushies are good fluids to use. Gelatin water (1 tablespoon of gelatin powder to ½ cup of water [4 ounces; 112 g]) can also be made. Other clear liquids to consider include the following: Tea Clear broth Apple juice (limited amounts) Gelatin Ginger ale

110

HEALTH PROBLEM	HEALTH CARE GUIDELINES	HELPFUL HINTS
	Fluids of thicker consistency and nutritional substance will be introduced into the diet when the child is able to accommodate them with no appreciable change in respiratory rate or mucus accumulation. Soft foods will be introduced next, to be followed by the usual dietary pattern for the child. As restlessness and anxiety decrease, the child's periods of rest and sleep will be prolonged. Usual patterns of sleep for the child will eventually be resumed.	As the child improves and appetite returns, other fluids and foods should be offered.
TONSILLITIS (SORE THROAT) *Tonsillitis:* Inflammation of the tonsils characterized by swelling with either patchy or disseminated redness of tonsillar tissue, leading to difficulty in swallowing.	Tonsillitis is an inflammatory condition that is usually caused by viral or bacterial invasion of the tonsils.	A "sore throat" (tonsillitis) is an infection of the tonsils, causing pain and difficulty with swallowing. Discomfort associated with sore throats can be minimized by providing fluids that are cool rather than hot, mild rather than spicy. As with other upper respiratory tract infections, avoid giving milk or milk products while the throat is extremely painful. Warm, moist compresses applied to the neck may provide some relief. Additional rest periods are recommended. Offer clear liquids frequently in small amounts, particularly if the temperature is elevated.
	Tonsillitis can occur as a single disease entity or in conjunction with other upper respiratory infections. Following are some signs and symptoms: 1. Low-grade fever to extremely elevated temperature, 99° to 104° F (37.2° to 40° C). 2. Swelling of tonsils, surrounding tissue, and adenoids. 3. Tonsillar tissue red and inflamed and often covered with white patches. 4. Sore throat most noticeable on swallowing.	
		Medical advice should be sought if the child has frequent bouts of tonsillitis or severe tonsillitis with an elevated temperature.
	Medical management is directed toward combating the infection and relieving respiratory distress. The therapies for tonsillitis will be similar to those discussed for respiratory problems such as laryngitis and laryngotracheobronchitis. A tonsillectomy may be necessary.	Hospitalization for the removal of tonsils (tonsillectomy) may be necessary if tonsillitis occurs frequently. (See Chapter 14, Tonsillectomy.)
Urinary tract infection *Urinary tract infection:* Inflammatory response to mechanical trauma, chemical irritation, or bacterial invasion, which may affect one or a number of the parts of the urinary system. The most common cause of urinary tract infection is a bacterial invasion.	Children of this age are prone to develop urinary tract infections for a number of reasons: 1. The length of the urethra is short, approximately 2 cm, thus presenting ready access for bacterial invasion. 2. The urethral location is close to the rectum.	Infection of the urinary tract (kidney, bladder, or urethra) is common in toddlerhood because the opening of the bladder is close to the rectum, and the tube leading to the bladder (urethra) is short. Infection often results from contamination from the bowel movement.

HEALTH PROBLEM	HEALTH CARE GUIDELINES	HELPFUL HINTS
Urinary tract infection—cont'd		
The high incidence of urinary tract infections noted in the toddler and preschool periods affect females more than males.	Toilet training affords many opportunities for contamination and irritation of the genitalia.	Wipe or cleanse the genitalia of girls from front to back. Children need to be taught and supervised to wipe themselves correctly. Toddlers may find it difficult to wipe correctly because the toddler's arms are short, and muscle control is limited.
	Urinary tract infections can be categorized by their location. *Urethritis:* Inflammation of the urethra.	Children might complain of pain on voiding (urination).
	Cystitis: Inflammation of the bladder and frequently associated with urethritis. *Pyelonephritis:* Inflammation of the pelvis of the kidney. *Ureteritis:* Inflammation of the ureter, which is usually found in conjunction with pyelonephritis, cystitis, or both.	Voiding may be more frequent, and the color, amount, and odor of the urine may change. Encouraging fluids above the usual daily requirements for this age will aid in ridding the body of the irritating substance.
	Urinary tract infections commonly involve the kidney, bladder, and urethra. Signs and symptoms will vary depending on the location and causative agent. Signs and symptoms of urinary tract infections can include low back pain, elevated temperature, burning on urination, frequency of urination, and discoloration of urine.	When a urinary tract infection is suspected, medical advice should be sought.
	Medical management is directed toward identifying and eradicating the causative organism.	In some instances, caretakers may be asked to collect urine specimens to bring to the physician or laboratory. (See Chapter 18, Urine Specimen.)
	Diagnostic tests such as urine specimens for culture, cystoscopy, and/or intravenous pyelogram, as well as other urinary tract function studies may be necessary.	Should the toddler require any diagnostic tests beyond a urine test, hospitalization will probably be necessary.

UNIT THREE

PRESCHOOL *initiating new experiences*

Children 4 through 5 years old continue to display a high energy level, but they seem to direct their energy into more controlled activities. Family members no longer view this child as a baby, but rather as an individual with a unique personality. The preschooler is eager to learn new tasks, start new projects, help with chores, and play with friends.

Preschool children are more settled and secure within the family than when they were toddlers. To a large extent preschoolers have learned what is expected of them and what they can expect of others in terms of daily routines, rituals, and traditions within the family constellation. However, it is well known that children will try to obtain permission for a treat from one caretaker and, if refused, race to another with a similar request. If a consistent, singular approach to requests, limit setting, and discipline is maintained, the preschooler gains a new level of self-control.

If foundations of trust and autonomy are well established, the child evidences eagerness to step outside the confines of the home. Preschoolers seek new adventures, but return to the security of the home and caretaker when confronted with situations beyond their ability to handle or control. Preschoolers demonstrate an ability to adhere to limits and remain within parameters that were previously delineated but will continue to need supervision and monitoring of activities. They are developing a sense of right from wrong.

Preschoolers' new physical and intellectual skills initiate enthusiasm in learning the *how to, why, what,* and *when* of daily experiences. They continue, as in toddlerhood, to assert themselves, but their desire to please makes them more amenable to suggestions and directions. They are "helpers." They enjoy helping with cooking, cleaning, gardening, building, and puttering. Caretakers will discover that these little "helpers" can follow instructions and will work alongside their role models for fairly long periods of time. Although preschool children appear to be "little adults," the 4- or 5-year-old can never be expected to perform as an adult or consistently conform to adult standards.

Preschoolers are more proficient in skills of eating, dressing, and bathing than in earlier stages of life. Bath and mealtimes can be very enjoyable. However, limited manual skills and knowledge hinder their ability to be left totally responsible for meeting these personal needs.

Children from 4 through 5 years of age are able to entertain themselves for long periods of time but enjoy being with others. Preschoolers can interact with two or three children of the same age. Their play is that of *give and take* rather than the parallel play observed in the toddler period.

Preschoolers are also developing their conversational skills. Many times these conversations become laced with imaginary friends, wild animals, ghosts, or scary adventures. These "tall tales" are usually based in part on stories they have heard on radio, television, or had read to them from books. The fabrication illustrates the child's beginning ability to conceptualize and demonstrate abstract thinking.

If the newly developed physical, mental, and social skills of preschoolers are encouraged rather than discouraged, their personalities will likely evidence enthusiasm for life.

CHAPTER 9

PRESCHOOL *4 through 5 years*

Endless bundles of energy might well describe 4- and 5-year-old children. Their physical and mental skills, coupled with their intellectual curiosity, keep them in constant motion. Running, climbing, jumping, turning somersaults, riding tricycles, and trying out skis and skates are but a few of the many motor skills in which these children will engage. Abstract thinking abilities enable them to experiment and question why things and circumstances are as they are. Inquisitiveness is directed toward the why and wherefore rather than just that it is there to be explored. Preschoolers love to play games. They can learn to follow rules, but as yet find it somewhat difficult to accept losing.

The enthusiastic personalities of 4- and 5-year-olds make them a delight to be with. Their untiring eagerness to perform tasks can easily tire and frustrate the caretaker. Preschoolers delight in helping the caretaker. They need opportunities to assist even though at times it could be accomplished more quickly by the caretaker.

Children of 4 and 5 often display the exuberance of childhood at one moment and the serious maturity of adulthood at the next. They try out many roles and engage in real mimicry of their role models. Preschoolers have definite ideas of who and what they will be when they grow up.

Four- and five-year-olds love to go on outings. They are usually a joy to have along, because they have developed and refined so many skills and talents. An increased attention span and the ability to sit still for long periods permit their inclusion at church services, restaurants, circuses, or other events.

The preschooler's ability to speak clearly and to express innermost thoughts and feelings sometimes presents a two-edged sword for caretakers. Since preschoolers are basically honest, many caretakers find themselves cringing when their darlings say such things as, "Look at that fat lady," or "Should I show everybody how I can stand up to go toity, Mommy?" Inevitably these statements are made in inappropriate times and places.

Knowledge of the expected performance and behaviors of 4- and 5-year-olds can provide caretakers with confidence to meet the needs of these growing children. The landmarks of growth and development of this preschool period are presented in conjunction with discussions of anticipatory guidance to be shared with caretakers.

GROWTH AND DEVELOPMENTAL LANDMARKS	**ANTICIPATORY GUIDANCE**

Biological

WEIGHT

The average weight gain for this period will range from 5 to 6 pounds (2.5 to 2.75 kg) per year.

By 4 years, the child will weigh between 35 and 40 pounds (16 to 18.2 kg).

By 5 years, the child will weigh between 40 and 45 pounds (18.2 to 20.5 kg).

Although ranges of normal weight are provided, it is important to remember that each child is unique.

Although a gain in weight is evident, it may be less noticeable than in previous periods because of the concomitant increase in height.

HEIGHT

The average gain in height for this period will range from 2 to 2½ inches (5 to 6.25 cm) per year.

By the end of this period most preschoolers will be approximately 4 feet (120 cm) tall.

Preschoolers appear to be thinner and taller than they are. This may be due to the more erect posture they can assume now that they have lost the pot belly posture of toddlerhood.

HEART RATE

The average heart rate for this age period will range from 85 to 110 beats per minute.

Heart rates must always be reviewed in relation to the child's emotional state and activity.

As children progress along the age continuum, the average heart rate becomes slower until it reaches the average adult rate of 60 to 100.

Cardiac rates increase when the cells of the body need additional food or oxygen as a result of illness, trauma, or stress.

Stress, illness, and intense activities alter the heart rate.

Pulse rates should be easily palpable at the wrist (radial artery).

The heart rate and rhythm should be consistent and easily discerned. Variations will be evidenced only with changes in activities. Arrhythmias should be monitored by health personnel.

RESPIRATION

The respiratory rate will continue to range from 20 to 30 breaths per minute.

Individual respiratory rates must always be evaluated in relation to the circumstances and activities in which the child is engaged.

The breathing pattern resembles that of the adult with the increased use of thoracic muscles.

The breathing pattern will be altered when the child is under exertion or stress.

BLOOD PRESSURE

Blood pressure readings for this age group approximate 85/60 mm Hg.

Both systolic and diastolic readings are readily auscultated.

Blood pressure readings will now be obtained during the well-child conference to establish a baseline of knowledge for future health conferences.

The readings will be altered if the child is fearful or anxious.

TEMPERATURE

The body temperature for this age continues to range from 98.6° to 99.6° F (37° to 37.6° C).

Body temperature fluctuates normally with the child's activity, hydration level, and environmental changes.

A child 4 years old can be taught to hold a thermometer in the mouth, under the tongue, and without biting down. *If there is any doubt that the child is unable to do this, then the temperature reading should be obtained either by the axillary or rectal methods.* In all events—stay with the child—never leave the child unattended while monitoring temperature.

Oral temperatures above 100° F (37.8° C) are indicative of fever and usually accompany infection and/or a pathological condition.

Fever may be detected when touching and observing the child's skin. The skin may feel warm, appear red (flushed), and evidence perspiration (even when the environmental temperature or activity of the child is not a factor).

Shivering may occur as the peripheral blood vessels dilate to permit elimination of body heat through cooling by room air. Panting-like respirations may likewise occur, a process by which evaporation of moisture from the lungs enables body heat to be eliminated.

GROWTH AND DEVELOPMENTAL LANDMARKS	ANTICIPATORY GUIDANCE

Temperatures indicative of a fever are as follows:
Oral, above 100° F (37.8° C)
Axillary, above 99° F (37.2° C)
Rectal, above 101° F (38.3° C)
For types of thermometers and procedures to be followed, see Chapter 18, Taking Temperatures with a Glass Thermometer.

HEAD

The shape of the head and facial contour will now approximate the adultlike features unique to this child.

Because the facial features so resemble those of adults, children are often referred to as "little adults." Adultlike features can mislead caretakers into expecting adultlike behavior on the part of the child.

HAIR

The texture, quality, and type (curly or straight) of hair is quite similar to that found during adulthood.

Children of this age become quite proficient at brushing and combing their own hair. Help is still required for achieving straight parts, braids, other involved styles, and shampoos.
Haircuts and trips to the barber or beauty salon are no longer viewed as threats, but are anticipated outings.

NOSE

The contour of the nose has achieved an adultlike appearance.
The specialized functions of the nose, ridding the nasal passage of mucus, warming and moisturizing inhaled air, and differentiating odors, are all highly developed.

Children of this age will voluntarily cleanse the nasal passages. They frequently upset caretakers by continuously "picking their nose."

MOUTH

Preschool children will have full sets of deciduous (temporary or baby) teeth.

The mouth is not only necessary for chewing and eating, but is extremely important for language development and expression of feelings.

By the end of this period, it is possible that some children may begin losing some of their temporary teeth, whereas others may be displaying the 6-year molars.
Adenoidal tissue usually reaches maximum size during this age period, although tonsils continue to grow until the school-age period.

Temporary teeth are replaced by permanent teeth. A displaced temporary tooth will not have a root but will closely resemble a kernel of corn.

EYES

Binocular vision should be evident.
If one eye lags behind or appears "crossed," the child should be seen by health personnel (ophthalmologist). (See Chapter 11, Squint.)

The eyes should work together as a unit.
Children who rub their eyes excessively, squint, tilt the head to one side, hold books close to the face while "reading," blink frequently, or who are unable to see readily with one eye may be exhibiting signs of serious eye problems. They should be evaluated by health personnel.

Children's visual acuity can be tested with Snellen eye charts. (Positional change of the big E or animal representation may be used instead of different letters of the alphabet as commonly used for adults.)

EARS

Hearing should be well developed and binauricular.
The specialized functions of the ear, differentiating sounds, assisting in balance, and cleansing the outer ear are all highly developed.

Preschoolers can clearly differentiate many sounds without difficulty. They hear equally well with both ears.

If the ear is intact structurally and functionally, a child should be able to hear everything from a soft whisper to very loud noises.
Gross hearing tests and fine hearing tests using tuning forks and bone conduction may be performed during well-child conferences.

Children who are inattentive, turn up the volume on the television, radio, or phonograph, or ask for repetition of items frequently may be providing caretakers with clues of hearing difficulties.

GROWTH AND DEVELOPMENTAL LANDMARKS	ANTICIPATORY GUIDANCE

Biological—cont'd

EARS—cont'd

During this period, children's ears appear to be placed lower on the head than in earlier periods. This appearance is related to structural changes that have modified and otherwise altered the shape of the head from round to more oval. The eustachian tube has increased in length.

Cerumen (earwax), a waxy secretion of the glands of the external ear (outer ear), frequently accumulates and can obstruct sound waves and impair hearing.

Children of this age will frequently have dark (yellow to brown) earwax (cerumen).

Caution: Avoid cleansing ears with cotton swabs or any other pointed articles. If a buildup of earwax is suspected by caretakers, children should be seen by health personnel to have it removed. Caretakers or children can damage the eardrum by trying to clean out earwax too vigorously.

TRUNK AND EXTREMITIES

Structural contours of the chest, back, and abdomen have changed from the pot belly, swayback lordosis of infancy and toddlerhood to the erect position of adults. Only a slight protrusion of the abdomen remains.

The spinal column is now straight. The thoracic, back, and abdominal musculature is more fully developed.

The chest contour now assumes adult proportions. The anteroposterior diameter of the chest is now smaller than the transverse diameter.

The contours of the arms and legs have become better delineated because of muscle development.

Preschoolers now resemble adults because of changes in bone and muscle development. Four- and five-year-olds stand erect with their backs straight. The pot belly of toddlerhood is replaced by a flatter firmer stomach (abdomen). Arms and legs have more contour because of muscle growth.

MOBILITY

Muscle development continues in an orderly head-to-toe fashion, but in the 4- and 5-year-old there seems to be greater emphasis on coordination of muscle groups in performing motor skills.

Motor skills that require greater agility include twisting the body, bending, lifting, climbing, reaching, and other combinations of arm and leg maneuvers (flexion and extension).

Improved fine motor coordination becomes evident as children of this age are more capable of building structures, taking things apart, and putting them back together again.

Children of this age manipulate small objects such as crayons, scissors, and paintbrushes with better dexterity than in earlier periods.

Eye-hand coordination has improved, but will not reach total refinement until well into the school-age period.

The mobility of the preschooler has increased because of the consistent rapid development of all muscles throughout the body.

Preschoolers struggle to learn to use tricycles, scooters, roller skates, or skis. They are enchanted with jungle gyms, merry-go-rounds, sliding boards, swings, or anything that involves running, jumping, and climbing.

Accident prevention is a prime consideration for this age. (See Chapter 10, Safety and Accident Prevention.)

The natural energy and ability of these children can be used constructively in and around the home. They can be encouraged to assist in setting tables, helping with simple chores, or pushing the grocery cart on shopping expeditions.

Additionally, this age child usually enjoys self-care activities such as bathing alone, brushing teeth, dressing, and undressing. Although quite self-sufficient, these children will need some supervision and assistance with buttons or zippers in the back of their clothes.

Some 5-year-olds can be taught to tie their shoes.

Psychological

DEPENDENCE-INDEPENDENCE

Preschoolers display many more independent behaviors than children in the toddler period.

Sex roles of the caretakers become very influential. At this time, it becomes apparent that the children are no longer attached only to a "mother" figure. Girls often become attached to a male family member and boys to a female member. Children will vie for the attention of the caretaker of the opposite sex.

An example of this increased independence is seen in the 4- or 5-year-old's ability to take care of toileting and dressing needs.

Preschoolers will imitate the caretaker to which they are exposed

Some 4- and 5-year-olds will become very attached to one family member or another. They will vie for the attention of this person (usually of the opposite sex) and become very possessive.

GROWTH AND DEVELOPMENTAL LANDMARKS	ANTICIPATORY GUIDANCE
This is the period of life when the groundwork for future sex-role orientation is developed. If caretakers feel competent in their own sex roles, they can assist and support their children in working through this period successfully.	If a preschooler expresses the desire to marry the caretaker, avoid ridiculing or laughing at the child's serious intentions.
Loss of a caretaker during this period can delay the foundation of sex roles for the future. Often children develop a sense of guilt or blame that they caused the death or the leaving of the caretaker.	Preschoolers who lose a caretaker (divorce, separation, or death) often believe they were responsible for the event. Preschoolers need opportunities to share or be reassured that the loss was not their fault.
By the end of the preschool period, both boys and girls are able to differentiate sexes and sex roles.	It is not at all unusual during this preschool period for children of opposite sexes to share the physical differences in their body parts through exposure, manipulation, and examination. Use the opportunity to help children understand the difference in their body parts and sex. Honestly answer any questions the preschoolers raise, then divert their attention to another activity.
Sex roles are demonstrated in preschoolers' play activities. Sex-role orientation varies with different cultures.	Children mimic what they see and hear. A great deal of knowledge is gained from television, radio, and records. Supervision of the programs to which children are exposed is desirable. Many comedy shows and cartoons depict life-styles that caretakers really do not wish to have their children emulate. The elements of love, security, and trust are rarely exemplified in modern day cartoons and comedies.
The ability to be granted increased opportunity for independent activities is evidenced through the preschooler's eagerness to please others, follow directions, and adhere to parameters of safety.	Preschoolers who evidence responsibility to perform tasks within assigned guidelines can be taught to cross streets safely and permitted to run errands beyond the home.
By the end of the preschool period, children have developed a rudimentary sense of conscience. Preschoolers can differentiate right from wrong, good from bad, and honesty from dishonesty. They are easily influenced and quickly confused by the adult standards to which they have been exposed.	Caretakers set examples their preschooler will follow. For example, if children see caretakers say something nice to someone, then just the opposite when the person is absent, mixed messages are given. If caretakers borrow items without returning them, this too provides negative role modeling.
The ideas of conscience, truth, and honesty are further developed through the child's exposure to spiritual or religious education.	

Social

SOCIAL AWARENESS

Preschoolers are more aware of their own role and place within the family constellation.	Preschoolers enjoy looking at photograph albums and identifying themselves, their relatives, close friends, and others. Children now identify themselves by name in pictures as opposed to the identification process commonly found in toddlers seeing themselves ("baby," "little boy," "girl and doggy").
Preschoolers can perceive and understand significant others beyond the confines of the home and the roles they play in society. Examples of these individuals include policemen, firemen, grocery store clerks, mailmen, ministers, garbage collectors, nurses, and physicians.	Caretakers can assist preschoolers in identifying and understanding the roles of firemen, policemen, nurses, and others by a variety of ways such as reading stories, meeting the people, or going places.
Preschoolers can learn and remember their telephone numbers and addresses.	Preschoolers can be taught that policemen, firemen, and mailmen will help them if they become lost. Caution children about speaking to, getting into cars with, or accompanying strangers on the promise of being given candy or gifts.
	It is essential to help children differentiate friend from foe.

RELATIONSHIPS

Preschoolers have developed strong bonds with their family members and close peers. In addition, they can establish relationships quickly and easily with many individuals in the surrounding community.	Four- and five-year-olds take for granted previously established relationships with family members as they become involved with others.
Peer relationships seem to become more important to preschoolers than maintaining and furthering close family relationships.	The fact that preschoolers no longer center their attention on the caretaker may be upsetting. The relationships that develop among peers is sometimes difficult for adults to understand.

GROWTH AND DEVELOPMENTAL LANDMARKS	ANTICIPATORY GUIDANCE

Social—cont'd

RELATIONSHIPS—cont'd

Exposure to nursery school and group activities assists preschoolers to grow in the physical and social realms of development.

Some caretakers may take advantage of nursery schools to provide opportunities for their children to socialize with other preschoolers. This is particularly helpful when there is only one child in the family.

Working caretakers find it necessary to place their preschoolers in a nursery school or day care center.

Some preschoolers enjoy nursery school—others do not. (See Chapter 10, Play and Activity.)

Preschoolers have many rare qualities, among which are forgiveness, forgetting, and the ability to focus on the positive aspects of their friends.

Preschoolers can be playing together happily, suddenly fight, separate, then the friendship resumes (sometimes only minutes later), and the bond between them seems stronger than ever.

Caretakers intervene with caution when preschoolers disagree because young children are able to forgive friends totally.

Children learn responsibility through the expectations of their behavior by others in the home. These expectations within the home lay the groundwork for the behavior that the children will demonstrate away from home.

The security object (blanket or favorite toy) continues to be very important to some 4- and 5-year-olds. As these children develop more friendships with peers and other individuals outside the home, the need for the security object fades.

Many preschoolers cling to a security object (blanket or favorite toy). Security objects fill a need in times of stress. Preschoolers give up the object on their own.

Some 4- and 5-year-olds continue to speak and play with imaginary friends. They are trying out new roles, refining patterns of interaction or behavior, or sharing feelings with a friend who does not question or criticize.

Imaginary friends are a normal occurrence in many children's lives. It is not necessary to agree that the friend exists, but let the child know that it is fun to have a make-believe friend.

LANGUAGE

Language development continues at a very rapid pace.

The typical 4-year-old has a vocabulary that ranges between 1400 and 1600 words.

The typical 5-year-old has a vocabulary well over 2000 words.

By the end of the preschool period, children will have added prepositions and prepositional phrases to their repertoire.

Language serves many purposes for 4- and 5-year-olds. It is more than just an accumulation of words and their meanings. Language becomes a means of expressing thoughts and feelings and sharing experiences and expanding relationships. Language assists preschoolers in expressing abstract ideas; helps them develop symbolic representations of that which they think they see, hear, or feel; and permits them to express their past experiences and their future plans for life.

Language is a learning process for preschoolers. Word usage (vocabulary) increases rapidly in the preschool years.

Four- and five-year-olds speak in complete sentences. In addition, they now speak of themselves using "I," "me," and "mine." They also use many other pronouns correctly and with ease.

Four- and five-year-olds want to learn about everything. Their intellectual curiosity has them questioning the how and why of past, present, and future events; time and space; and birth and death. Caretakers may not know all the answers.

This is an excellent time for children to be taken to a library where they see the many books and other printed materials available for learning. Libraries also provide opportunities for 4- and 5-year-olds to attend special programs and story times. Children in nursery schools often take class trips to libraries, museums, zoos, or other places of interest.

Books for preschool children should be sturdy, small enough to be easily handled, and contain large print and pictures. Preschoolers are attracted by stories of children, animals, machines, and real life situations of which they have some knowledge.

LEARNING

Cognitive (knowledge) learning and psychomotor (skills) learning are extremely dominant in this period of life.

When children learn new skills, they need time to practice on their own. The 4- and 5-year-old must be permitted to make mistakes, to try again, and even again if necessary. Experience is a great teacher.

Children learn from people with whom they interact. New experiences, both inside and outside the home, expand their knowledge.

Outings that stimulate learning for 4- and 5-year-olds can include visits to a library or zoo, going to a shipyard, visiting a museum, riding on a bus or train, taking walks through the woods, going fishing, or attending the theater for musical and drama performances.

GROWTH AND DEVELOPMENTAL LANDMARKS	ANTICIPATORY GUIDANCE

The preschooler's attitude and desire to learn are influenced by the behavior of the caretakers.

Preschoolers are learning about time and space. They have the ability to understand the meaning of short periods of time such as "after lunch" or "before supper." But the distant future, such as "next summer" or "next year," has little meaning.

Their language begins to try to connect the ideas of time and space to their world. For example, "Tomorrow I'll be bigger."

Four- and five-year-olds are becoming aware of the fact that they and objects occupy space. Children of this age can be seen attempting to sit in a stroller or carriage and find they no longer fit.

Through imaginative play preschoolers demonstrate their understanding of numbers. Four- and five-year-olds recognize the presence of more than one object in any one place and know the difference between those which are smaller or larger. They play with money; they have some idea of its importance in purchasing items (this is seen by playing store), but they do not have the capacity to understand its true value. Four- and five-year-olds may delight in collecting money in a container (to them it makes no difference what kind of money), and they become quite possessive of it. They realize a difference between a lot and a little and do not hesitate to let other individuals in their environment know that it is theirs.

Preschoolers learn through songs and rhythm games that they hear on television, radio, records, in movies, or at church.

Children of this age can be heard singing to themselves and seen mimicking rhythm in their body movements.

Group experiences help preschoolers learn songs and games.

Although preschoolers learn many activities, behaviors, and skills through mimicry, imitation, and trial and error, there are many things they need to be taught.

Teaching always involves more than just telling. Teaching frequently requires demonstration, repetition, and assistance.

Although 4- and 5-year-olds strive to reach adult standards, adults must remember the limitations of these children's abilities. Praise for their endeavors encourages children to strive for future goals.

CHAPTER 10

HEALTH MAINTENANCE FOR PRESCHOOLERS

Four- and five-year-olds are usually healthy and energetic. Each day is filled with new learning experiences. They have become more aware of their changing body shape, size, and contour. They can use their bodies with greater agility and have increased confidence in their physical skills. Trusting in their own abilities (both mental and physical) may thrust them beyond safe parameters.

Having learned self-care activities in toddlerhood, preschoolers believe that they can handle the responsibility for their own care, such as bathing, dressing, toileting, sleeping, and eating. By 5 years, naps are rarely taken, nighttime sleep ranges from 9 to 12 hours, and periods of wakefulness continue to expand.

Preschoolers are often so busy they forget mealtimes and often use tactics to delay sleep time. Although toilet training has usually been completed by this period, accidents occur because the 4- and 5-year-old waits too long before responding to the need for elimination.

Eagerness to learn and the desire to demonstrate newly acquired skills seem to occupy the 4- and 5-year-old's every waking minute.

Keeping preschoolers healthy requires caretakers to monitor their activities, enforce mealtimes and sleep times, and maintain standards of good health. Consistency on the part of the caretaker is the key. Preschoolers can be expected to conform to the established family routines. Discipline and limit setting continue to be an important facet for the development of a healthy child.

Accident prevention is still an extremely important task of caretakers during this period. Explanations, warnings, and setting limits are useful tools that caretakers now have at their disposal to assist them in keeping their children accident-free. Four- and five-year-olds have the ability to conceptualize and do abstract thinking.

The need for health supervision for the four- and five-year-old rarely exceeds two visits per year. A major focus for health visits during preschool years is the maintenance of immunization levels. Progress in every realm of development is also evaluated.

Chapter 10 will discuss helpful hints associated with areas of concern related to the maintenance of healthy preschoolers.

AREAS FOR CONCERN	HELPFUL HINTS

Health conference

The health care conference continues to offer health personnel opportunities to assess a child's growth and development, supervise health, and assist caretakers in learning more about their children.

Safety guidelines, health protection principles, and suggestions for anticipatory guidance should be a basic component of every health care conference.

Most preschoolers will be seen at least once each year.

Preschoolers will remember previous visits for health supervision. If preschoolers are reluctant to go to the health conference because they fear painful or intrusive procedures, caretakers *should never lie to the children* by offering false reassurance that they will not be hurt. The bond of trust continues to be reinforced with truthful statements, although it may be difficult for the caretaker to insist that the visit must be made.

Health history (reviewed and updated)

The examiner will ask about infections, illnesses, injuries, and other stressful situations that have occurred since the last visit.

Information will be requested regarding the possibility of the toddler having been exposed to any communicable disease.

The family history will be reviewed for health problems (congenital, familial) that may have significance for the child's health.

It is helpful if the caretaker brings a record of any injuries, illnesses, or stressful situations that have occurred to the preschooler since the last visit.

The health history is brought up to date during the physical examination.

Health assessment: physical examination

Emphasis will be placed on gathering data related to growth and development. The information will be gained more rapidly because of the 4- and 5-year-old's increased ability to cooperate.

Height, weight, and vital signs will be measured.

Examiners gather data on gross and fine motor skills by asking children to climb onto the examining table, by permitting them to listen to their chests with the stethoscope, or by asking them to perform a specific hand-eye coordination skill.

Examinations of the eyes, ears, nose, mouth, and throat will be included. Examiners will measure the child's participation and reactions when checking visual and auditory abilities.

Visual acuity, accommodation, and control of eye muscles are checked during eye examinations. Ask the child to follow an object such as the examiner's finger as it is moved to the left, right, up and down, and close to the child's nose. Binocular motion should be present. If one eye tends to deviate in the opposite direction of the other eye it usually is indicative of weak eye muscles. This is a common eye problem in children and should be treated immediately. (See Chapter 11, Strabismus.)

Eye accommodation may be tested with a flashlight. The pupil will constrict when the bright light is brought into focus.

The examiner may use an ophthalmoscope to assess the inner structure of the eye.

Assessment of the ear includes physical examination of the ear and ear canal and assessment of hearing.

The audiometer is a machine that can determine a child's hearing acuity through the identification of sounds at various pitches.

Preschoolers are usually cooperative during the routine health assessment. They will open their mouths, stick out their tongues, turn their heads, stand erect, walk, and in general perform the body maneuvers when asked to do so.

Examiners usually assess many body functions with only one or two tests.

Four- and five-year-olds have the ability to close one eye and read with the other. Many preschoolers can identify the letters of the alphabet. Special eye charts with pictures of toys and animals are available for use with children who do not read.

Children of this age will usually enjoy "playing hearing games with the examiner" such as repeating words or sounds that they hear, signaling when they hear something or when they do not, or following directions whispered just to them.

AREAS FOR CONCERN	HELPFUL HINTS

Health assessment: physical examination—cont'd

When an audiometer is not available, the examiner may use less definitive methods to test hearing. A bell, tuning fork, the examiner's voice, gravel, and sandpaper are but a few of the "noises" that can be used to provide samples of sound with different volume or character.

A bone conduction test using a tuning fork is often used. Vibrate the tuning fork and place it just behind the child's ear on the bony prominence. The child should be able to hear the tone or pitch of the tuning fork.

Visual and/or hearing difficulties should be treated as soon as possible because intellectual and cognitive development depend on these two senses.

Auscultation and palpation of the chest, back, and abdomen are performed while the child sits and lies on the examining table.

Reflexes are tested throughout the examination.

The skeletal structure and musculature are evaluated while the child sits, stands, climbs, and walks.

The examiner gathers information related to many body functions as the child sits, stands, walks, or otherwise cooperates with the examination.

Health assessment: mental and social examination

Mental capabilities of preschoolers are evaluated by the ease with which they perform the various maneuvers or tasks requested.

Communication skills are assessed by the child's responses to questions asked by the examiner.

A child's sociability is also evaluated through response to questions asked and the ease with which a health assessment is performed.

Permit preschoolers to answer questions directed to them. Permitting children to respond enhances the assessment.

Four- and five-year-old children, if given the freedom to socialize and become comfortable with the examiner, will permit a more thorough and thus more reliable health assessment to be performed. The more comfortable children become with the examiner, the easier and more pleasurable will be future health visits.

Health protection

Preschoolers will usually have completed their initial series and booster immunizations.

Most preschoolers only require booster immunizations just prior to attending school.

If an accidental injury predisposes the child to the possibility of tetanus, a tetanus toxoid injection may be given.

If the child has *not* been immunized, the initial series of immunization will be instituted. (See Appendix A.)

Immunization is required for entrance to public schools in many states.

Health promotion

The health conference usually includes discussions and/or a review of the following topics: dentition, nutrition, elimination, sleep and rest, play and activity, safety and accident prevention, discipline, sibling rivalry, sex education, masturbation, and hospitalization.

When caretakers make appointments for health supervision visits, remind them to jot down any questions of concern they may have regarding their preschooler's health.

DENTITION

The preschooler has a complete set of deciduous (temporary) teeth. Dental care is essential during this period because caries (tooth decay) is widely prevalent.

Foods containing large quantities of simple carbohydrates should be avoided because they are important factors in the development of caries.

Children should visit the dentist twice a year to maintain the "baby teeth." Baby teeth maintain the natural arch of the mouth. First visits to the dentist have usually occurred in toddlerhood.

Preschoolers can be taught and expected to brush their teeth thoroughly twice a day (toothbrushing habits are best established in toddlerhood).

Avoid offering candy and other foods containing refined sugars because they contribute to cavity formation.

AREAS FOR CONCERN

HELPFUL HINTS

Some 5-year-olds may begin to lose their temporary teeth, although the majority of children begin this process around age 6. The central incisors are usually the first teeth to be lost.

Accidents involving the teeth are common. Teeth can be chipped, totally dislodged, or pushed back into the gum line. If the teeth are lost or chipped, no action is usually necessary. If the teeth have been driven back into the gum line, dental evaluation is necessary. (The central incisors are most frequently involved.)

Although the loss or chipping of a temporary tooth is unfortunate, it will not affect the development or eruption of permanent teeth.

When temporary teeth are driven back into the gum line, there may be large amounts of bleeding. Application of cold wet washcloths and slight pressure will usually control the bleeding quickly. The child will be frightened and quite anxious immediately after the accident. Calm reassurance on the part of the caretaker is helpful.

It is necessary that a dental evaluation be performed to determine if injury has occurred to the permanent teeth. Removal of the temporary teeth may be necessary, although temporary teeth often return to their original position without treatment.

NUTRITION

Preschoolers typically eat three meals a day plus snacks.

Caloric requirements vary, depending on the child's size and activity. Most preschoolers need 35 to 40 calories per pound of body weight.

Four- and five-year-olds needs will range between 1500 and 1800 calories a day.

The nutritional intake for the preschooler should reflect selections from each of the four basic food groups.

Milk and milk products—1 to 1½ pints of milk a day.

Preschoolers will usually eat more food than toddlers. A rule of thumb for children's serving sizes would be one level tablespoon per year of age (4-year-olds might be offered 4 level tablespoons of potatoes). Huge portions (adult size) frequently depress children's appetites.

Milk products include ice-cream, puddings, and cheese. Milk is also included in prepared foods such as mashed potatoes, cream sauces, or soups. Preschoolers enjoy puddings and custards so well that it is not necessary to overly sweeten these foods.

Encourage preschoolers to drink milk with their meals as opposed to drinking an entire glass as soon as they sit down at the table. Taking large amounts of fluid just prior to eating will depress appetites.

Meats—two servings a day (each serving approximately 2 ounces).

The meat category includes all types of meat, poultry, and fish. Other food items such as eggs, legumes (dried peas, beans, or lentils), nuts, and peanut butter may be substituted.

Preschoolers, like toddlers, enjoy meals with finger foods. Hard-boiled eggs, peanut butter sandwiches, hot dogs, chicken, and hamburgers in a bun are but a few of the protein-rich foods that preschoolers enjoy.

Portion sizes should be remembered: one egg, one hot dog, one drumstick, one tablespoon of peanut butter and about one half to two thirds the average hamburger will provide an adequate serving for most 4-year-olds. *Encouraging children to eat more or to clean up their plates may lay the groundwork for being overweight (obese) in the future.*

Vegetables and fruits—four or five servings a day.

Preschoolers typically favor fruits over vegetables. They also seem to prefer raw to cooked fruits and vegetables. Raw fruits and vegetables provide excellent snacks and should be encouraged over candy and sweets.

Raw fruits and vegetables cut into small finger-length strips permit children to manipulate them easily.

Four- and five-year-olds may eat a whole piece of fruit, but more often than not their appetites will be satisfied after they have consumed only a portion of the fruit.

AREAS FOR CONCERN	HELPFUL HINTS

Health promotion—cont'd

NUTRITION—cont'd

	Carrot sticks and pickles seem to be favored over celery, green beans, or cucumbers, partly because the latter are often stringy and/or contain seeds.
	Cooked vegetables such as corn, peas, or beans are better received if served as single items rather than mixed together or in casseroles or stews.
Bread and cereals—four servings a day.	This category includes all breads, cereals (cooked and ready to eat), pastas (rice, macaroni, noodles, and spaghetti), cakes, crackers, and cookies.
	Preschoolers can be expected to eat cereal or toast for breakfast, have a sandwich or soup with crackers at lunch, and some form of pasta at night. They often eat dry cereals or crackers as snack foods and not as part of a meal.
	Reduce sweetened bread items such as cake, cookies or presweetened cereals. As noted in the discussion of dentition, high concentrations of sugar encourages cavities.
Preschoolers, like toddlers, have tremendous developmental needs for proteins, vitamins, and minerals. In addition, they require more calories in the form of carbohydrates than did toddlers.	
Four- and five-year-olds have a keen sense of taste and are attracted by the color and odor of foods.	
Mealtime is a period for socializing and/or learning good eating habits.	Caretakers are role models. Patterns demonstrated in the selection, quantity, and manner of eating performed by adults will be quickly imitated by 4- and 5-year-olds. If the preschooler notes that a favorite caretaker refuses vegetables, the preschooler too will refuse vegetables.
	Mealtime should be pleasant. The dinner table is not the place for all of the faults, crimes, or misdemeanors of family members to be aired.
Four- and five-year-olds are capable of participating in selecting, preparing, and serving meals.	Children 4 and 5 years old enjoy being helpers and can carry out directions quite well.
	Permit 4- and 5-year-olds to serve their own portions. Some spilling may occur; this is not done deliberately, and caution should be exercised in giving assistance when necessary. The use of admonitions such as "Don't be clumsy" or "Don't spill" are negative and indicate that the caretaker expects the child to spill. Providing affirmative statements such as "You may serve yourself," or "Help yourself to the amount you would like, I'll hold the bowl for you" displays the caretaker's confidence in the child's abilities. Rudimentary though they are, situations like these provide opportunities for children to demonstrate initiative, independence, and responsibility.
Appetites of children are affected by fevers, illness, injury, emotional stress, fatigue, dental caries, or overeating between meals.	Investigate episodes of poor eating. Children eat less when they have a fever, are hurt, under stress, or have snacked all day.
New foods should be added gradually.	Although certain foods were refused in earlier periods of life, they should be tried again now.

ELIMINATION

Bowel and bladder control become established during this period of life.	Just as each child develops at a unique rate, so toileting controls vary with each child. Each child develops a specific pattern of elimination.
Preschoolers will ask to go to the bathroom, and most can care for their own toileting needs.	Appropriate words for toileting should be taught and used consistently. Avoid babytalk, slang, or offensive words. The caretaker is the role model the preschooler mimics.
Some preschoolers may have wetting accidents during the day. These accidents are usually associated with delayed response to an elimination need because of play activity.	When toileting accidents occur, avoid overreacting or making the child feel guilty or ashamed. The child's assistance in cleaning up or changing clothes or bed linen can be permitted and encouraged.

AREAS FOR CONCERN	HELPFUL HINTS
Some preschoolers may have difficulty with enuresis (nighttime bedwetting). Enuresis may be due to stress, sound sleep, excess fluid intake, environmental temperature change, tension, or illness. If an illness is suspected, seek medical advice.	If accidents persist over prolonged periods of time, make sure there is no physical reason for the occurrence.

SLEEP AND REST

Sleep patterns are usually well established by the preschool period. Four- and five-year-olds require less sleep than toddlers. The typical 4-year-old will sleep 10 to 12 hours at night. The typical 5-year-old will average 9 to 11 hours at night. Although 4- and 5-year-olds rarely take naps, their needs for rest periods remain high. It is not unusual for preschoolers to need 12 to 14 hours of sleep and rest every day.	Ideally 4- and 5-year-olds should have their own beds (and when possible, their own rooms). Preschool children need help in establishing and maintaining consistent patterns of sleep and rest. If a consistent pattern is maintained, they will go to bed quickly with little fuss or fanfare. Adherence to a consistent routine can be expected of the preschooler. A quiet time before bedtime is helpful in calming children and preparing them for sleep. It may be helpful to maintain a soft night-light in the room or in the hallway so that if nightmares occur, the child will awaken to that which is familiar and readily identified.
The imagination and fantasies of preschoolers may predispose them to dreams and nightmares.	Assurance and support from the caretaker when nightmares occur will help the child realize that it was just a bad dream and not real. The caretaker's presence at times like these deepens the child's trust.

PLAY AND ACTIVITY

Preschoolers learn and develop their physical, emotional, and social skills through play. Preschoolers' patterns of play will reveal their capabilities and limitations.	Four- and five-year-olds reflect the behaviors and attitudes of the people who are around them through their play activities. Preschoolers usually enjoy developing their physical skills. In particular, they will delight in the following:

Tricycles or other pedaling devices
Merry-go-rounds
Teeter-totters (seesaws)
Swings
Skates and scooters
Sliding boards
Swimming pools
Catch and throw games
Gymnastics, trampolines

A preschooler's sense of balance is still somewhat immature; therefore there will be falls, tumbles, and many minor accidents. Caretakers must teach principles of safety before permitting a 4- or 5-year-old to be around playground equipment unaccompanied. Some principles to emphasize would include the following:

1. Walk around swings. Never walk in front or in back of swings because the occupants cannot control the swing's path, nor stop it, nor see people in their path.
2. Walk around, never under a teeter-totter.
3. Climb onto merry-go-rounds when they are fully stopped and hang on tightly at all times when they are in motion.
4. Sit on the sliding board and slide down feet first.
5. When playing catch, avoid hitting others. Be sure that the person to whom you are throwing the ball is aware of the ball.
6. Swimming. (See Chapter 7, Play.)

Trampoline usage requires supervision by caretakers.
Babysitters and others entrusted to care for preschoolers need to know and maintain the rules of safety for play.

Solitary play during this period continues to be very important because it permits the children to refine skills and use their imagination and creativity. Playing alone eliminates competition and permits the child to test out skills without criticism.	Preschoolers need time to be alone. Playing alone may take the place of a nap or rest period because the activities are usually less strenuous than playing with others.

AREAS FOR CONCERN	HELPFUL HINTS

Health promotion—cont'd

PLAY AND ACTIVITY—cont'd

Four- and five-year-olds frequently create an imaginary playmate who becomes real to them.

Imaginary play or an imaginary friend need not be discouraged because they fill a need at this time. Caretakers can acknowledge that it is fun to have an imaginary friend to confide in or talk to or play with, but that this friend is imaginary. The imaginary friend or playmate becomes less important to the child as the child develops new friends in the neighborhood, church, parks, or school settings.

Preschoolers enjoy playing with other children.

Parallel play (two or more children engaged in the same activity within the same physical area, but not exchanging ideas or equipment) becomes less apparent during this period than in toddlerhood. Preschoolers enjoy *group play*.

Group play involves two or more children performing tasks together. Frequently group play is highly creative and imaginative because children imitate and expand on activities of daily living to which they have been exposed.

Children this age will build things with blocks or boxes. They will use chairs or boxes to imitate buses or trains. They will play house, assigning roles and tasks similar to those seen in their homes. They will pretend to be in church or in school and will try to perform dances and songs seen and heard there or on television or radio.

Gross motor and fine motor skills are constantly being refined and further developed.

Four- and five-year-olds need opportunities to socialize with other children, but they also need opportunities to use their large muscles in activities of running, jumping, climbing, twisting, and stretching.

Preschoolers need to engage in activities requiring the fine motor skills such as drawing, sewing, doing puzzles, reading books, cutting, pasting, and dressing, including snapping, buttoning, or even zipping clothes.

Preschoolers' play will frequently involve getting dirty. Dress children in clothing that can tolerate hard usage and be laundered frequently.

Providing preschoolers with opportunities to socialize, equipment they can manipulate, time to be creative, and including them in home activities will provide excellent learning experiences.

Nursery school or other preschool experiences can be valuable. Structured experiences with supervision (adults educated to enhance the learning experiences of children), with children their own age, and with materials and equipment designed for use by children of this age can certainly potentiate levels of achievement in all spheres of learning.

Children should be introduced to nursery schools gradually. At the first visit, the caretaker can anticipate staying the entire time and remaining in the child's view. At the second or third visit, the child may permit the caretaker's absence for part of the time or all of the time. Establishing and maintaining the parameters of leaving and returning can be assisted through the trust relationship built since infancy between the child and caretaker. Many children love nursery schools; some hate it. For those who dislike nursery school, it may be helpful to withdraw them until they are older.

Some caretakers must rely on nursery schools because of work schedules. Children of all ages learn to adapt or adjust to consistent routines. When a child resists attending nursery school, it may be due to a problem at the school, health problem, or desire to spend more time with the caretaker. Explore each possibility.

Children's ideas of the how, what, when, and why of life experiences are exemplified by play. Male and female roles, as well as the expectations of others in regard to adult and children's behaviors, are learned through exposure to real live people and those on television. These roles and behaviors are evidenced in and through children's play.

Observations of children's play can reveal positive and negative attitudes.

Play reveals the inner thoughts, concerns, emotions, and even fears of 4- and 5-year-olds.

128

AREAS FOR CONCERN	HELPFUL HINTS

Children express their feelings better through their activities than through verbal expression.

Television viewing time should be monitored and restricted.

Although language development has increased by leaps and bounds, it is still difficult for 4- and 5-year-olds to express their thoughts and feelings in words.

Avoid using television as a substitute for play. Although television can entertain, teach, and reinforce ideas taught in the home, there are too many inappropriate programs on television for preschool viewing. Playing with siblings, adults, other relatives, and peers is more advantageous to a child's healthy development than hours of passive observation of television. Children need time with caretakers when the caretaker can focus totally on them.

SAFETY AND ACCIDENT PREVENTION

Accident prevention for preschoolers is as great a concern as it was for toddlers, although the circumstances have altered. Whereas toddlers had limited mobility, innate curiosity, and the desire to investigate everything and anything, the preschooler's world is much broader. Abilities, skills, and intelligence factors have increased. Curiosity has been replaced by contemplative inquiry. Preschoolers persist in their examination and manipulation until they have satisfied their need to know the what and why of the situation.

Safety measures can now be taught because preschoolers are able to learn rules and regulations.

Health professionals might remind caretakers of potential danger areas inside and outside the home.

Accidents do occur during the preschool period, despite the most thorough precautions. Efforts are geared to reducing their incidence.

Childproofing efforts are now directed toward teaching the child as well as decreasing hazards. Childproofing environments becomes impossible because preschoolers are no longer confined to their home and yards.

Preschoolers are able to learn safety rules and regulations. Teaching safety to the 4- or 5-year-old often becomes an enjoyable task for the caretaker.

Anticipate situations and objects that are potentially dangerous. Although it is impossible to anticipate every area of danger, the following categories should be considered:
  Traffic crossings
  Matches and other flammables
  Unattended vehicles
  Motor-driven machinery
  Wells and other bodies of water
  Stored liquids
  Abandoned appliances
  Abandoned buildings

Danger lies in the child's intent to test and experiment.

Preschoolers are likely to pick up a book of matches (not to eat or taste them as would the toddler) but to strike them and watch them burn. They may experiment further with fire by exposing different substances or objects to the flame to see if they too will burn.

Four- and five-year-olds can manipulate keys in ignitions and push-button switches with ease. When left unsupervised and in proximity to these kinds of equipment, preschoolers will test their abilities and may unfortunately injure themselves as well as others.

Safety measures *must be taught* and never left to chance.

Family discussions on safety measures are helpful. Preschoolers can appreciate and understand dangerous situations without having to experience them. Caretakers can build on the concepts learned in toddlerhood. For example, expand the ideas of "burn" and "hot" to teach the dangers of matches, candles, and other flammables. It may be wise to permit a preschooler to light and blow out matches while being supervised. This method was used by one of the authors (S.P.) with several children at different times (her own plus nieces, nephews, and neighbors). Large kitchen safety matches were used. The burnt matches were then used to create a cross that was lacquered and hung in many of the children's rooms. Inevitably, someone got a singe burn, or the matches burned too far. The children learned that matches are useful, dangerous, and to be used with caution.

AREAS FOR CONCERN	HELPFUL HINTS

Health promotion—cont'd

SAFETY AND ACCIDENT PREVENTION—cont'd

The preschooler's sphere of operation is no longer confined to the home and yard. Four- and five-year-olds often have access to entire neighborhoods, parks, fields, and woods.

Preschoolers learn the rules and principles of safe practice if opportunities are offered repeatedly.

Preschoolers need to know their limits and that those which have been set will be enforced.

Safety education begins in the preschool years. Areas of safety include the following:
1. Procedures used when crossing streets.
2. Methods used for escaping from a burning home.
3. Rules and procedures used for fire alarm boxes.
4. Rules for swimming or boating.
5. Areas that are potentially dangerous in and around the home as well as in the community.
6. Dangers in regard to strangers.

Testing children's abilities to perform when exposed to certain dangers assists caretakers in identifying their children's capabilities, as well as relieving the anxiety of caretakers. Some examples include simple safety drills, fire drills, and street crossings.

Another helpful aspect in this educational process is to be certain that preschoolers have learned their full names, addresses, and telephone numbers.

DISCIPLINE (LIMIT SETTING)

Discipline must be consistent. Preschoolers can be expected to adhere to limits that have been set and to adapt their behavior to the expectations set by adults.

Children need to know where they can go and what they can do. It is not enough to tell children once that they are not to go out of the yard or cross a street. Preschoolers need brief explanations along with clear concise directions.

The physical parameters for safe exploration and play need revision as children demonstrate responsibility for their behaviors and new capabilities.

When preschoolers are unable to conform to the established guidelines of adult expectations, it may be necessary to mete out punishment.

Preschoolers need to know their limitations. Caretakers must be consistent in expectations of behavior.

The type and extent of punishment should be explained to preschoolers prior to the infraction of rules. They will know in advance what to expect if they do not obey the rules.

It is extremely important for caretakers to listen carefully to their children's explanations of their misbehavior. Inappropriate misbehavior may well prove to be the child's efforts to do something nice, such as pouring milk from a gallon bottle and dropping it, creating a mess.

If children have learned that caretakers believe in and trust them, it is likely that there will be little reason to lie or try to deceive caretakers in their explanations of misbehavior.

Four- and five-year-olds are developing a conscience and learning right from wrong. They need guidelines and limits imposed on their behavior. Adherence to guidelines assists them in developing their own method of self-control.

Children need and really want rules and guidelines. When children are disciplined, they may express physical distress or shout words that indicate they dislike caretakers, but these phases quickly pass.

SIBLING RIVALRY

Sibling rivalry is still present and often quite evident in the preschool period. The defense mechanisms described in the toddler period will also be manifested in the preschooler but the behavior observed will often be quite different.

The toddler's *hostility* is usually quite open and direct (name calling and hitting), whereas preschoolers attempt to hide their hostility (may drop the bottle or bump the baby rather hard).

Caretakers should recognize the preschooler's bid for attention when acts of hostility, anger, or frustration are noted toward brothers or sisters.

AREAS FOR CONCERN	HELPFUL HINTS
Preschoolers may offer their feelings through comments such as "I don't know why you always have to carry that baby" or "No one ever has time for me."	Help preschoolers adjust to and accept new siblings by including them in activities. Set aside time just for them and reassure them that they are loved.
Sibling rivalry of a different nature often occurs as preschoolers attempt to imitate abilities noted in older siblings. If the younger child cannot compete or perform as well, envy, jealousy, or frustration may result.	Remember to include each child to reduce feelings of envy and despair.
	Helping children understand that each person is unique and has special talents must be started early in life and reinforced in the home setting. Helping children develop their own talents reduces sibling rivalry and assists preschoolers to develop their own creativity.
Regression to infantile behavior occurs among preschoolers only when they feel really threatened by the presence of a newcomer or inferior to the achievements noted in others.	As children are praised for their capabilities and accomplishments, a positive sense of self-worth will emerge.

SEX EDUCATION

Sex education actually begins in infancy when children begin to identify their body parts. This eduation expands in toddlerhood as children learn to name their body parts and especially when they begin the toilet training process. Children should be taught body parts in correct terminology.	If caretakers could express words describing the male and female genitalia as easily as they can describe the nose, fingers, and stomach, much of the mystery and mystique associated with sex education could be averted. The use of correct terminology cannot be overemphasized. Correct terms can be learned by children, although this does not mean that the functions which organs serve is understood or that the functions even need to be explained at this time.
Sex education during this period introduces children to the meaning of being boys and girls and men and women. Presenting this material from the point of loving, caring, and trusting relationships is a focal point.	The role models provided by caretakers and other adults will teach preschoolers the attitudes and feelings generated between and among males and females much more than verbal descriiptions.
	Long involved explanations of where babies come from or how they got into mommy's tummy are to be avoided. Caretakers can answer questions simply, concisely, and honestly. Realize that preschoolers have limited knowledge and experiences. They are seeking new knowledge and clarification of old ideas.
	We are reminded of the little boy who asked his mother where he came from. After she went through the lengthy explanation of daddy planting a seed in her tummy and how it grew and turned out to be him, the child was very impressed. He turned to her and said, "Wow, wait till I tell Georgie—he only came from Chicago!"

MASTURBATION

Masturbation: Self-manipulation of the genitalia.

Expect self-investigation of all 4- and 5-year-old boys and girls.	Caretakers need to understand that the child who is found "playing with himself/herself" is only rediscovering a body part. This self-manipulation (masturbation) is a normal pattern of sexual development.
	The behavior of the child is not as important as the way in which caretakers respond to the behavior. If caretakers could respond to this type of self-investigation as they do when children spend time in manipulating and trying out new skills with fingers and toes, then children will not view particular body parts as being shameful or less than desirable.
	This behavior can be diverted by engaging preschoolers in other types of activity.
	Masturbation at this preschool age is a pleasurable often self-consoling activity but is not to be confused with sexual arousal.

AREAS FOR CONCERN	HELPFUL HINTS

Health promotion—cont'd

HOSPITALIZATION

Preschool children may have to be admitted to hospitals because of trauma, infection, illness, or elective surgery.

If hospitalization is elective, prepare the preschooler for this experience. Preparation can be achieved through simple, honest explanations and play. Many children's books are available that describe what it is like to be a patient in a hospital. Role playing has also proved beneficial in that it capitalizes on the preschooler's imaginative and imitative play patterns. Hospitalization experiences can be enacted by caretakers, preschoolers, and others playing the roles of the health care workers with whom the child will come in contact.

If the child attends a nursery school, the teacher should be informed. Reinforcement of the preparation for hospitalization can be achieved through play with peers at school.

Preschoolers may still need a security object brought from home.

Preschoolers can be involved in packing their own suitcases for this adventure. Permit them to bring security objects.

It is helpful if the caretaker(s) and health care worker together acquaint the child to the physical surroundings: the room, bed, place to store clothes and toys, bathroom, playroom, and those areas which the child can freely explore.

In addition, health care workers should inform the caretaker and child as to which areas are "off limits." Caretakers must maintain these safety standards.

Provide explanations to preschoolers prior to performing new procedures.

Whereas explanations of procedures were given primarily to caretakers in previous stages of life, the 4- or 5-year-old child is capable of understanding some abstract thoughts and should be included in these discussions.

The explanations should be kept simple. Children must be told truthfully the procedures to be performed and whether there will or will not be pain.

Preschoolers will accept separation from caretakers more readily than toddlers; however, hospitalization will still be a frightening experience. Crying and some resistance can be expected during the hospitalization process and with all procedures.

Preschoolers aim to please adults; however, their ability to cooperate under stress such as during painful or intrusive procedures is limited. Health care workers are advised to have assistants available to help immobilize the preschooler during painful procedures.

Preschoolers are trying to cooperate even when screaming and resisting certain procedures. Shaming the child or threatening additional punishment because of this behavior does not help the child.

Four- and five-year-olds fear mutilation of body parts. Hospitalization during this period may compound this fear.

The type of reassurance and support given to the child by caretakers and health care workers can do much to alleviate the fears of the child during the entire process of hospitalization.

If hospitalization resulted from acts by preschoolers that they were cautioned against, feelings of guilt may also occur.

If hospitalization occurs because of a preschooler's act, avoid compounding the guilt through statements such as "I told you not to do that—now look what you've done!"

The preschooler's abilities should be used by health care workers. Four- and five-year-olds are self-reliant in terms of their feeding, bathing, dressing, and toileting needs, but will require supervision and some assistance.

As in toddlerhood, regressive behavior can be expected on the part of the preschooler. Hospitalized children want and need to be babied. The preschooler's appetite may change drastically during hospitalization. Offering small amounts frequently and in small containers will prove more successful than giving large amounts at one time.

Health care workers can capitalize on the preschooler's desire to please and ability to conceptualize and cooperate, especially when fluid intake must be encouraged. These children will readily respond to games such as "tea parties" and stars on the intake sheet for accomplishment.

During hospitalization, praise should be offered when the preschooler tries to meet the expectations of others. That cooperation was not always at the level expected is not as important as that the child tried. Initiative will be rewarded and guilt avoided.

CHAPTER 11

HEALTH PROBLEMS OF PRESCHOOLERS

The testing and investigative nature of 4- and 5-year-old children predispose them to potential accidents and hazards. Expanding social contacts expose the preschool child to infections and communicable diseases.

Falls and burns are some of the more common accidents in and around the home. Injuries of all magnitudes occur to preschoolers while riding in motor vehicles. The special car seats available to infants and toddlers are not appropriate for the preschooler who is too large for a car seat and too small for a seat belt.

The typical health problems of this period of life are the same as those of the toddler period: colds, sore throats, ear infections, bites, stings, accidents, and allergic responses. Discussion of those problems will not be repeated. (See Chapters 5 and 8.)

Discussion in this chapter will be directed to communicable diseases and strabismus. Health care guidelines and helpful hints will be provided for the caretaker.

HEALTH PROBLEM	HEALTH CARE GUIDELINES	HELPFUL HINTS

Communicable disease

Communicable disease: A disease that spreads by direct or indirect contact with causative agents or sources of infection.

TRANSMISSION OF DISEASE

An individual acquires a disease by direct contact, indirect contact, vectors, or combinations of the three.

Direct contact: Contact with the infected person, body excretions, or discharges from open lesions or wounds.

Diseases that can be spread from persons or objects to other people are called *communicable diseases.*

The prodromal stages (that period of time prior to the manifestations most characteristic of the disease) differ with each communicable disease. Communicability of the disease is frequently high during this period.

Physical signs noticeable during the prodromal and/or the early stage of an illness include a change in behavior (lethargy or irritability), slightly elevated temperature, reddened eyes, runny eyes or nose, decreased appetite, and even a sore throat.

All communicable diseases do not have prodromal stages with noticeable signs and symptoms.

Some communicable diseases are manifested by the presence of a rash or lesions and are highly communicable when there is weeping or drainage from the lesions.

Developing illnesses in children are often indicated by early signs and symptoms. Preschoolers will sometimes clue the caretaker to the onset of illness with phrases such as, "my throat scratches," "my tummy hurts," or "I don't feel good." Additional clues include the preschooler's desire to take a nap or a change in behavior such as whining, crying, or fighting.

Preschoolers who enter nursery school programs or day care centers frequently develop one communicable disease after another, until their bodies develop the ability to fight off some of these infections.

The caretaker who notes changes in the behavior of the child or the child's playmates and who suspects an illness can take steps to isolate that child from others and perhaps stop the spread of disease. This is as important within a family as between families.

Indirect contact: Use of contaminated eating or drinking utensils, bed linen, toys, or other such objects.

Health teaching about communicable disease should emphasize the periods of communicability and the modes of transmission.

Children who use their own toothbrushes, eat only from their own plates, and use only their own handkerchiefs have been taught principles of health, although they do not understand how disease spreads. They will need reminders and reinforcement of these principles, especially when they spend time away from home with their friends.

Vectors: Insects or other animals that transfer the causative agent from one host to another.

BODY RESPONSE TO EXPOSURE TO COMMUNICABLE DISEASE

Body response to exposure to communicable disease is resistance or acquisition of the disease.

134

HEALTH PROBLEM	HEALTH CARE GUIDELINES	HELPFUL HINTS
Immunity: Resistance of the body to an infectious disease agent or its toxins.	*Humoral antibodies:* Circulating antibodies (immunoglobulins: IgA, IgG, and others) that respond to many infectious agents.	Children can be assisted in developing the ability to resist certain infections (immunity).
1. Acquired immunity is induced resistance to disease through the introduction of antibodies or substances that trigger the production of antibodies.	*Cell-mediated antibodies:* Defense mechanisms at the cellular level that are called into play when humoral antibodies are ineffective. Immunization should be started when the infant is 2 months old, since at this time the immune system is mature enough to respond to artificial stimulation by toxoids or vaccines. (See Appendix A for recommended schedule for immunization.)	Immunity (resistance to disease) can be obtained in several ways. Active immunization is receiving material (orally or by injection) that stimulates the body to produce antibodies (having had the disease also usually produces active immunity to it).
a. Active immunity results from production of antibodies by the body as a result of either having had the illness or having received attenuated (weakened) organisms through injection or oral routes. Active immunity usually has long-lasting effects.	1. A toxoid is a toxin treated by chemical or heat to reduce its deleterious effects without destroying its ability to stimulate the production of antibodies. Examples include diphtheria toxoid and tetanus toxoid.	
	2. A vaccine is a suspension of attenuated (weakened) or killed microorganisms (bacteria, virus, or other infectious organisms). Following are some types of vaccines with examples of diseases:	
	a. Killed bacteria—typhoid, pertussis	
	b. Attenuated virus—measles, mumps, rubella, poliomyelitis, smallpox, tuberculosis	
	c. Killed virus—poliomyelitis	
	Most active immunity is attained through artificial stimulation requiring more than one administration. (See Appendix A.) Combinations of vaccines and toxoids may be administered. (See Appendix A.)	Active immunity cannot be attained by having just one injection of vaccine; a series of injections must be given. (See Appendix A.)
	The sequence of immunization is extremely important to attain adequate levels of immunity, although it is not necessary to start the series over if it has been interrupted for any reason.	Active immunity, once attained, usually has long-lasting effects.
b. Passive immunity is derived from injections of ready-made antibodies that usually provide protection from 6 to 8 weeks.	The following antibodies are ready made and provide short-term passive immunity:	Passive immunization is injection of material that actively fights certain disease organisms (acquired passive). Newborn babies received some defense materials (antibodies) from the mother during the pregnancy (natural passive).
	1. Gamma globulin (prepared from pooled human serum)	
	2. Immune serum globulin (ISG) (prepared with serum containing antibodies that are specific to an illness)	
	3. Antiserum or antitoxin (usually prepared from animals)	
2. Natural immunity is an innate resistance to disease, antibodies already present in the blood.		
3. Passive immunity is derived from antibodies passed through the placenta from the mother to the infant. It provides protection from birth through approximately the third month of life.		Passive immunity, whether natural or acquired, is always short lived.

HEALTH PROBLEM	HEALTH CARE GUIDELINES	HELPFUL HINTS
Communicable disease—cont'd		
Susceptibility: Lack of resistance to an infectious disease agent or its toxins.		Children who have not developed antibodies cannot resist disease (susceptibility).
Susceptibility to disease is rarely because of only one factor.	Because of their immature immunological systems, infants through 1 year of age are at high risk for acquiring disease.	
1. Age is a factor in an individual's susceptibility to disease.	In certain periods of life, individuals have greater exposure to illness.	
	Infancy: Upper respiratory tract and gastrointestinal tract infections.	Newborns should not be exposed to individuals known to have communicable diseases, since newborns have little resistance.
	Preschool period: Communicable diseases.	Preschool children are at a stage of life when they are more prone to exposure to communicable disease because of their increased sphere of socialization. Preschool children will frequently introduce a communicable disease into a family.
		At each period of the child's life, caretakers need to be alerted to the increased likelihood of exposure to infectious or communicable diseases.
	Toddler period: Infectious diseases and beginning exposure to communicable diseases.	As toddlers enter the social stream, there is a greater chance that the child will be exposed to individuals with illnesses.
	School-age period: Communicable diseases, viruses.	As children enter school settings, there is an increased likelihood that they will be exposed to children with other types of infectious disease.
	Adolescence: Venereal diseases and other infectious diseases.	
2. Nutrition and nutritional status may affect the individual's ability to resist disease.	The individual's nutritional status should be carefully assessed for the quality and quantity of dietary intake.	A healthy nutritional state provides a child with a good beginning defense against disease. Knowledge of basic nutritional needs for each age group is essential. (See Chapter 10, Nutrition.)
	The health history and physical examination will aid in the assessment of nutritional status.	
	Inadequate nutrition alters the body's ability to respond to or resist the effects of exposure to infectious disease.	
3. The health status, the ability of individuals to resist and fight infectious diseases, may be altered by the presence of physiological and/or psychosocial deviations.	The internal cellular response to infectious agents may be altered in an individual who has an acute or chronic health problem. Thus the individual's resistance to disease will be less than normally expected.	Children with known health problems should receive medical attention when they are exposed to infectious or communicable diseases.
	A child's natural ability to resist illness may be decreased through the use of certain medications such as prednisone, cortisone, or corticosteroids. Caretakers whose children are taking these medications should be warned of the dangers of exposure to individuals with infectious or communicable diseases.	If a child who is receiving corticosteroid therapy is exposed to individuals with an infectious or communicable disease, medical attention should be sought immediately.

HEALTH PROBLEM	HEALTH CARE GUIDELINES	HELPFUL HINTS
	Children whose body defense systems are lacking or impaired must also have their activities with other individuals monitored. *Caretakers must be alerted to the dangers of exposure of their children to individuals with communicable disease.*	
	Communicable diseases such as chickenpox or measles, which are usually not life threatening to children, may well have serious consequences to children whose bodies lack the ability to fight infection.	
4. Environmental conditions can predispose individuals to infectious and communicable diseases. Some of those environmental factors include housing, sanitation, climate, and/or geographical location. Exposure to infected individuals, contaminated objects, rodents, insects, or flies predisposes individuals to contracting disease.	It is essential to gather exposure possibilities and environmental data in health histories.	Environmental factors that may lead to disease include poor housing conditions, inadequate plumbing facilities, climate, and the presence of rodents, insects, or flies.
	Infectious or communicable diseases occur when the host is susceptible, a causative agent is present, and the environment is conducive for transmission of disease.	
a. An agent is that which causes the disease, such as the organism. It can also refer to a lack or absence of something the body requires, such as nutrients.	The host's susceptibility can be decreased and/or resistance increased by the following factors: 1. Immunization 2. Optimum health and nutritional status	
b. The environment is where the individual resides, works, or otherwise spends time.	Environmental factors, if known, can often be mediated to decrease favorability for disease transmission, such as draining ponds to decrease the breeding of mosquitos.	Reduce or eliminate exposure to individuals known to have an infectious or communicable disease.
c. The host is the individual.	Knowledge of disease prevalence patterns alerts health care workers to the probability of an increased incidence of a disease and the organism associated with it. For example, some communicable diseases are seen more often in the spring.	Plan family outings during the spring months with caution to avoid those groups or situations where the possibility for exposure to communicable or infectious disease increases.
	Identification of susceptibility to tuberculosis is done through tuberculin testing at specific periods in a child's life (at 1 year of age and before entering school).	Tuberculin testing may be performed more often than the recommended schedule if there is reason to believe the child has more potential for exposure to tuberculosis than the average.
Immunization: The process of rendering an individual immune to specific illnesses.	Recommended schedules for immunization to measles, mumps, rubella, diphtheria, pertussis, tetanus, and poliomyelitis are given in Appendix A.	Immunization provides protection against the following diseases: Measles (rubella) Mumps (parotitis) German measles (rubella) Diphtheria Whooping cough (pertussis) Lockjaw (tetanus) Infantile paralysis (poliomyelitis)

HEALTH PROBLEM	HEALTH CARE GUIDELINES	HELPFUL HINTS
Communicable disease—cont'd *Immunization*—cont'd	Health workers must reinforce the need and desirability of immunization for infants, toddlers, and preschoolers. Reactions and risks associated with immunizations are minimal compared with the possible severity of the disease(s) and its sequelae. Continuous health teaching on the desirability of immunizations is necessary because the myth still exists that "having the disease provides better immunization than an injection."	There is no immunization for the following diseases: Chickenpox Colds Meningitis
1. Informed consent is the right of the caretaker to know both the benefits and risks associated with immunizations.	Health workers must be able to provide information about the benefits and risks of immunizations clearly and in terms the caretakers can understand, but without causing needless alarm (e.g., "Certain reactions to this immunization can be expected, such as redness and swelling at the site, irritability, and fever, but these reactions are usually less harmful and of shorter duration than those associated with the disease itself.")	Before immunizations are administered, health workers should share with caretakers the benefits and risks associated with the procedure. Raise questions and seek understanding of each and every immunization to be administered.

2. Contraindications are circumstances or conditions that suggest delay or total omission of the immunization(s) because of the increased risk of dangerous sequelae.	Health professionals should keep in mind that the following conditions or states of health warrant deferment or total elimination of the immunization:
	  1. Fever
	  2. Acute illness
	  3. Children receiving immunosuppressant drug therapy
	  4. Immunodeficiency disease
	  5. Children who have allergic responses to eggs and egg products or who have eczema
	  6. Children who may have received immune serum globulin or transfusions (blood or plasma)
	  7. Girls who may be pregnant
	Smallpox vaccinations are no longer routinely administered. Health care workers who administer them for a specific reason need to remember to ask if there are any individuals in the home who may have eczema or other allergies because they could acquire a generalized vaccinia if in contact with the vaccine.
		Health care workers need to be kept up to date on the child's recent health problems and/or therapies.
		Immunizations cannot be given if the child already is ill, is receiving specific medicines, or who has allergies to eggs and/or egg products.
		When deferment or omission of immunization may be necessary, inquire as to the reason.

3. Common reactions to immunization include the following:
 	
  a. Redness and/or swelling at the site.
	The health care professional should suggest or provide the following information when immunizations are administered:
	  1. Redness and swelling are usually of short duration.
		Ask the health care professional if the child might experience any reactions after immunization. Request advice.
		Children can be dressed in clothing that covers the injection site, but does not constrict. This may reduce discomfort and/or irritation and distract the child from aggravating the area.

HEALTH PROBLEM	HEALTH CARE GUIDELINES	HELPFUL HINTS
b. Elevated temperature (fever).	2. Antipyretics, tepid sponge baths, and increased fluid intake are often recommended.	If the child has a fever (elevated temperature), avoid milk and milk products, but increase fluid intake by providing juice, soup, or gelatin.
c. Irritability.	3. Alert caretakers that a temporary change in behavior is likely.	Keeping the child quiet and avoiding overexertion or excessive stimulation may reduce the amount of irritability that accompanies illness.

BODY REACTION TO COMMUNICABLE DISEASE

The body's reaction to communicable disease is the response of the individual to a specific disease(s).

Some of the more common responses to communicable diseases will be described. This list of reactions is not meant to be all inclusive or descriptive of combinations of reactions that occur with each and every disease. For example, certain communicable diseases typically produce a rash, whereas others produce fever and irritability but no rash.

1. Temperature variations may range from 100.4° to 105° F (38° to 40.6° C) and persist for different lengths of time or recur periodically.

Health professionals must be alert to the fact that febrile states may precipitate convulsions. Caretakers must be informed about measures that should be used to decrease body temperature and thus reduce the risk of febrile convulsions.

Methods that can be used to decrease elevated temperatures include increasing clear fluids, giving tepid sponge baths, and decreasing activity.

2. Rashes are peculiar to each disease, but may vary in nature, appearance, and longevity.

Health care professionals must be able to recognize and describe various rashes by the following criteria:
1. Appearance.
   a. Macular: Flat, colored lesion of the skin.
   b. Papule: Raised circumscribed lesion that may have different variations of red colors.
   c. Vesicle: Raised blisterlike lesion filled with fluid.
   d. Pustule: An infected lesion that is elevated and contains purulent material.
2. Onset and sequence. The onset and sequence of the spread of rashes is peculiar to each communicable disease and frequently is the key to disease identification.
3. Nature and characteristic of the lesions. Some rashes stay at the macular stage, whereas others progress from macular to papular to vesicular and pustular. The latter two are frequently associated with intense itching and concomitant scratching.

When seeking medical advice about rashes they observe on their children, caretakers should provide the following information:
1. Appearance:
   Flat, raised, blistered, or if the rash has variations such as some flat and some blistered.
2. Color.
3. Location: Chest, face, trunk, arms, or legs.
4. Onset and sequence of rash: Where it started and how it spread over the child's body.

If a child has a rash that is accompanied by blisters (vesicles) and itching, it would be helpful to keep the fingernails cut short to reduce the possibility of infecting the lesion.

HEALTH PROBLEM	HEALTH CARE GUIDELINES	HELPFUL HINTS
Communicable disease—cont'd BODY REACTION—cont'd	Health care workers should provide treatment protocols for rashes that itch, to reduce the possibility of secondary infections.	Caretakers may obtain prescriptions that can reduce itching. Specific lotions, creams, or soothing baths may also be available. (See Chapter 8, Allergies.)
3. Signs and symptoms may occur when the disease process involves the tissue and membranes of the central nervous system.	The extent to which central nervous system tissue and membranes are involved will determine the severity of presenting signs and symptoms. Mild forms of the disease may be evidenced by behavioral changes characterized by lethargy and/or irritability. As the extent of the disease progresses, signs and symptoms such as involuntary movement of muscles, drowsiness, prolonged wakefulness, whining or a piercing cry, tremors, convulsions, and even coma may exist. Hospitalization would be required. Additional signs and symptoms might include nausea, vomiting, headache, and dizziness. Medical management is directed toward the following: 1. Relieving the irritation to the central nervous system 2. Preventing injury from convulsions. 3. Providing adequate rest by decreasing environmental stimuli. 4. Preventing complications from further invasion into brain tissue.	Caretakers usually know their children's behavior patterns better than anyone else. Behavioral changes that are not consistent with the usual need further investigation. Caretakers should seek medical advice for the following symptoms in their children: 1. Excessive drowsiness or the child is difficult to arouse. 2. Uncontrolled shaking (tremors) or twitching of arms and legs. 3. Sudden forceful (projectile-type) vomiting episodes. 4. Headache that does not disappear. When seeking medical advice, briefly but succinctly describe the behavioral changes that have been noticed in the child.

4. Sequelae: conditions that follow or result from a disease.
  a. Secondary infections are infections by a different organism superimposed on the one already present.
  b. Secondary disease is a disease that occurs after the original disease.
	Communicable diseases may have similar, although unique, aftereffects, or complications.
	Raised lesions are prone to the invasion of other organisms because of aggravation of the site through bumping, bruising, or scratching.
	An individual's resistance to disease may be reduced while resisting or recovering from a primary illness, thus making that individual more susceptible to other new organisms.
		Maintain efforts to prevent the child from irritating the rash. Keep fingernails short and dress the child in loose-fitting clothing.
		Limit the sick child's exposure to other individuals because they may have infections of which they are unaware.

c. Complications are conditions that are superimposed on the original disease that affect or modify the recovery.	Complications vary with each disease. They may affect any body tissue or organ, thus compounding the primary effects and outcome of the disease.	During the period of illness and/or recovery, new signs or symptoms may emerge that indicate complications, another infection, or another disease.

HEALTH PROBLEM	HEALTH CARE GUIDELINES	HELPFUL HINTS

Strabismus (squint or crossed eyes)

Strabismus: A deviation of the eye in which lack of muscular coordination limits binocular vision because the optic axes cannot be directed on the same object.

Strabismus may be caused by many factors, including heredity, trauma, illness, or eye muscle paralysis.

Following are some types of strabismus:

1. Unilateral (monocular): The deviation is always noticed in the same eye.
2. Bilateral (accommodative): Disorder related to the ability of the eye to accommodate and converge.
3. Alternating: Either eye may be the fixed eye while the other deviates.
4. Convergent (internal squint) esotropia: Deviant eye turns inward.
5. Divergent (outward squint) exotropia: Deviant eye turns outward.

Children with strabismus receive faulty visual images. Either the child sees two different images (diplopia) or learns to use only one eye and ignore the image of the affected eye. The affected eye becomes weakened from disease, resulting in amblyopia.

Treatment varies.

Patching the stronger eye forces usage of the weakened eye.

Glasses and/or eye exercises may correct the condition.

Surgery on the eye muscle may be necessary.

Crossed eyes (squint) are eye conditions in children that must be rectified before age 6, or permanent visual problems may occur.

It is not uncommon for young infants to display "crossed eyes" at times. Crossed eyes that persist beyond 6 months will need treatment. *Children do not outgrow this condition.*

Caretakers can be very helpful to health personnel through their description of the eye movement, that is, the direction of movement, involved eye, and periodicity or constancy of the condition.

Children with squints (crossed eyes) will frequently tilt their heads or close one eye to bring clarity to objects they are trying to see.

Children with this health problem may appear clumsy or bump into objects because they lack the depth perception that is achieved through binocular vision.

Children must be encouraged to wear eye patches consistently, although they may feel out of place among their friends.

Glasses and eye exercises must be used consistently, or these treatments will have limited value.

Eye exercises can be enhanced by incorporating elements of play while exercises are performed. The basic exercise is maintained, but the objects used for visual contact could be hand puppets doing different maneuvers.

Children through 5 years of age may have difficulty keeping glasses in place due to the lack of prominence of the bridge of the nose. Attaching an elastic band to the earpieces of the glasses provides additional support to hold the glasses in place.

Children's glasses should have shatterproof lenses. Even with continued diligence on the part of the caretaker and frequent reminders for the child to be careful, there will be times when glasses will be broken, mislaid, or lost.

UNIT FOUR

CHILDHOOD *getting involved*

Children 6 through 12 years old continue to meet new challenges, both physical and intellectual. They are self-motivated to achieve. A carefree zest for life and a love of learning are typical at this stage of development.

Maturation of the central nervous system and development of the musculoskeletal system have enhanced physical and intellectual capabilities. School and schooling become the hub of the child's existence. Competition and recognition seem to be two of the major ingredients in the child's struggle to achieve. School-age children tend to measure their abilities and accomplishments to those of peers and adults. It is important that children be reminded to compare their achievements with their own past performances rather than with the achievements of others.

Encouragement for the attained levels of performance reached by the 6- through 12-year-old is extremely important for the continued development of a positive self-concept. Children who focus only on their limitations and failures are likely to develop a negative self-concept.

Although family bonds and ties exist, children in this age period are influenced by many external factors. Whereas caretakers' values, opinions, suggestions, and beliefs were accepted without question by younger children, now caretakers often feel displaced from their 6- through 12-year-old child's sphere of influence by outsiders (peers, friends, teachers, and even strangers). Some of the values and beliefs the children espouse are frequently in direct conflict with those of caretakers. Caretakers also frequently deplore their children's choice of friends, language, and habits.

The need for friendships and close personal friends becomes more apparent in this period of life than in any previous developmental phase. The naivete and trusting attitudes of the younger school-age child foster the sharing of intimate thoughts and desires with others, including strangers. As the child grows older and experiences numerous interpersonal relationships, the naivete disappears, but the need to share innermost thoughts and feelings continues. As a result, close friendships developed in this stage of life frequently endure throughout a lifetime. Friendships influence the school-age child's choice of dress, language, groups, and organized activities.

School-age children enjoy the informality and the feeling of belonging that are inherent features of a gang. Gangs are frequently groups of similar-age boys and girls who either live in the same neighborhood, attend the same school or church, or have a similar interest. Gangs function under loose rules that frequently change. Rules and regulations become more important as the child progresses through the school-age period.

During this period, more formal groups, such as Little League, bands, book clubs, or scouts, attract children's attention. These formal groups have pre-established goals.

Gangs, formal groups, school friends, and family all can assist the school-age child to develop a sense of responsibility. School-age children can be expected to care for themselves, their belongings, and their room, as well as to help around the home. By the end of this period of life, the school-age child realizes that outcomes of behavior are determined by the choices made. As they enter adolescence, they will have developed the concept of industry if they received positive reinforcement for their attempts and achievements.

CHAPTER 12

SCHOOL AGE TO PREADOLESCENCE
6 through 12 years

The child from 6 through 12 years seems to be in a relatively calm period of life. During this time, children continue to grow and develop, refine new skills, and seem to have limitless amounts of energy. Their time, talents, and energy, unlike previous periods, seem directed to specific goals, both personal and group.

The intellectual skills of children in this age period permit involved abstract thinking, as well as the ability to follow complex step-by-step procedures. Games with multiple directions, rules, and strategies are thoroughly enjoyed by most school-age children. Game rules are strictly adhered to, and children learn to accept losing.

Individuals entering the school-age period enjoy group activities in which both sexes participate. The sex of the individual is less important than the shared interest. During this period of life the groups tend to exclude one sex or the other. New heterosexual relationships begin to emerge by the twelfth year.

Interest is evidenced in many facets of life, al-though the dominance of the athlete versus bookworm or extrovert versus introvert becomes apparent. School serves both educational and social purposes. The need for companionship and structure continues in the summer months as these children select camps, vacation Bible schools, music lessons, and/or swim clubs.

The school-age child frequently seeks out ways and means to make money. Typically, they transfer the skills learned at home into money-making endeavors in the community, such as mowing lawns, babysitting, raking leaves, or shoveling walks. Boys and girls frequently acquire paper routes or attach themselves to a "Hire the Kid" community program.

By the end of this period, many children have started a second growth spurt, with concomitant secondary sex changes. At about the same time, group activities change to more social outings, and the stage is set for the heterosexual relationships and problems of adolescence.

GROWTH AND DEVELOPMENTAL LANDMARKS	ANTICIPATORY GUIDANCE

Biological

WEIGHT

The average weight gain will range from 5 to 7 pounds (2.3 to 3.2 kg) a year.

By age 12 the average weight would be 78 to 85 pounds (35.4 to 38.6 kg).

The typical weight gain pattern for girls is usually slightly less than that for boys.

Each child has a unique pattern of weight gain. Some children will gain more than the average, whereas others will gain less. Caretakers and children of this age frequently establish battlegrounds over adequate meals and mealtimes.

A growth spurt for both height and weight can be expected just prior to the teen years. Girls tend to begin this rapid growth period earlier than boys.

HEIGHT

The average increase in height during this period will be about 2½ inches (6 cm a year).

Since many children experience the second major growth spurt of their lives during this period of development, an average height would be atypical and meaningless.

As children enter this age period, they may appear thin and lanky. This school-age period seems to provide time for bodies to fill out, the growth rate to stabilize, and more adultlike features to emerge that are unique to each child.

HEART RATE

The average heart rate for this age period will range from 60 to 100 beats per minute.

Variations in heart rates (pulse) depend on many factors. The pulse rate should always be viewed in relation to the child's state of health, activity level, and the presence or absence of environmental stress.

As noted in previous chapters, the average heart rate decreases with age and during this period continues to approximate the heart rate of the adult.

Variations in heart rate and rhythm are noted when the child is at rest, active or under stress, or ill. A prolonged rapid heart rate (tachycardia) or prolonged slow heart rate (bradycardia) may be indicative of disease or a health problem.

Abnormal sounds or arrhythmias noted during health conferences should be further monitored by health personnel.

Pulse rates are easily palpable at the wrist (radial artery). Children enjoy "taking their own pulse."

Following extreme physical activity, it is not uncommon to observe pulsations at the sides of the neck or temple area of the forehead.

RESPIRATIONS

The average respiratory rate for children of this age period ranges from 18 to 30 breaths per minute.

Respiratory rates do vary among children. Individual respiratory rates must always be viewed in relation to the circumstances and activities in which the child is engaged.

A sustained and significantly increased respiratory rate (tachypnea) may be indicative of infection or disease. A sustained decreased respiratory rate (bradypnea) may be indicative of a central nervous system problem.

BLOOD PRESSURE

Systolic blood pressure readings for this period of age range from 90 to 108 mm Hg, and diastolic blood pressure readings range from 60 to 67 mm Hg.

Blood pressure readings are readily obtained at both brachial and popliteal sites of 6- through 12-year-old children. A blood pressure reading should be recorded at each health conference.

Blood pressure readings are typically taken on children of this age.

Blood pressure readings vary with each child.

TEMPERATURE

The body temperature continues to range from 98.6° to 99.6° F (36.6° to 37.6° C).

Temperature readings can now be readily obtained orally, since children of this age can cooperate and follow directions extremely well.

Fever may be detected in the school-age child in the same manner as in the preschool child. (See Chapter 9, Temperature.)

GROWTH AND DEVELOPMENTAL LANDMARKS	ANTICIPATORY GUIDANCE

HEAD

Head size, shape, and circumference continue to approximate the adult features unique for each child. Head circumference will be approximately 21 inches (52.5 to 54 cm) by age 12.

By the end of this period the size of the brain will be that of the adult.

The mandible (jaw bone) increases in size (extending forward), thus providing space for the eruption of permanent teeth.

Facial features become more pronounced. The adult appearance will make more evident certain family characteristics.

The receding chin of early childhood disappears. As the jawbone increases in size, the chin becomes more prominent.

HAIR

The texture, quality, and type of hair (straight or curly) is characteristic of the hair of adulthood. The color may change by becoming darker with age or lighter when exposed to the elements.

The luster of the hair may be indicative of the child's health status.

Activation of the sebaceous glands in the late school-age period causes changes in the odor and appearance of the hair.

Children from 6 through 12 can be held responsible for their own grooming, but might need reminders about washing their hair. The average frequency for shampooing is once a week.

Children can be reminded that hair retains odors from the environment and that it might become more greasy because of the action of sweat glands.

Hairstyles during this period are influenced by peers, fads, and trends. Caretakers should not be surprised if, by the end of this period, an inordinate amount of time is spent by both boys and girls in hair grooming.

NOSE

The nose develops adult shape and function during the preschool period. Nose size will be comparable to that of an adult.

MOUTH

Loss of deciduous (temporary or "baby") teeth and gain of permanent teeth are two of the most striking features of this period of growth and development.

A typical pattern of eruption of permanent teeth is similar to that of the temporary teeth, starting with the upper central incisors. (See Chapter 13, Dentition.)

Dental caries continues to be a major health problem of this age group. (See Chapter 13, Dentition, Nutrition.)

Halitosis (bad breath) may occur as a result of oral, dental, or systemic health problems.

Children 6 through 12 can be expected to perform oral hygiene measures on their own.

Unusual dryness of the lips or a change of color or moistness of the tongue and/or inner linings of the mouth may be indicative of a health problem. Should this occur, seek advice from health personnel.

Breath odor is usually nonoffensive. Bad breath (halitosis) may indicate a health problem, and advice should be sought from health personnel.

EYES

Binocular vision is well established. Eye-hand coordination has developed to an optimal state and is essential for all further intellectual and manual skill integration.

Visual acuity should be 20/20. If acuity is 20/40 or worse, the child should be referred to an ophthalmologist for evaluation and treatment. Normal vision is considered to be 20/20. This refers to the ability of the subject to see from a distance of 20 feet objects that a normal person would see from 20 feet. Acuity of 20/40 indicates that the subject can only see from 20 feet objects that a normal person can see from 40 feet.

Three typical problems of vision found in the school-age child include astigmatism (distortion of the curvature of the lens), hyperopia (farsightedness), and myopia (nearsightedness).

Symptoms commonly associated with visual problems in children include headache, vertigo, blurred vision, frowning, eyestrain, inability to clearly distinguish objects in the distance, or holding books close to the face when reading.

Children with visual difficulties should have their vision evaluated annually.

Visual difficulties are frequently identified in the school setting by the child, teacher, or school nurse. The inability to see the blackboard, squinting, rubbing the eyes, headaches, or holding books close to the face are some outward (overt) signs directly related to visual difficulties.

Caretakers may notice the same signs, but also a change in the child's disposition, learning ability, or a lack of interest in attending school. These somewhat obscure clues (covert) are often overlooked as manifestations of either a visual or hearing problem.

School health screening programs may provide the first evidence that a physical problem exists. Do not disregard suggestions and recommendations made for children to have further eye examinations.

GROWTH AND DEVELOPMENTAL LANDMARKS	ANTICIPATORY GUIDANCE

Biological—cont'd

EYES—cont'd

Visual problems continue to develop both during this period and adolescence because of the growth and developmental changes that are occurring. It is therefore essential that children have an annual eye examination.

The popularity of contact lenses today may lead caretakers to request these lenses for their children. The use of contact lenses rests with the ophthalmologist, but should not be considered until the child is capable of total care of the lenses. Improper placement and/or care can result in permanent eye damage.

EARS

Binauricular hearing is well established. The differentiation of sound pitch (frequencies—low to high) and level of intensity (decibels—soft to loud) is most acute during this period of life.

Audiometric screening should be included in the health conference conducted prior to entry into school.

During audiometric testing normal hearing ranges between 500 to 5000 Hz at 20 decibels. Normal frequencies used in human speech range from 1000 to 5000 Hz. Individuals who are unable to detect frequencies within the normal range at 20 decibels require further evaluation.

Two types of hearing loss, conductive and sensorineural, can be identified through the use of an audiogram.

Several infections or diseases that occur during the school-age period can cause hearing loss or impairment either because of the disease process itself or the sequelae following the disease.

Evidence is accumulating that the bombardment of sound observed through use of stereo equipment turned to full volume can cause irreparable hearing damage.

School health screening programs frequently provide the first evidence that a hearing problem exists.

Frequently the signs or symptoms of hearing problems are covert. Caretakers and/or teachers may notice a change in the child's disposition, attentiveness, or even attendance. These somewhat obscure clues are often overlooked or attached to possible causes other than the physical one of hearing difficulty. The screening tests in school may consist of audiometry testing but the conditions under which they are performed are not as reliable as when done by an audiologist. Do not disregard suggestions made for the child to have further evaluation.

TRUNK AND EXTREMITIES

Structurally school-age children resemble adults. They stand erect, with their backs straight, shoulders held back, and abdomen flat. Pelvic tilts are absent. They look like miniature adults and have lost their last "baby" features.

Maturation of the musculoskeletal system continues, with ossification of the long bones.

The contour of the legs and arms has become well delineated. The legs appear much longer and straighter than in previous periods of life.

Deviations in the physical structure of the trunk and extremities can occur as a result of disease or nutritional problems.

School-age children stand erect. They have lost the "paunch" and swayback of earlier years. Adults often view them as miniature adults. Although they resemble the adult, they do not have the ability or experience to behave as a mature adult.

MOBILITY

Neuromuscular development continues throughout the school-age period. Refinement of both gross and fine motor skills is evident as the child becomes more coordinated and graceful.

Motor skills become more precise. The child seems better able to control every motion. New skills are learned quickly—old skills become second nature. Manipulative skills requiring finely tuned eye-hand coordination now can be achieved with relative ease.

Fine motor ability increases, and the domination of left- or right-sidedness becomes apparent.

Children's abilities are reflected in their activities. The 6- and 7-year old-child enjoys the less complex games of hide and seek, kick ball, and hopscotch. The 8- through 10-year-old seems to enjoy competitive games with more rules and strategies, such as football, baseball, or soccer. Also in evidence would be the attempts to help with constructive or creative activities around the house. Painting, sewing, and crafts of all kinds attract the 6- to 12-year-old.

Opportunities are necessary for the refinement of both gross and fine motor skills.

SECONDARY SEX CHARACTERISTICS

The appearance of secondary sex characteristics usually occurs toward the end of the school-age period in both boys and girls. The pattern of progression is orderly and sequential.

It is believed that maturation of the brain and neuroendocrine system triggers the development of secondary sex characteristics and changes in the body configurations.

Maturing body changes (secondary sex characteristics) that uniquely characterize male and female begin in the late school-age period.

Changes in personality frequently accompany the physical changes brought about by hormonal influences in the late school-age period. Boys and girls demonstrate noticeable changes in behavior and attitudes. "Moodiness," "laziness," "clumsy," and "obnoxious" are some of the labels given to these children.

GROWTH AND DEVELOPMENTAL LANDMARKS

ANTICIPATORY GUIDANCE

The anterior pituitary gland stimulates the secretion of gonadotropic, adrenocortical, and somatotropic hormones. Each of these hormones is directed to specific target areas responsible for skeletal growth and sexual changes (Fig. 12-1).

Children are powerless to stop physical changes. They are often unaware of the personality changes.

Acceptance of the changes provides support and is helpful to the development of a positive self-image in these young people.

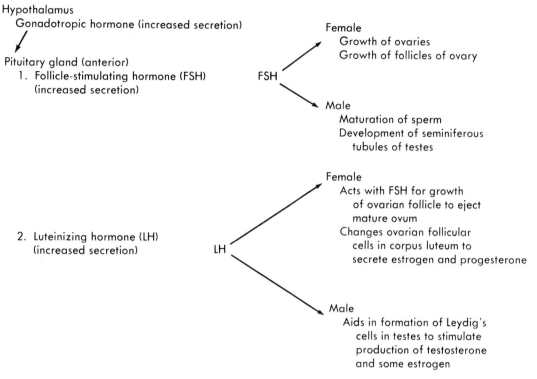

Hypothalamus
    Gonadotropic hormone (increased secretion)

Pituitary gland (anterior)
    1. Follicle-stimulating hormone (FSH)
       (increased secretion)

FSH

Female
    Growth of ovaries
    Growth of follicles of ovary

Male
    Maturation of sperm
    Development of seminiferous
       tubules of testes

    2. Luteinizing hormone (LH)
       (increased secretion)

LH

Female
    Acts with FSH for growth
       of ovarian follicle to eject
       mature ovum
    Changes ovarian follicular
       cells in corpus luteum to
       secrete estrogen and progesterone

Male
    Aids in formation of Leydig's
       cells in testes to stimulate
       production of testosterone
       and some estrogen

Estrogen: Major secretion from ovaries
       responsible for secondary sex changes in females

Testosterone: Responsible for development of secondary
       sex changes in male

Fig. 12-1. Hormones that stimulate secondary sex changes in reproductive system of males and females.

The gonadotropic hormone stimulates the ovary in the female to secrete estrogen and the testes in the male to secrete testosterone. Simultaneously, the cortex of the adrenal gland is stimulated to secrete estrogen and testosterone. An excess of either of these two hormones (estrogen and testosterone) will determine the predominance of female or male sex characteristics.

Psychological changes associated with the changing body and growth spurt of the preadolescent will be further discussed in Chapter 13, Sex Education.

The somatotropic hormone is primarily responsible for the growth of muscles, bones, and other tissues. Decreased stimulation of this hormone at the end of puberty brings about fusion of the epiphyseal ends of long bones and retards skeletal growth.

The usual physical changes expected in puberty for both boys and girls will take place if secretion of the sex hormones is in appropriate proportions and amounts.

The typical pattern of change for girls is as follows:

1. Secondary sex characteristics develop from ages 9 to 12.
2. Hips become broader; the transverse diameter of pelvis increases.
3. Breasts become tender and enlarged.

Hips in girls naturally become broader. Many girls complain about becoming "fat," even though their weight has not changed, when they notice they must purchase larger sizes of slacks.

Breast development becomes noticeable. Girls become conscious of the changes in the size of their breasts.

GROWTH AND DEVELOPMENTAL LANDMARKS

Biological—cont'd

SECONDARY SEX CHARACTERISTICS—cont'd

4. Pubic hair begins to appear (at first the hair is straight and later becomes kinky and darker).
5. Vaginal changes are occurring. The mucosal lining thickens, and the pH level changes from alkaline to acid.
6. Nipple and areolar pigmentation changes occur.
7. Axillary hair becomes noticeable. In some girls, the menses precedes the appearance of axillary hair; in others, the reverse is true.

8. Menstruation (menses) occurs.

9. Body hair becomes darker, coarser, and is especially evident on the legs.

A spurt in skeletal growth is noticeable early in the appearance of the secondary sex characteristics. The legs grow longer and straighter. There is a notable increase in muscle masses throughout the body.

Cessation of skeletal growth in girls usually occurs after the menstrual cycle is well established.

The typical pattern of change for boys is as follows:

1. The development of secondary sex characteristics begins at ages 11 to 14.
2. The testes and penis begin to enlarge.
3. Pubic hair begins to appear (at first the hair is straight but becomes kinky and dark).
4. The penis increases in length and size.

5. Breast changes become evident.

6. Voice changes become noticeable.

7. Nocturnal emissions, or "wet dreams," (ejaculations) may begin.

8. In some boys, nocturnal emissions precede the appearance of axillary hair; in others the reverse is true. Axillary hair and fine facial hair appear (especially noticeable on the upper lip).
9. Body hair.

ANTICIPATORY GUIDANCE

A significant change in body stance and carriage can be noticed in boys and girls of this later age period who are developing secondary sex characteristics. In younger years, both boys and girls carried books and lunch boxes hanging from arms that were extended and backs that were straight. Now girls hunch their shoulders and cradle their books across the front of their chests. (Perhaps this is an attempt to hide the presence or absence of budding breasts.) Boys on the other hand stand straight with shoulders back, chest out, and often walk with a swagger.

It is important for young pubescent girls to have a brassiere.

Pubic hair becomes noticeable. Monthly periods (menstruation) will occur soon.

Hair develops under the arms (axillary hair). Girls should be informed of the need for extra care and cleanliness of the underarm, particularly after axillary hair appears. Deodorants should be encouraged.

Caretakers should be alerted to the fact that many girls will experience menstruation earlier in life than in their own generation.

Invariably girls grow taller sooner than boys of similar age. This fact causes tremendous concern to members of both sexes.

Physical changes in boys usually occur 1 year later than in girls.

Changes in the size and appearance of the penis, testes, scrotal sac, and pubic hair are very important to boys. Delayed genital growth may cause concern and even embarrassment. Boys should be reminded of individual differences in growth spurts. For those boys whose genital growth has accelerated, the use of athletic supports is highly recommended.

Breast changes are evidenced in both boys and girls during the growth spurts, although the breast enlargement is usually temporary in boys.

Most boys are aware that voice changes will occur, but the actual event sometimes proves embarrassing.

Inform and reassure boys that "wet dreams" (ejaculation) are *normal* and part of the growth pattern of reproduction. Involuntary erection of the penis is also normal, although sometimes a disturbing facet of becoming a man.

Alert boys to the need for extra cleanliness because of axillary hair growth and increased sweat gland activity. Encourage boys to use deodorants.

Some boys will have an abundance of body hair, others will not, this is frequently a familial characteristic. Body hair is not an indication of sexual maturity. Boys often accentuate chest hair by wearing open shirts with their chests exposed.

As facial hair appears, many boys become preoccupied with it and spend hours in front of the mirror anticipating their first "shave."

GROWTH AND DEVELOPMENTAL LANDMARKS	ANTICIPATORY GUIDANCE

Skeletal growth becomes noticeable some time after secondary sex characteristics are noted, but usually before nocturnal emissions begin. Of particular note are the following:

1. An increase in the length of the long bones.
2. A significant increase in muscle mass and strength occurs that is much greater than in girls.

3. An increase in shoulder and chest breadth.

Skeletal growth in boys often continues through the late teens and into the early twenties.

Boys whose growth spurt is delayed become concerned and may exhibit changes in behavior (either withdrawing or acting out). Boys whose growth spurt is accelerated frequently feel self-conscious and out of place.

A lack of coordination and adaptation to physical space related to skeletal growth and muscular mass is noticeable. Boys who earlier seemed agile and graceful now trip over their feet, upset milk, bump into doors, and appear clumsy in general.

To emphasize the increased height and accentuated shoulder breadth, boys now carry their bodies erect, shoulders back, chests out, and walk with a swagger.

Psychological

DEPENDENCE-INDEPENDENCE

Six- through twelve-year-olds believe themselves to be independent and self-sufficient. They tend to be oblivious of their dependency on others for shelter, food, clothing, and money. The early years of this period indeed seem "carefree."

School-age children demonstrate industry through their productivity and creativity.

The ability to do abstract thinking and follow complex directions permits them to assume greater amounts of responsibility.

Dependability of the school-age child is directly related to the sense of honesty (conscience) and trust developed in earlier periods of life.

Caretakers at times lose patience with the school-age child's inability to see chores that need doing or understand that money stretches only so far. By the end of the school-age period the typical 12-year-old is much more aware of the reality of finances and the responsibilities of being a productive member of a family.

Intent on productivity and creativity, the school-age child needs help in becoming a more responsible individual.

Provide opportunities for school-age children to demonstrate dependability. Permit them to perform tasks that require effort, knowledge, and ability without hovering over them. This gives children a sense of accomplishment and willingness to accept more responsibility in the future.

Tasks that children are expected to perform should be those children enjoy, not just the tasks caretakers do not wish to do.

The tasks, chores, or responsibilities that children are expected to perform should be discussed and mutually agreed on with caretakers.

School-age children are eager to have increased opportunities for independent responsibilities.

Caretakers are role models and taskmasters, but they should not set standards for achievement beyond the capabilities (physical and intellectual) of their children. Acknowledgment of children's successful undertaking provides them with a sense of achievement and a renewed desire to please. Caretakers are the key figures in molding the dependability aspects of children's personalities and will influence the way in which children respect authority and regulations outside the home.

Allowance

Allowances are that portion of the family budget set aside for the financial needs of each of the individual family members. Most families use this term primarily in relation to the children of the family. The allowance should not be construed as payment for specific chores or as a part-time gift, but rather as the opportunity for each family member to plan and budget certain known finances. Each family member must be a contributing member, willing to take on and meet responsibilities.

Allowances and other financial concerns are always a potential source for controversy among family members. The way in which an allowance is perceived is crucial. Allowances can be as simple as a small sum awarded weekly to provide some financial leeway for fun for each child, or they can be complex, taking into consideration the following expenditures:

School lunches
Church offerings
Savings
Entertainment
School supplies
Clothing costs

151

GROWTH AND DEVELOPMENTAL LANDMARKS

Psychological—cont'd

DEPENDENCE-INDEPENDENCE—cont'd

Establishment of the allowance should be a shared experience among the family members who are involved.

Each family sets its own rules and guidelines for both the establishment of allowances and the items to be covered by the allowance.

INTERDEPENDENCE

Children develop increased awareness of being members of different units: family, church, school, community, and world. They discover the need for cooperative efforts to achieve and/or maintain the goals of the unit. Confidence in themselves permits them to be contributing members of each unit. The hierarchical order of each unit becomes self-evident. Knowledge and acceptance of the individual's position or place within each unit can enhance or diminish that individual's sense of worth, productivity, and/or achievement.

Success in a group is sometimes contingent on productivity and the ability to interact with others within that group.

Qualities and responsibilities of leadership and membership within groups are learned in this age period.

The ability to reach leadership status depends on factors other than just the ability to lead.

Children imitate the behavior of those adults with whom they frequently associate and of those adults they respect, but might not often see.

ANTICIPATORY GUIDANCE

The allowance is usually the basic cornerstone for future financial accountability. Each person must learn to budget time and money. Allowances provide children with the opportunity to become financially responsible.

Provide guidance in the handling of money, but be prepared to permit children to make mistakes and to learn from their mistakes.

Some children spend all of their money on something important to them, neglecting to save money for their lunches. Obviously the child should not starve, but contingent plans can be available that help the child through the crisis, but also get the point across meaningfully. For example, carrying a basic lunch consisting of a sandwich, piece of fruit, and beverage, providing no extra money for sweets or other snacks, may help the child. Experiences such as this may be the impetus for seeking employment outside the home, such as mowing lawns, pulling weeds, washing windows, baby sitting, or delivering papers. Industry should be encouraged.

Allowances need to be reviewed annually as the needs of the children change.

Too often, caretakers eliminate the allowance when their children become proficient in earning money. They may undermine the child's desire to be self-sufficient. As in the mutual discussions concerning allowances and items to be covered by it, so too discontinuation of the allowance should be discussed and mutually agreed on. Typically, the need for an allowance ends with graduation from high school, although some families continue the practice as long as the children attend school.

Involve children in family discussions and plans that affect them. Some examples include vacation plans, allowance allocations, or the choice of chores. Care must be taken to avoid involving them in those decisions beyond their capacities, such as the total family budget, family planning, or family relocation.

Encourage children to strive to achieve in their school endeavors. The acquisition of knowledge, skills, and abilities is indeed the work of the school-age child, similar to play being the work of the toddler and preschooler.

School activities provide formal education and offer children opportunities to work with others to achieve common goals, (e.g., bands, athletic games, or other projects). The foundation for cooperative ventures, however, begins in projects associated with the home.

Children quickly learn their position in a group, partially as a result of their own abilities and partially because of socioeconomic factors.

The potential for each child will differ. Every child needs assistance in recognizing and developing their talents and abilities.

Some children may wish to become leaders, whereas others are content to be followers. Help the child develop the role they select.

The ability to work with others is a learned skill. This ability to interact and develop relationships is as important as innate talents of intelligence or skills.

Caretakers must be consistent in modeling those behaviors they wish their children to emulate. It is not enough to say, "Do as I say, not as I do," since children pattern after that which has been demonstrated—"Actions speak louder than words!"

GROWTH AND DEVELOPMENTAL LANDMARKS	ANTICIPATORY GUIDANCE

Social

SOCIAL AWARENESS

Some children become aware of societal demands and expectations early in life (preschool). Many children do not become aware of these demands until they enter school. A child's awareness of position and importance within the family unit is now tested in units in society. Just as the child had to establish an identity, role, and position within the family, these activities must be repeated in each unit in the larger society. Each unit in the larger society will view the child differently.

The need to socialize with others is of paramount importance to school-age children. Provide opportunities for social experiences.

Involvement in societal units provides opportunities for comparison of abilities to those of peers and adults. As children become more sure of themselves in relating to and with others, they will seek more opportunities to socialize.

The way the child is perceived by individuals in other settings may well be different than the way the child is perceived by family members. The "little demon" or "peachy pet" at home may prove to be just the opposite in another situation. Learning the rules and meeting the expectations of others is as important in social settings as it is in the home.

Acceptance by members of different groups is important to the children. If, within the group, children are permitted to learn from their mistakes, they will become more secure and continue to contribute to the goals of the unit. Achievement within the group enhances the child's sense of industry and further builds the sense of self-worth and autonomy.

Group participation provides avenues for cooperative effort with others. Through group interaction, children learn to express viewpoints and differences of opinion and to recognize that although opinions may vary, each person's participation will influence the progress of the group. Positive experiences will foster children's ability to socialize and their desire to enter new social situations.

The need to achieve as an individual now often becomes subsumed in the need to reach a group goal.

Negative experiences in social settings may discourage future group participation and instead foster a sense of inferiority.

RELATIONSHIPS

The school-age child has many more opportunities and abilities to develop relationships with others than in previous periods of life.

Relationships with and among family members remain important, but the need to relate with peers and others is a most striking feature of this developmental stage.

Caretakers find it difficult to believe and accept the fact that the school-age child still loves and respects them, when so much of the child's time, conversation, and endeavors are directed toward or shared with individuals outside of the family. Maintaining dialogue with children helps caretakers remain abreast of children's interests and concerns.

It is difficult to know whether it is the relationship with others that determines the behavior, language, and dress styles, or if these factors determine the type of relationships that exists. It appears that the child's personality and behavior change with the group in which they are observed.

The need for acceptance pervades every relationship, thus conformity to the expectations of others becomes a priority to the child. This conformity is frequently evidenced in language (slang phrases), dress codes, hairstyles, and/or other activities.

Caretakers frequently become hypercritical of their children's choice of friends, dress codes, hairstyles, and/or language. Permitting independent choices on the part of the child in these realms is just as important as learning to make choices in other aspects of life.

Early in the school-age period, groups of neighborhood children frequently form gangs. These gangs tend to be loosely structured and consist of both boys and girls. The activities of the gang range from impromptu ball games to backyard dramas or small money-making endeavors. The cohesiveness of the group (gang) is quite fluid.

Gangs are an important part of the school-age child's life. Gangs can be quite productive and enhance individual growth by providing opportunities for group interaction, leadership, and cooperative ventures.

GROWTH AND DEVELOPMENTAL LANDMARKS	ANTICIPATORY GUIDANCE

Social—cont'd

RELATIONSHIPS—cont'd

The leader role changes frequently, rules come and go, and the primary focus seems to be that of having fun while being part of a group.

At 9 or 10 years of age the group structure of gangs changes. Boys and girls drift apart into same-sex groups. Entrance to the new group is now quite dependent on being a member of the same sex, although frequently membership also requires active participation on the part of caretakers as well. (See Chapter 13, Play and Activity.)

Athletic ability, intellectual pursuits, or artistic bents now frequently influence membership in organizations.

Caretaker's interests may influence some group activities selected by their children. Avoid overinfluencing children's choices of activities.

Caretakers often become involved in community groups, such as scouting, because of their children's activities.

By the end of the school period, heterosexual relationships again become important. Once again groups of boys and groups of girls get together to have fun, such as roller skating parties, picnics, neighborhood cookouts, or dance parties. Individual dating patterns emerge from these group-related outings.

Encourage group activities in the late school-age period because they help establish baseline behaviors for future boy-girl relationships.

Although peer relationships take precedence with 6- through 12-year-old children, relationships with adults also become extremely important.

Children who have moved from identifying with the parent of the same sex to the parent of the opposite sex will shift their attachment to adults outside of the home. The attachment can be identified as "hero worship." Typically, teachers, coaches, or famous people, such as presidents, actors, or professional athletes, become the targets for the hero worship.

Caretakers frequently feel rejected as a role model or person of worth as school-age children enter the stage where they reach out to other adults for guidance and direction. Caretakers may have difficulty in accepting this shift of attachment. This is a normal phase of development and is of relatively short duration. Hero worship provides children with goals or directions for their own future achievement and should not be discouraged.

The adult-child relationship is different from that of the peer relationship. The easy give-and-take among peers gives way to a relationship in which children no longer perceive themselves as equal. This adult-child relationship contains elements of admiration, adulation, and emulation. Frequently, children place adults on a "pedestal" and hold them in high esteem. Children bend over backwards to gain their favor or be acknowledged. A smile, a pat on the back, or a kind word will "make the child's day."

Through the relationships developed with family members, peers, and significant others, children refine their concept of self and the roles they will perform in society.

LANGUAGE

Conversational skills now become developed and refined with each interaction. Children quickly learn to adapt words and voice in tonation to each social setting. Slang, curse words, and secret codes that may be approved language with peers are found to be inappropriate when used with adults.

Encourage communication and sharing of the day's events. Speaking with children and not down to them enhances family relationships and maintains channels of communication that are necessary for the difficult years of adolescence.

Children will quickly parrot slang and curse words heard in the home, on television, in school, or among friends.

Children evidence ability to adapt well to learning two languages concurrently when both languages are spoken in the home, for example, English and Spanish.

When two languages are spoken in the home, bilingual skills should be encouraged. Pride in the ability to carry on cultural values should be fostered. When children first learn to speak, bilingual exposure may delay language formation, but by the time the school years are reached, bilingual exposure often enhances learning.

LEARNING

Education takes on more formal aspects. Specific times and places have been established where children are to be educated by people prepared to teach, and learning is the expected end product. School provides a ready-made channel for the industrious school-age child.

Play was the work of children through the preschool years, now education becomes the work of the school-age child.

During this period of schooling, children's abilities to conceptualize and think in abstract terms permit them to understand more fully the concepts of time (present, past, and future), space, depth, size, structure, and distance.

GROWTH AND DEVELOPMENTAL LANDMARKS	**ANTICIPATORY GUIDANCE**
Logic in thinking permits them to do mathematical computations, follow complex sets of instructions, and recognize when errors have been made. The school-age child will attempt a difficult task repeatedly, trying to achieve mastery.	Caretakers should stay abreast of the courses and extracurricular offerings in each school and should, if necessary, express both their positive and negative concerns about the offerings.
Children will also learn from the mistakes they make.	
Principles of cause and effect, right from wrong, and choice with accountability are acquired in this period. Competition, collaboration, and cooperation are learned behaviors that are enhanced by projects both within and outside of the school setting.	
Informal learning continues in projects found at home or in the neighborhood, but every child is expected to learn the curricula taught in the schools.	
Some individuals learn best by doing. For them the only real learning is that achieved outside of the classroom. Emphasis on "book learning" in school can lead to feelings of inferiority and loss of self-worth in these children.	Caretakers might help the child see how projects being developed at home can be incorporated into school studies or how the learning from the school's courses can be applied to improve the talents being developed outside the school environment.
Children who do not achieve well in school may seek attention in a variety of ways, such as cheating, clowning, playing hooky, creating disturbances in the classroom, or bullying others.	Children need assistance in achieving their potential.
Television has become a vital force in the education of children. Fine programs developed specifically to meet the learning needs of children can be found on many stations and at a variety of times. The influence of unrestricted television on the minds and lives of those who watch it by the hour has not been researched.	Television can have a tremendous impact on children and provide untapped avenues for the promotion of health education.
The effects of loud volume, varying intensities of light, and programs dealing with violence are presently being researched.	Children's television viewing needs supervision and discussion. Caretakers might be dismayed by the interpretations of an actor's behavior as perceived by the child.

CHAPTER 13

HEALTH MAINTENANCE FOR SCHOOL-AGE CHILDREN

Children from 6 through 12 years of age continue to be relatively free of disease. Visits to health care workers for health maintenance are usually limited to annual preschool checkups or physical examinations that are required for admission to camping programs.

Adaptation to the requirements of school and to the behavioral expectations of teachers and others may prove difficult for children. Some children may fear leaving home or being separated from caretakers.

Continued contact with large groups of children exposes school-age children to many communicable diseases. They frequently develop one illness after another until immunity becomes established.

Nutrition continues to be a major area for concern in this period of life. Six- through twelve-year-old children readily adapt to the established meal patterns of home and school. Children may miss or be late for meals because of their absorption in other affairs. Strong food preferences develop during the school years. Children demonstrate an increase in appetite and the desire for "junk" foods and frequent snacks.

Although necessary, long uninterrupted hours of sleep are often difficult to build into their busy lives. Naps and rest times were abandoned by or during the preschool period. There never seem to be enough hours available to accomplish all of the projects, tasks, and fun school-age children try to pack into each day.

Schoolchildren are quite capable of caring for their own body hygiene. Patterns of bathing, washing hands, and brushing teeth established in earlier periods now frequently are ignored, forgotten, or put off as other activities take precedence.

This relatively healthy period of life is coupled with the inexperience of youth. The school-age child has the ability and desire to explore vast areas of the community. The need to do the same things as their peers often places children in unfamiliar situations. Children value the opinions of their peers and often try potentially dangerous exploits to avoid being considered cowardly ("chicken"). Accident prevention becomes a major thrust. The responsibility for accident prevention, however, now shifts from caretakers and other adults to the children themselves.

Sex education begun in younger years now takes on a greater emphasis as physical differences in boys and girls become noticeable. Children need to understand the normality of menstruation, nocturnal emissions, and the appearance of secondary sex characteristics.

This chapter focuses on the areas of concern for maintenance of healthy school-age children. Helpful hints are also provided for each topic.

AREAS FOR CONCERN	HELPFUL HINTS

Safety

School-age children are particularly vulnerable to accidental injuries because of their increased ability to explore areas beyond the home, investigative curiosity, inexperience with potential hazards, and lack of caution.

Although school-age children are learning to conceptualize, they lack the ability to see dangers in situations that contain similar elements. They may know that matches should not be lit around gasoline, but might not know that matches should not be lit near inflammables such as lacquer and film.

Principles of safety and accident prevention must be introduced and reinforced at every possible opportunity by all responsible adults. Children can and must learn that they are responsible for their own actions.

Potential hazards should be discussed in health care conferences, in the school, through the media, and in the home. Topics might include the following:

1. Street play (ball games of all types, tag, bikes, skates, and skateboards). The desire to participate in games with others and/or the need for space in which to perform activities frequently lead children to play in the streets. Involved and engrossed in their own activities, children neither see nor hear vehicular traffic.

2. Flammable substances (matches, kerosene, gasoline, paint thinners, film). Children frequently try to use flammable substances in their creative endeavors.

3. Ponds, quarries, or other unknown bodies of water. The desire to swim, dive, and show off has led to death by drowning or paralysis from striking heads against pond bases.

Safety consciousness can be developed in children 6 through 12 years old. Safety consciousness is developed from knowledge, role models, and experience.

The adage "Do as I say, not as I do" is not only trite, but almost totally worthless. If children see caretakers and other adults mow the grass without shoes, ride in cars without safety belts, or use new equipment without reading instructions, then they will follow those examples.

Discussion of safety can be included in mealtime topics. Focus on positive aspects of safety; avoid digression to individual acts of carelessness, foolishness, or other transgressions.

Caretakers and community leaders bear the responsibility for providing safe places for children to play. All too often parks are designed for the young child's activities or organized sports. Parks lack places for 6- through 12-year-olds' spontaneous endeavors. City streets quickly become their playground.

Skateboards, bikes, and minibikes all require space and special knowledge. Children need to know the rules of the road and secure licenses before they are permitted to ride in the streets.

Bike riders must adhere to the rules of all vehicles. Following are some of the rules that are most commonly violated:
1. Obeying stop lights or signs.
2. Riding on the correct side of the road.
3. Riding single file.
4. Carrying adequate lights and reflectors when on the road at night.

The care exercised by adults with inflammable substances will be imitated by children.

Review the meaning of the words flammable, inflammable, and combustible. Discuss the need for careful storage of substances such as paint thinners, gasoline, kerosene, or oils. Helping children understand the volatile nature of each helps prevent accidents.

Children love water. Once they know how to swim (even beginning strokes), they venture into all depths of water with a total lack of fear or caution.

Quarries are especially enticing and extremely dangerous:
1. They are easily entered but difficult to exit. Slippery jutting rocks on the sides of the quarry make it precarious for entering or exiting water.
2. They are rarely supervised.
3. They contain cold deep water. The depth of the water prevents the tired swimmer from touching bottom.

Unknown bodies of water such as ponds, lakes, rivers, reservoirs, bays, and streams bear similar risks, since the depth may vary, and supervision is lacking.

The rules of water safety (Chapter 7) are of little help when children swim or play in unsafe waters.

157

AREAS FOR CONCERN	HELPFUL HINTS

Safety—cont'd

4. Mines, caves, and construction sites. The desire to explore, dig, be private, or build leads children to places like these without the knowledge of risk associated with rotting wood, shifting sand, or cave-ins.

5. Equipment (tractors, mowers, hedge cutters, tree trimmers, construction equipment, stoves, irons, blenders, electric mixers, or chopping machines of all types). The desire to know coupled with the desire to use machinery causes many serious permanent injuries, particularly to arms, legs, hands, and feet.

Children will explore and investigate construction sites, caves, and abandoned mines. Their lack of experience and knowledge about the capacities of wooden structures or the movement and weight of earth, rocks, and minerals places children at a disadvantage.

Children will be as attracted to construction equipment as they are to cars, motorcycles, and farm machinery. Children *can and must* be taught to respect machinery from babyhood on. They should not be permitted or encouraged to sit in the driver's seat of cars, tractors, or motorcycles. They should be discouraged from pushing buttons, pulling levers, and turning knobs, since they have neither the knowledge nor capacity to deal with the machine should they get it to start.

Every year children are maimed or killed and property destroyed when they start cars or tractors or mowers inappropriately.

Health conference

Health conferences continue to provide health care workers with the opportunity to assess the health status of the child, determine progress, and provide counseling and teaching on health.

Health conferences are usually limited to examinations needed prior to the return to school each year. The conference usually consists of updating the health history, a physical examination, immunizations (if needed), and health education or counseling.

Health history (reviewed and updated)

The examiner will raise questions to both the caretaker and the child. The child's responses aid the examiner in assessing and evaluating progress made by the child in both physical and psychosocial development.

Provide the health care worker with information related to any injuries, illnesses, or stress-related incidents that altered the child's health status since the last visit.

Permit children to answer the examiner's questions, adding information as needed.

Health assessment: physical examination

The pattern of the physical examination may be much the same as that performed in previous health visits.

Vital signs for temperature, pulse, respiration, and blood pressure will be obtained. Height and weight will be measured.

The examiner will involve the child in several simple exercises that demonstrate flexibility, agility, and ease of movement of the skeletal structure. The curvature of the spine becomes a primary focus of the examination.

Assessment of the reflexes at the knees, elbows, and feet is included.

Caretakers and school-age children are usually quite knowledgeable about health care examinations by this time.

The temperature will now be taken orally instead of rectally.

Children can follow the directions and complete maneuvers requested of them with relative ease. These movements provide valuable information in regard to structural development.

Examination of the feet and toes sometimes causes giggling or laughter on the part of the child and a natural desire to pull the foot away. The examiner is really not tickling the foot, but testing a particular reflex that provides information as to nerve growth.

An examination of the eyes, ears, nose, and throat will be performed.

Examiners solicit children's cooperation through simple explanations and directions.

Auscultation and palpation of the chest and abdomen are included.

Examination of the genitalia during this period is limited to the external structures.

It is essential in males that examiners check the scrotal sac for the presence or absence of testes (testicles). Testes, when palpated, are usually about 1 cm in diameter through pubescence. The left testis usually hangs lower in the scrotal sac than the right.

Most children enjoy being able to follow directions and participate in eye, ear, nose, and throat examinations without hesitation.

Examination of private areas (genitalia) may be the most difficult for the child because of embarrassment more than discomfort.

158

An inguinal hernia and/or hydrocele may be found during this examination. These conditions require medical referral and treatment. Inguinal hernias require immediate follow-up because they can become incarcerated, leading to intestinal obstruction (Chapter 5).

Privacy and minimal exposure of body parts should be maintained by the examiner throughout the entire examination process.

Health assessment: mental and social evaluation

These aspects of development are evaluated through the child's responses to questions and ability to follow directions.

Health protection

Children whose immunization series are incomplete may receive booster injections. (See Appendix A.)

Health promotion

Health promotion in the school-age child covers the areas of dentition, nutrition, elimination, sleep and rest, play and activity, discipline, sex education, and hospitalization.

DENTITION

The loss of deciduous (temporary or "baby") teeth comes to an end during this age period, and the eruption of the permanent (secondary) teeth occurs.

A characteristic of the early school period is the child who is missing two front teeth.

School-age children are capable of caring for their own oral hygiene needs.

Visits to the dentist should be annual.

NUTRITION

School-age children continue to require more calories per pound of body weight than do adults. School-age children usually need 35 calories per pound of body weight each day.

A basic rule for caloric needs of the school-aged child is 1000 calories, plus an additional 100 calories for each year of age.

    6 years old—1600 calories
    7 years old—1700 calories
    8 years old—1800 calories
    9 years old—1900 calories
    10 years old—2000 calories
    11 years old—2100 calories
    12 years old—2200 calories

Actual caloric needs depend on the weight and activities of each child.

Children in this age period are constantly exposed to many different groups of people who may carry communicable diseases. Protection from many of these diseases is provided through immunization.

School-age children lose their "baby" teeth (deciduous teeth). The 6- to 9-year-old seems to gain particular enjoyment in wriggling or drawing attention to loose teeth.

Once the tooth is out, many families participate in a "tooth fairy" ritual. The child places the tooth under the pillow at night and in the morning finds the tooth gone and some token or object in its place.

When more than one front tooth is missing, some children become quite self-conscious and avoid smiling. Other children revel in the absence of two front teeth, since it provides opportunities for whistling and/or spitting through the new opening.

Caretakers may need to supervise or remind children to brush their teeth.

By the end of this period, most children can go to the dentist's office alone.

Avoid purchasing or serving foods that are high in calories, oils, and salt but low in needed nutrients, such as presweetened cereals, candy bars, chips, cookies, and cakes.

Fresh fruits, which provide natural sweeteners and less highly concentrated sugars, and fresh vegetables provide interesting snack foods.

AREAS FOR CONCERN	HELPFUL HINTS

Health promotion—cont'd

NUTRITION—cont'd

Using the formula in Chapter 7, Nutrition, daily fluid requirements for the school-age child can be determined.

6 years old—1500 ml*

7 years old—1600 ml

8 years old—1700 ml

9 years old—1800 ml

10 years old—1900 ml

Over 10 years—2000 ml minimum

The following guidelines may be used to calculate if daily fluid requirements are being met by the school-age child:

1 cup (6 ounces†) = 180 ml

1 juice glass (4 ounces) = 120 ml

1 drinking glass (8 ounces) = 240 ml

1 Popsicle = 90-100 ml

1 small Dixie cup = 100-120 ml

Fluids include milk, juices, water, gelatin, soups, puddings, and ice cream.

Avoid coffee, tea, and carbonated beverages because they lack needed nutrients.

School-age children require three meals per day plus snacks.

Children continue to require diets that include foods from each of the basic four groups. Children who were required to try new foods since infancy usually enjoy a greater variety of foods than children who were not encouraged to do so.

Include selections daily from each of the four basic food groups. The following amounts are recommended daily:

Milk and milk products—1 to 1½ pints (0.5 to 0.7 L)

Milk products that school-age children seem to enjoy most include cheese, milk shakes, and ice cream.

Milk and milk supplements are part of most school lunch programs, providing at least half of the daily needs.

Meats—two to three servings (each serving approximately 3 ounces; 84 g)

School-age children continue to enjoy "fast foods" and finger foods such as hot dogs, hamburgers, chicken, or peanut butter sandwiches.

Small portion sizes are more likely to encourage children to eat and to ask for second helpings.

Vegetables and fruits—four to five servings

Raw fruits and vegetables continue to be preferred over those which are cooked.

Continue to encourage fruits and vegetables for snacks rather than highly sweetened foods.

Bread and cereals—four to five servings

School-age children frequently neglect or forget breakfast. Insist that something be eaten for breakfast. Cereal, which takes longer to eat, could be replaced by a slice of toast with peanut butter, a cheese sandwich, or even a hard-boiled egg. Children may take these foods to eat on their way to school.

Because of the skeletal growth needs toward the end of this period, the body requires more calories, proteins, vitamins, and minerals (in particular iron and calcium) than in earlier years.

Meats, enriched cereals, breads, and green leafy vegetables provide a variety of foods high in iron. Iron is needed for growth of bones. Milk and milk products continue to be major sources for calcium. Many experts in nutrition now recommend less than 1 quart (0.95 L) of milk per day and encourage supplementing the diet with fish, dark green vegetables, and egg yolks.

Table manners, etiquette, and socializing are important aspects of the mealtime.

Table manners and etiquette can be taught during mealtimes. Table accidents of spilling and dropping decrease during this period. Eating too rapidly and placing large amounts of food into the mouth at one time present new problems.

Caretakers' comments such as, "Don't eat so fast," "Stop putting so much food in your mouth," and "Can't you eat right" have negative connotations.

---

*1 milliliter is equal to 1 cubic centimeter.

†1 ounce is equal to 30 milliliters.

AREAS FOR CONCERN	HELPFUL HINTS
	Use of statements such as, "I can't understand what you are saying when you talk with your mouth full of food" and "Eating slowly helps food to be digested more easily" may have a more positive influence in changing the undesirable behavior.
	The pattern established in the home will be the basis for mealtime behavior practiced in the future both at home and away.
	Eating in restaurants can now be an enjoyable family experience. School-age children enjoy socializing and can accept the delay of the meal.
Boys and girls can be involved in meal selection, purchase and preparation of foods, and cleanup operations that accompany these endeavors.	Encourage participation of both sexes in meal planning and preparation. Six-year-old children can learn to prepare simple basic meals for themselves and for the family. Breakfasts are usually the first meals attempted—lunches follow. By the end of the school period it is not unrealistic for each child to have a repertoire of menus and recipes from which the child can assume full responsibility for preparation of specific meals.
	Participation in grocery shopping, menu planning, and meal preparation provides opportunities to learn principles of budgeting and nutrition.
School lunch programs usually provide well-balanced meals. Many schools today are experimenting with lunch offerings that incorporate the foods sold in "fast food" restaurants. This dietary plan includes hamburgers, french fries, pizzas, and is supplemented by vegetables, soups, and salads.	Meals at school or at a friend's home expose children to different cultures, rules of etiquette, and food preparation.
	Caretakers become exasperated when they hear children refuse foods they used to like with statements such as, "Billy doesn't eat our food." On the other hand, caretakers are delighted when their "picky" eater starts trying everything because "Billy says I'm crazy not to eat, cuz it's delicious."
Principles of nutrition are often emphasized in the classroom.	
Television and other media continue to have an impact on the food preferences of children.	School-age children are less influenced than in preschool years by the recommendation of television stars to eat certain foods.
	Other advertising gimmicks such as premiums obtained through boxtops or proof-of-purchase seals attract the 6- to 9-year-old. Caretakers will often be bombarded by children's requests to purchase these foods.

ELIMINATION

Patterns of elimination, unique to each child, are well established before the school years.	Some children experience changes in their elimination patterns because of the constraints of the schoolroom. The alteration (whether diarrhea or constipation) is usually a temporary condition. If the child enoys school, the adaptation is made very quickly.
Children usually have a daily bowel movement, although this varies if eating habits change or illness occurs.	Adding additional fruits, vegetables, or other roughage foods to the diet can reduce problems of constipation. Reducing the intake of fruits, vegetables, or other roughage foods often remedies diarrhea.
The frequency of urination will depend on the child's bladder capacity, sphincter control, and fluid intake. The frequency with which the 6- through 12-year-old child voids (urinates) may vary from four to eight times a day.	Most school-age children empty their bladders four to eight times a day.
	Some children are able to retain urine for long periods of time, whereas others need to urinate every 2 hours. Children who void more often than expected or continue nighttime bed-wetting could have a physical problem or could be reacting to stress (such as starting school, making good grades, meeting new people, or an additional sibling).

161

AREAS FOR CONCERN	HELPFUL HINTS

Health promotion—cont'd

SLEEP AND REST

Patterns for sleep are well established and unique to each child. The hours of sleep needed by children during this period decrease from those of the preschool period.

The hours of sleep needed each day will vary with the activity and health status of the child. A minimum number of 8 hours a day is recommended.

Naps and rest periods have been eliminated by most children in this period of life.

Maintaining routines of expected sleep time minimizes the problems of caretakers. The 6- through 12-year-old can find many good reasons for delaying the hour for sleep. A good show on television, an extra homework assignment, not sleepy, or "I can sleep late tomorrow" are among the most common excuses.

To facilitate sleep, caretakers may find it helpful to reduce stress at bedtime by encouraging quiet activities, a light snack, or a warm bath.

Sleep may be interrupted by dreams and nightmares.

PLAY AND ACTIVITY

Play continues to be an important factor, but it often ranks second in importance to schoolwork in the continued development of the child.

Play continues to provide the child with opportunities to expand physical, social, and emotional skills.

Play with others is much more cooperative than in previous periods. Play provides opportunities for the fine and gross motor skills and coordination of development.

Set times for schoolwork and household chores are advisable, but free time for play is equally important. Play time is not wasted time. Many skills, abilities, and relationships are developed and refined through play.

Activities of the school-age child center around bicycles, skates and skateboards, ball games of all sorts, swimming, and camping.

Although children have been taught the principles of safety and consideration of the rights of others, they often need frequent reminders.

School-age children demonstrate great agility and a keen sense of balance. A great amount of time is devoted to games and activities that involve the large muscles. Opportunities for development of the fine muscles should also be encouraged.

Complex motor activities such as jumping rope, playing marbles or jacks, roller skating, balancing acts, and acrobatics now are easily learned by most school-age children. These activities provide opportunities for further development of both large and fine muscle control.

Fine muscle coordination is further refined through activities such as painting, drawing, constructing models, penmanship, and working on jigsaw puzzles.

Cooperative ventures include team sports, sidewalk sales, booths, or backyard dramas.

Play takes on a competitive nature not seen before in previous periods of life. Some children excel in competitive play and constantly seek out these types of opportunities. Other children may seek activities that stress cooperation and participation without the emphasis on competition.

It is important to allow children to develop their own talents. Avoid pressuring them to conform to other people's expectations. Children might not enjoy certain activities as much as their siblings, parents, or other relatives.

Although competition and competitive sports abound, it is helpful if caretakers avoid emphasizing the need to win. Children enjoy participation. The caretaker's attitude in relation to winning and/or losing carries over to the child. Children seek approval and aim to please.

The school-age child needs some time for individual pursuits to refine talents, test abilities, and further identify personal capabilities.

School-age children in general have an overwhelming need to be with the "gang" or with their special friends.

As in former periods, children need time to be alone.

If a child is usually alone and rarely plays with others, caretakers should find ways to encourage involvement in group activities with other children.

Close bonds between the caretaker and child can be maintained by finding a time (each week) to do something together. These special times are remembered in adulthood.

AREAS FOR CONCERN	HELPFUL HINTS

DISCIPLINE (LIMIT SETTING)

Limit setting continues during the school-age period, although the parameters of approved limits will be changed as children demonstrate increased senses of responsibility and accountability.

Consistency in the expectations of children's behavior is important. Children from 6 through 12 learn to capitalize on those areas where caretakers lack agreement. The 6- through 12-year-old manipulates one caretaker against another to gain approval of new exploits.

Caretakers may have to mete out punishment when children do not adhere to previously established and understood rules.

Children in this age period need and want rules. Consistency in the application of the rules fosters their trust in others.

Rules and regulations that govern organizations in society such as schools also mold the school-age child.

The rules and regulations of society help young people learn that with freedom comes responsibility. An individual's rights end when they impinge on the rights of others.

Be realistic in the rules established for children. Revise the rules as children grow older to permit greater freedom, provided they have demonstrated responsibility.

Present a united front in the limits on behaviors that will be accepted and approved. Avoid disagreeing about these limits in front of children. Every family establishes its own rules. These rules might be centered around mealtime, bedtime, chores, schoolwork, and curfew.

Deliberate disobedience warrants retribution. First, be sure it was deliberate disobedience.

Support the established rules and regulations of society and expect that children will adhere to them as well. As in the family, if children are exposed to adults who do not obey expected rules, the children will not either. Some examples of common breaches include breaking traffic rules, disregarding authority, and mistreating or degrading others.

Punctual attendance, completion of homework, and attentiveness during school hours are expectations to which children can adhere.

Children need to know and feel secure that caretakers and school personnel work cooperatively and collaboratively to assist the children's growth and development.

SEX EDUCATION

The reproductive system of both females and males will be reviewed in this discussion. Although it is neither our intent nor our belief that children 6 years of age need to know all of the following information, by 12 years of age many children will have developed both secondary and primary sex characteristics and thus need much of the information.

Sex education continues in this age period as before with simple, honest explanations to children's questions. By the end of this period, both boys and girls are well aware of many major differences between the sexes.

Children developing secondary sex characteristics who do not raise any questions about body changes are receiving information or misinformation elsewhere.

The 6- through 12-year-old needs truthful and factual information about body parts, functions, and the changes occurring in themselves and individuals of the opposite sex.

Some parents can provide sex education without difficulty, others may need help from health professionals or school personnel. During health care conferences, health care personnel should review these topics with the caretaker and child.

Sex education should begin in the home. Learning about the parts of the body and how they function is fascinating, normal, and natural. If caretakers start the process in infancy and toddlerhood, they simply continue adding to the child's stockpile of information.

Knowledge about reproductive systems is usually passed to uninformed individuals by members of the same sex. Thus grandmothers, mothers, aunts, sisters, and girl friends share the information about menstruation (monthly period) with girls. Grandfathers, fathers, uncles, brothers, and boy friends share information about nocturnal emission and ejaculation with boys.

It is better for children to receive answers to questions about body parts and the differences between boys and girls from their loved ones than distorted versions, half truths, myths, and misinformation from others.

Children continue to be curious about their bodies and will raise questions. If caretakers feel comfortable when answering questions about body changes, sex functions, and reproduction, the trusting, sharing relationship previously established becomes reinforced. If, however, caretakers and/or health personnel are uncomfortable when speaking on this topic of sex education, a major line of communication disruption occurs. This may influence caretaker-child relationships in later years.

AREAS FOR CONCERN	HELPFUL HINTS

Health promotion—cont'd

SEX EDUCATION—cont'd

The appearance and order of the secondary sex characteristics described in Chapter 12 can be one of the first topics discussed. The name, location, and function of each part of the reproductive system could be included in the discussion.

Caretakers can use those special times spent alone with each child to discuss topics such as the changing body.

Use of correct terminology in describing the sex organs of the human body maintains a sense of dignity and purpose. Avoid giving the impression that portions of the body cannot be addressed unless degradingly or with sick humor attached.

Female external sex characteristics

Breasts: Breasts (mammary glands) are located on the anterior chest wall and are relatively equal in size, shape, and firmness.

The breasts are composed of glandular and fatty tissue. The glandular tissue consists of lactiferous ducts and lobules that produce milk after pregnancy. The fatty tissue provides the material substance of the breast's shape and contour (Fig. 13-1, *A*).

The size of the breasts varies with each individual. Breast size, small or large, usually causes distress in girls.

The female's shape takes on softer lines and contours, and breast tissue develops somewhere between 9 and 13 years of age. Shortly thereafter (usually between 10 and 14 years of age), internal changes begin to occur.

Girls who are beginning to develop breasts will start discussing these events with adults they trust and/or with friends. The discussions with adults typically begin in the form of questions. Discussion with friends centers on pooling or sharing all the information (truth, fiction, myth, and untruth) they have gleaned from people, books, movies, and television.

Each breast has a reddish area called the *areola* at its center. The nipple, located in the center of the areola, has contractile and erectile qualities. These qualities permit ready access for the breast-fed infant following pregnancy (Fig. 13-1, *B*).

Girls become aware of the erectile reaction of the nipple to changes in temperature, activity, or friction. Knowledge that these reactions are normal may reduce discomfort or concern on the part of the child.

As breasts increase in size, brassieres should be worn to provide support. Breast tissue does not contain muscles, and if not supported postural change and discomfort may result.

Menstruation usually begins after breast development becomes noticeable and before hair develops under the arm. Because the exact date of onset cannot be predicted, it is advisable that the pubescent girl be knowledgeable about menstruation and carry the appropriate equipment with her. Some pubescent/adolescent girls may enter the new stage of womanhood quite young (9 to 11); others may not begin menses until quite late (14 to 16). In either event, both groups are still within the normal range. (See Menstruation.)

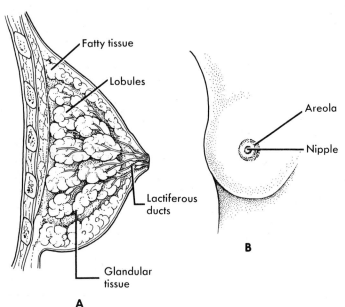

Fig. 13-1. Female breast. **A,** Cutaway view. **B,** Straight view.

Pubic area: Fleshy area covering the pubic bone and external genitalia, readily identified as the triangular portion at the base of the abdomen and extending between the legs to the rectal area. By the end of the adolescent period, the pubic area is usually covered with hair (referred to as pubic hair) (Fig. 13-2).

AREAS FOR CONCERN

Vulva: External portion of female reproductive system.

Labia majora (major lip): Larger outer fold, usually covered with pubic hair.

Labia minora (minor lip): More delicate inner fold.

The forward upper juncture of the labia covers the *clitoris*. The clitoris is an erectile-type tissue that responds to external stimulation.

The inner linings of the labia contain mucus-secreting glands that provide lubrication.

Located just beneath the clitoris is the *urethra* (external meatus of the urinary system).

Beneath the urethra lies the *vagina* (vestibular canal to the cervix), the canal from the external genitalia to the uterus. The walls of the vagina are muscular and fibrous. Mucous membranes line the vagina. The lining secretes a substance that becomes slightly acidic, thus providing some protection from invasion by organisms located in the external genitalia.

Two small glands (Bartholin's glands) that are located one on each side of the vagina secrete mucus. The precise nature of Bartholin's glands is not known, although they are activated and provide additional lubrication during coitus (intercourse).

The labia join together at the base to partially fold over and cover the vagina. The tough, membranous tissue covering the vagina is called the *hymen*. There is a growing practice among health professionals to incise this tissue early in a child's life to facilitate menstrual flow and reduce the trauma sometimes associated with intercourse in later years (Fig. 13-2).

HELPFUL HINTS

Between the legs of girls is a double fold of tissue (vulva) that protects the female reproductive system and urinary excretive system.

The outer fold (or lip) covered with pubic hair is called the *labia majora*. The inner fold (lip), which is less thick, is called the *labia minora*. These lips join together at the front and cover an area called the *clitoris*. The clitoris, which can be described as a small triangular piece of tissue that has about the same firm consistency as the tip of the nose and is sensitive to manipulation.

The labia also fold over the area called the *urethra*. The urethra is the name given to the external opening through which urine is excreted.

The labia partially cover the next opening called the *vagina*. The vagina is the external opening from which the menstrual flow is discharged. The vagina provides the passageway for the birth of a baby.

The partial covering over the vagina (hymen) is membranous. In some females this membrane may cover the entire vaginal opening and need to be incised.

Old wives' tales of the past inferred that an intact hymen is a sign of virginity. Some young girls have an intact hymen until intercourse occurs. Others maintain an intact hymen even through pregnancy, as the stretching capacity of the opening is great in some women and almost nonexistent in others.

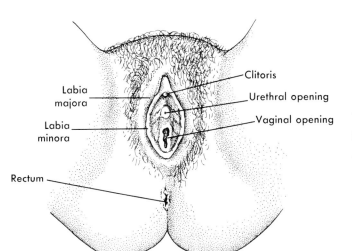

Fig. 13-2. External female genitalia.

Health promotion—cont'd

SEX EDUCATION—cont'd

Female internal sex characteristics (Fig. 13-3)

Ovaries: Two almond-shaped female sex glands approximating the size of walnuts located in the lower abdomen, one on each side of the uterus. The ovaries produce ova (eggs) and hormones (estrogen and progesterone).

Female sex glands (ovaries) produce eggs (ova) needed for the development of a new baby.

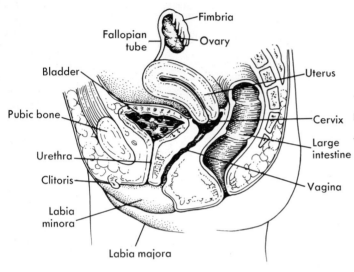

Fig. 13-3. Cutaway view of internal female genitalia.

Fallopian tube(s) (oviducts or uterine tubes): Hollow tubes that extend laterally from the uterus toward the ovary.

The portion of the tube with frondlike projections close to each of the ovaries provides access to the uterus for the mature ova (egg) released by the ovary.

During reproduction, spermatozoa (male seeds) and ova (female egg) meet, and fertilization usually takes place within the fallopian tube.

The fertilized ovum continues down the tube to the uterus, where it will attach itself to the uterine wall and continue to develop as a new infant.

The fallopian tubes are canals through which the egg (ova) travels from the ovaries to the uterus.

AREAS FOR CONCERN	HELPFUL HINTS

An unfertilized ovum reaches the uterus but does not attach to the uterine wall. It is discharged from the body through the vagina during menstruation (Fig. 13-4).

Uterus (womb): Pear-shaped, hollow organ of the female designed to accommodate the growth of a child. Located within the lower abdomen (pelvic area), the uterus consists of the following connective, muscular, and mucoid tissues:
Parametrium—Outer covering of fatty connective tissue.
Myometrium—Inner layer or muscular wall.
Endometrium—Innermost mucosal surface.

The womb (uterus) is the protective internal pouch that encases a developing infant during pregnancy.

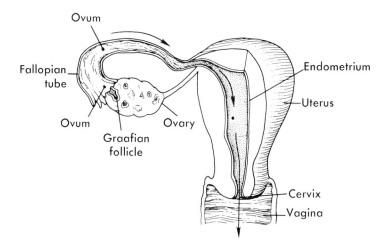

Menstruation begins with the development of an egg (ovum) in a follicle of an ovary by stimulation from the pituitary gland. The average menstrual cycle is 28 days. Following are the stages of the cycle:
Stage I: The pituitary gland releases estrogen to thicken the endometrial lining of the uterus. This takes place during the first 14 days of the cycle.
Stage II: The ovaries release both estrogen and progesterone, which prepares the endometrium for implantation of a fertilized ovum. This stage takes place during the last 14 days of the cycle.
Stage III: If fertilization of the ovum does not occur, the pituitary gland/hypothalamus is triggered to decrease secretion of follicle-stimulating hormones (FSH) and gonadotropins.

Fig. 13-4. Menstruation. Unfertilized ovum (egg) is discharged from body with uterine lining.

The lining of the uterus goes through a cyclical change (usually monthly) called *menses* (menstruation).

Menstruation, commonly called "monthly," occurs cyclically.
There are few events more distressing to young girls than the advent of menstruation when they have not been prepared either mentally or physically.
Common mistakes made regarding information about menstruation include the following:
1. Keeping it a mystery.
2. Giving all the information at one time.
3. Waiting too long to share the knowledge.
The guidelines that follow might help caretakers explain the beauty and rhythm of the menstrual cycle:
1. Be knowledgeable of body parts and their functions starting in infancy and continuing throughout the life cycle.
2. Provide honest responses to children's questions.
3. Provide opportunities for sharing.
4. Avoid giving more information than is requested.
5. Seek indications of the child's understanding through open-ended or clarifying questions.
6. Provide books and illustrations for elaboration on menstruation.

AREAS FOR CONCERN	HELPFUL HINTS

Health promotion—cont'd

SEX EDUCATION—cont'd

Menstruation: A cyclic discharge of bloody material from the uterus. Occurs at fairly regular intervals, usually every 28 to 35 days from onset of puberty to menopause.

The average age for onset of menstruation is 10 to 14 years, and the duration is unique for each female. The average length of flow is about 4 to 5 days. Some females may flow 7 days; others may flow only 2 to 3 days.

Menstruation is primarily the outcome of decreased progesterone level, resulting from the effects of an unfertilized ovum.

Menstruation is the body's response to ridding itself of material the body cannot use at that time and can store no longer. This is somewhat similar to urination or defecation, where waste products must be eliminated because the body can no longer use them or store them. Although urination and defecation can be somewhat controlled (either hastened or delayed) by the individual, this is not true for menstruation, which is controlled by activities within the body.

Menstruation occurs cyclically, usually every 28 to 35 days and is governed by substances called *hormones*.

The onset of menstruation usually occurs between 10 and 14 years of age.

Until the menstrual pattern is established, there may be irregularity in onset as well as quantity and length of flow. Once the pattern of menstruation is established there may be variations of onset and quantity of flow that may result from changes in emotions, climate, or living conditions.

Each month the lining of the womb (uterus) begins to adapt to the day when pregnancy occurs. The ovaries produce eggs (ova), which they release (usually one at a time, once each month).

Normally ovulation (periodic ejection of an ovum from a ruptured mature graafian follicle of the ovary) takes place at the midpoint of each menstrual cycle (average fourteenth day). A corpus luteum then develops within the ruptured follicle that secretes progesterone and estrogen (hormones that prepare the endometrial lining of the uterus for implantation of the fertilized ovum). Estrogen is the major hormonal secretion from the ovaries and is responsible for secondary sex characteristics of the female (Fig. 12-1).

Ovulation, when it occurs, will alternate between the two ovaries.

The increased blood supply and tissue structure of the uterine wall (endometrium) are not needed for the growth of a fetus and are discharged from the body as waste material.

The egg (microscopically tiny) travels down a tube (fallopian tube) to the uterus. If the egg, during passage through the fallopian tube, does not come in contact with male seed (spermatozoa) it will not be fertilized or implant itself into the uterine lining.

The prepared innermost lining of the uterus and the unfertilized egg will be shed from the body. This shedding is what is known as *menstrual flow*.

Menstrual flow resembles blood in that it is red and may contain some clotted material. An unnerving aspect of menstruation is that females cannot make it start, stop, or control how long it will flow or the amount that will be discharged.

Menstrual flow is not uncontrollable bleeding because it *is not* blood that is being shed.

Menstrual flow usually lasts from 4 to 5 days. During the period of flow it is necessary to wear some form of sanitary protection to prevent soiling of clothing. Sanitary protection varies; younger girls find a belt and pads or liners quite comfortable; adolescents and older women may prefer to use tampons or other devices worn internally to provide protection. (Recent research has demonstrated a danger of illness and death [toxic shock syndrome] associated with the continued use of tampons.)

AREAS FOR CONCERN	HELPFUL HINTS

Sometimes the following alterations in menstruation occur:

1. Amenorrhea—menstruation does not occur at puberty. Correction of this condition may require administration of hormones, but needs to be brought to the attention of a physician.

If menses (menstruation, monthly periods) do not begin (amenorrhea) by the late teenage years, the young lady should have a gynecological examination by a health care worker.

When menses first begins, it is quite typical to have an irregular cycle. Sometimes the times between periods may be short or long, or an entire cycle may be skipped. Cycles become regular within 1 year. If irregularity persists beyond that time, consult health personnel.

2. Dysmenorrhea—pain with menstruation. Some discomfort is to be expected, but acute discomfort requires medical evaluation. There may be a relationship between anxiety, emotional tension, or stress and menstrual discomfort.

A myth still perpetuated today suggests that menstruation is always accompanied by pain or discomfort, referred to as *cramps* (dysmenorrhea). Although it is true that the muscles of the uterine wall may contract and relax more frequently during menses than at other times of the cycle, many females feel no discomfort at all. Some women notice a feeling of being bloated, others notice a headache, some speak of being more tired, and still others notice they are more edgy or irritable. These changes in behavior may also be clues that menses is about to begin.

Should painful cramps occur, it is helpful to know that these sensations are usually of short duration (1 to 4 hours). Some females find the following suggestions helpful:

1. Get extra rest.
2. Apply a warm water bottle to the lower abdomen for 20 minutes and repeat if necessary.
3. Assume a knee-chest position for 10- to 20-minute periods.

If the abdominal discomfort is severe or protracted, consult health personnel.

3. Menorrhagia—excessive bleeding or prolonged duration. This condition requires immediate medical evaluation and treatment.

Menstrual flow typically lasts 4 to 5 days and consists of a bloody discharge containing some clotted material. The average flow requires changing the pad or tampon about every 2 to 3 hours on the first day, and less frequently on successive days. The flow diminishes and changes from a bright red to dark brownish red color. If the flow stays bright red, increases in amount, and persists, consult health personnel.

Health promotion—cont'd

SEX EDUCATION—cont'd

Male sex characteristics

Breasts (inactive, nonfunctional mammary glands): Breasts are located on the anterior chest wall, and are equal in size, shape, and firmness. Breast tissue of males is usually slight to nonexistent, although there may be some deposition of fatty tissue. Lactiferous glands do not develop due to the excess production of androgen (male) hormones.

Each breast has a reddish area called the *areola* at its center. The nipple, located in the center of the areola, has contractile and erectile qualities as in the female (Fig. 13-1).

Pubic area: The triangular, fleshy portion at the base of the abdomen, covering the pubic bone, and extending between the legs to the rectal area. By the end of the adolescent period the pubic area is usually covered with hair (referred to as pubic hair) (Fig. 13-5).

During early adolescence (puberty) when the male hormones have not yet taken charge, the breasts of some boys enlarge. Knowledge of the temporary nature of this phenomenon can relieve the young man's anxiety.

During puberty, males develop hair over the fleshy tissue at the base of the abdomen above the penis and extending down between the legs (pubic hair).

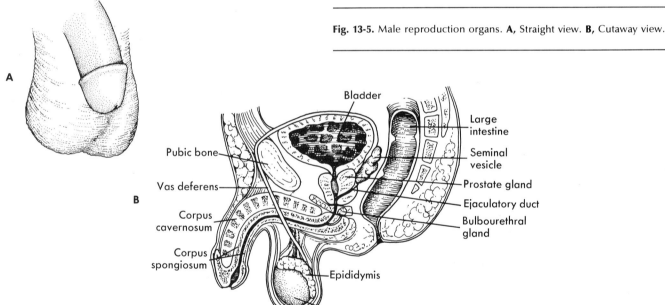

Fig. 13-5. Male reproduction organs. **A,** Straight view. **B,** Cutaway view.

Penis: Male organ that serves two major functions, urinary excretion and coitus (intercourse).

The penis, located at the base of the pubic arch, is a cylindrical structure consisting of three columns of erectile tissue and covered by skin.

Corpora cavernosa: Two lateral columns of erectile tissue.

Corpus spongiosum: The third, innermost column of erectile tissue that contains the urethra, a canal which permits excretion of urine from the bladder or the emission of semen from the testes during ejaculation.

The penis serves two functions, urinary excretion and transmission of male seed (sperm).

During puberty, the size and length of the penis increase.

170

AREAS FOR CONCERN	HELPFUL HINTS

Glans penis: A cone-shaped head at the tip of the penis covered by a loose skin hood called the *prepuce* (foreskin).

Smegma, a lubricant, is secreted from tissue beneath the prepuce.

Excision (circumcision) of the prepuce (foreskin) is performed on most males shortly after birth for hygienic and cosmetic purposes. The Jewish faith requires circumcision of all males.

The urethral meatus (opening) is usually located centrally at the tip of the glans.

The length and overall size of the penis varies with each individual but does not determine reproductive capacity.

If a young boy has not been circumcised, daily retraction of the foreskin (prepuce) must be continued because the lubricant (smegma) that is produced must be cleansed away.

Many young males, particularly pubescents and adolescents, suffer feelings of inferiority because the size of their penis does not measure up in size or shape to those of their peers. Reassurance that size is not a reflection on manhood or reproductive abilities can be quite helpful.

Scrotum: Saclike structure located posterior to the penis and suspended from the base of the pubis.

The scrotum consists of skin, dartos (muscular tissue), fascia (cremasteric, spermatic, and infundibular), and the tunica vaginalis.

The sac consists of a double pouch, separated by a septum, each side containing a testis, or testicle (male reproductive organ), and spermatic cord.

The spermatic cord (a structure extending from the inguinal ring to the testis) has ducts (that permit the egress of mature sperm from the testes), nerves, and blood vessels.

The saclike structure (scrotal sac) containing the male sex organs lies exterior to the body. This sac, found between the legs and at the base of the abdomen, increases in size during the school period. The sac and its contents are vulnerable to injury and should be protected during physical sports by wearing a scrotal support (jock strap).

Testes (gonads): Male organs (two) of reproduction, located in the scrotal sac, which produce spermatozoa and the male hormone testosterone.

The position of the testes in the scrotum is not fixed, since each is connected to the abdominal wall by a cremasteric muscle. These muscles can draw the testes close to the abdominal wall during cold weather or permit the testes to move from the abdominal wall to the lower portion of the scrotal sac during warm weather.

Each testis consists of approximately 250 segments. Each segment contains one to three highly convoluted tubules that can produce mature spermatozoa. The sperm leave the tubules and are stored in the epididymis located at the top and behind each testis. During ejaculation, the sperm leave the epididymus through the vas deferens to the urethra (Fig. 13-5).

Gonadotropic hormones are released by the hypothalamus, which in turn triggers the pituitary gland to secrete FSH and luteinizing hormone (LH).

In the male, FSH is responsible for the development of the seminiferous tubules and the maturation of sperm. LH is responsible for formation of Leydig cells in the testes. Dying cells stimulate production of testosterone and with FSH are responsible for spermatogenesis and development of secondary sex characteristics.

In addition, testosterone from the adrenal gland promotes development and maturation of the male sex organs (penis, scrotum, and testes) (Fig. 12-1).

Male sex organs (testicles) produce male seeds (sperm), which are needed in the formation of a new baby.

AREAS FOR CONCERN	HELPFUL HINTS

Health promotion—cont'd

SEX EDUCATION—cont'd

The internal structures that secrete fluid known as semen are the seminal vesicles and prostate and bulbourethral glands.

The seminal vesicles are connected to the ductus deferens and lie just behind the bladder neck. These two saclike structures secrete a thick vesicular fluid that makes up part of the semen.

Surrounding the neck of the bladder and urethra is the prostate gland. This gland secretes a thin, slightly alkaline fluid that also becomes part of the semen.

On each side of the prostate gland are two pea-size glands known as the *bulbourethral,* or *Cowper's,* glands. They secrete a viscid fluid and form part of the seminal fluid through ducts that empty into the urethral wall.

Ejaculation (expulsion of seminal fluid) is a reflex response to nerve impulses from the glans penis that stimulate the ductus deferens (excretory duct of the testes) and seminal vesicles. Spermatozoa (male reproductive cells) form part of the testicular secretions. Simultaneously, nerve impulses to the ischiocavernous and bulbocavernous muscles cause the penis to become erect. Erection of the penis usually precedes ejaculation.

Expulsion of testicular and seminal fluid occurs in two stages:

Stage I: Secretions and semen from the bulbourethral and prostate glands and seminal vesicles enter the urethra. Secretions from the prostate gland precede those of seminal vesicles.

Stage II: Expulsion of the contents is made possible by contraction of smooth muscle of the ductus deferens and the increased glandular secretions.

Nocturnal emission (wet dreams): Involuntary expulsion of seminal fluid during sleep.

Noctural emission is indicative of a maturing male reproductive system, undergoing changes necessary for future procreation.

Wet dreams (nocturnal emissions) happen at night to most pubescent/adolescent males. Wet dreams are involuntary discharges from the penis of a thick, whitish, mucoid substance called *semen* (seminal fluid). Semen in the young male is made up of secretions from the sex glands (prostate), plus plasma and cells.

Noctural emissions (wet dreams) are the result of the development and maturation of the male's sex glands. In the young man this seminal fluid does not contain mature sperm. Nocturnal emissions are not under the control of the male, any more than the time of menses is under the control of the female. When the emissions first occur, they can be quite embarrassing or confusing to the young men.

The adolescent might think that this discharge is a result of masturbation, sex fantasies, or a serious physical flaw in his makeup.

Pubescent males should be prepared by adults (parents, health personnel, or others) for these occurrences before they appear and should be reassured that it is normal.

Hospitalization

Children in the school-age period are hospitalized most frequently because of accidental injuries, tonsillectomies, adenoidectomies, herniorrhaphies, or appendectomies.

If hospitalization is a planned event, school-age children are capable of understanding the reason for being hospitalized and what is expected of them.

Six- through twelve-year-olds may need to be hospitalized because of injury.

Hospitalization for the school-age child may be a planned event, such as removal of tonsils or repair of a hernia. At these times, prepare the child as thoroughly as possible by explaining the following:

172

AREAS FOR CONCERN	HELPFUL HINTS
Honest explanations in understandable terms prior to hospitalization will assist children in adjusting and accepting this experience.	1. Why they must go to the hospital. 2. What will be done to them. 3. How long they might be there. Be honest and truthful, even in regard to those procedures that will be painful. Children's confidence and trust in caretakers becomes further established with truthful explanations.
School-age children usually know the location of external body parts but do not know the locations of all internal body parts. For example, they may know the location of the tonsils but not the location of the kidneys.	Children's levels of understanding about their own body parts can be determined by providing them with an outline drawing of a human body and asking them to draw in and label the external and internal body parts.
Six- through twelve-year-olds usually adjust to hospitalization with ease.	
Rules, regulations, and parameters of safety need to be reviewed with the child and the caretaker. Children will investigate and manipulate equipment within the environment. Behaviors expected of children must be enforced by caretakers and health personnel.	Children need to know the rules and regulations of the hospital. Caretakers can help children learn and abide by the rules.
Children of school age need to be informed where they can place their belongings, where the bathroom facilities are located, who is to be their nurse, and how to get in touch with the nurse when necessary.	
Adjustment to hospitalization occurs when children begin to feel secure and comfortable.	
School-age children are capable of following directions and performing tasks in regard to their own personal hygiene, grooming, and eating and should be permitted (when possible) to be independent in these activities.	Children need to remain as independent as possible, even when hospitalized. Caretakers are advised to avoid overindulgence or reduced expectations of behavior because the child is sick.
Procedures that require several steps can be understood by this age child. Participation should be encouraged when at all possible.	When procedures must be performed, children need simple explanations and directions. Reinforcement by the caretaker(s) often helps obtain compliance from the child.
Children can be expected to learn and master new tasks (such as giving their own insulin injections).	When procedures must be learned for continued use at home, the directions and explanations need to be given repeatedly.
School-age children try to cooperate with intrusive procedures. However, even though they try to hold still, at the last moment they are often unable to do so. It may be necessary to immobilize the child until the procedure has been completed. Truthfulness about and the ease with which intrusive procedures are completed foster a sense of trust between the child and health personnel.	The school-age child fears intrusive procedures more than younger children but tries to cooperate. Children should be offered one opportunity to cooperate, but if difficulties ensue, they should then be assisted. This recommendation is made based on the belief that if the procedure can be accomplished quickly and with minimal trauma, this same or similar procedures can then be repeated more easily with total cooperation.
The need for privacy cannot be overlooked for school-age children. They are aware of body changes and become easily embarrassed when exposed. Privacy should be considered during baths, toileting times, and when examinations or procedures are being performed. *Dignity and privacy are as important to school-age children as they are to adolescents or adults.*	Children 6 through 12 begin to crave privacy. Exposure of body parts unnecessarily is to be avoided.
Prolonged hospitalization limits social relationships with peers and hinders school performance. Visiting regulations should facilitate the social relationships so important to the school-age child.	Many hospitals have liberal visiting hours and visitor policies. If the hospital does not permit liberal visitation, exceptions might be sought if the hospitalization period will be extensive. Children need peer support as much as adults need their friends and loved ones to help them through their trying times.
School performance can be fostered through private tutoring, school programs within the hospital, friends who share homework assignments, and projects that can be done during the hospitalization.	Many schools have programs or tutors to assist children who are hospitalized for extended periods of time. Inquire whether these services are available.

CHAPTER 14

HEALTH PROBLEMS OF SCHOOL-AGE CHILDREN

Children 6 through 12 years of age usually enjoy good health. Accidents of all types continue to be the cause of most of the major health problems, although communicable diseases and infections may be prevalent.

Accidents that occur are frequently associated with sports, vehicles, and/or machinery. Cuts, lacerations, sprains, broken bones, and even concussions are commonly encountered. After emergency treatment, the care of the child usually continues at home. Many of these events are temporary inconveniences and are often quickly forgotten by the school-age child.

Children in this period often forget to eat meals or overeat "junk" foods. Dietary habits such as these predispose them to problems such as anemias, dental caries, or constipation. Continued poor nutrition can contribute to future health problems such as acne or gastrointestinal tract illnesses.

School-age children are susceptible to conjunctivitis (pinkeye), plantar warts, and athlete's foot. Improperly maintained pools, common towels, and community bathhouses or showers seem to be important factors in the spread of these illnesses.

This chapter will focus on health problems that have not been discussed in previous chapters. Each health problem will be reviewed, and health care guidelines and helpful hints will be included.

HEALTH PROBLEM	HEALTH CARE GUIDELINES	HELPFUL HINTS

Anemia (tired blood)

Anemia: A symptom of a disease or disorder of the blood in which there is a reduction in hemoglobin, decreased number of red blood cells (erythrocytes), or decrease in total blood volume (packed red blood cells).

Anemia is present when the hemoglobin level is less than 13 to 14 g of packed red cells per 100 ml of blood for males or 11 to 12 g of packed red cells per 100 ml of blood for females.

Tired blood (anemia) is the term used to describe a condition where there is (1) an insufficient number of red blood cells or (2) a decreased oxygen and/or nutrient content within the blood cell.

Anemia can result from the following:
1. Large amount of blood loss (hemorrhage).
2. Poor nutrition.
3. Production of immature red blood cells.
4. Destruction of red blood cells.

Anemias that occur from blood loss (usually associated with some form of injury) are quickly rectified by healthy children once fluid volume is restored and needed nutrients are made available to the body.

Anemia may be a result of the following:
1. Injury or trauma with loss of a large quantity of blood (hemorrhage).
2. Poor dietary intake, especially iron (iron deficiency anemia).
3. Impaired bone marrow function.
4. Excessive blood cell destruction.

As a result of anemia, there is a decreased oxygen supply to the body.

Symptoms of anemia are often vague. Fatigue and decreased energy level may be the first indicators.

Children averaging 8 to 10 hours of sleep a night who are tired, weak, or lie down during the day without a caretaker's suggestion may have anemia.

Prolonged fatigue and weakness should be investigated.

As the anemia progresses, skin and mucous membranes become pale (pallor). Pallor is most evident in the conjunctiva of eyes, palms of hands, and fingernails.

The body compensates for oxygen need by increasing the respiratory, cardiac, and metabolic rates.

Anemia is diagnosed through microscopic examination of blood samples. The shape, size, color, and number of red blood cells, as well as the hemoglobin level, can be determined by the following:
1. Mean corpuscular volume (MCV)
   a. Normocytic—normal or average size of red blood cell
   b. Macrocytic—larger than normal size red blood cell
   c. Microcytic—smaller than normal size red blood cell
2. Mean corpuscular hemoglobin concentration (MCHC)
   a. Normochromic—normal color and hemoglobin concentration of blood
   b. Hypochromic—decrease in color and hemoglobin concentration of blood
   c. Hyperchromic—increase in color and hemoglobin concentration of blood

Medical management and treatment is directed toward diagnosis of the anemia and institution of appropriate measures to rectify the problem.

Laboratory tests may be needed. A finger prick may be all that is needed, although at times additional blood studies may be required. It may be necessary for the caretaker to hold the child firmly while the procedure is being performed.

HEALTH PROBLEM	HEALTH CARE GUIDELINES	HELPFUL HINTS
Anemia—cont'd		
The most common type of anemia in childhood is *iron deficiency anemia*.	If anemia is a result of poor iron intake, recommendations wll be made for caretakers to provide adequate amounts of iron, protein, vitamin B_{12}, and other vitamins and minerals through adjustments in the child's diet and supplementary mineral/vitamin preparations. The following measures may be instituted: 1. Encourage those foods which are high in iron, minerals, proteins, and vitamins.	The most common type of anemia found in children is related to a lack of iron in the diet. Become concerned if the child consistently omits one or more of the basic four food groups. Although it is not possible for caretakers to be with children all the time, they should encourage their children to eat a good basic diet, consisting of the four basic food groups. (See Chapter 13, Nutrition.) Encourage those foods known to contain large quantities of iron, protein, and minerals. *Milk, although a good source of protein and minerals, lacks iron.* Caretakers can increase the value of the milk by adding an egg and preparing a milk shake.
	2. Encourage rest. This decreases cardiac effort and metabolic rate, thus sparing energy.	Children who have anemia, however, may need more rest than they wish. Caretakers can find ways to make rest periods more enjoyable by providing paint-by-number pictures, radios, record players, television, or books.
Conjunctivitis (pinkeye)		
Conjunctivitis (pinkeye): Inflammation and infection of the thin membrane lining the eyelids and covering the eyeball.	Infection of the lining of the eyelid and covering of the eyeball can be identified by redness, excessive tearing, thick mucoid drainage, itching, and irritation.	Caretakers may first identify pinkeye (conjunctivitis) in the child when there is noticeable eye discharge, or the child is unable to open the eyelid because of caked discharge.
Causative agents may be a virus, bacteria, or an allergic response (chemical or physical). Conjunctivitis may occur at any age in the life cycle.	Viral or bacterial infections can be transferred easily from one eye to the other. Pinkeye spreads easily among children and/or family members.	On close inspection, the eyeball appears red and inflamed. The child may rub the infected eye frequently and spread infection to the other eye. Explain the importance of not rubbing the eye. If the child is too young to understand, measures to keep the child from bending the arm and getting the hands to the face might need to be instituted. Children may become anxious and fearful when they wake up in the morning and cannot open their eyes because of dried discharge sealing their eyes shut. Application of a moist washcloth will help soften and loosen the crusts.
	Causative agents are identified by microscopic examination and a culture of the eye discharge.	Pinkeye *requires* medical management.

176

HEALTH PROBLEM	HEALTH CARE GUIDELINES	HELPFUL HINTS
	Inflammation of the lining of the eyeball can cause corneal ulcerations, leading to impaired vision. Medical management should be sought when an eye infection is suspected. Medical management is directed toward eradication of the source of infection and comfort measures. Antibiotic ointments are usually prescribed.	Pinkeye is highly contagious; therefore reduce contact of the infected child with others. Remember to keep this child's wash cloths, towels, and bedding separate from other laundry. Avoid permitting the child with pinkeye to swim in pools with other people, since this infection can be easily spread from one person to another through the water. If children swim in neighbors', friends', or relative's pools, caretakers are well advised to be sure the owners of the pools maintain high standards of hygiene and maintenance.
School phobia *School phobia:* Refusal to attend school.	School phobia is typically a symptom of an underlying condition of overdependency rather than a disease. Symptoms include reluctance to leave the caretaker, reluctance to leave home, refusal to attend school, and truancy. Somatic complaints or disorders, such as headaches, feeling tired, nausea, vomiting, and vague gastrointestinal tract complaints, are used as excuses to remain home.	Reluctance or refusal to attend school (school phobia) is usually a fear of leaving the caretaker and home. Some children express this reluctance as fear of school, the teacher, or the other children. Investigate the situation. After clarifying that indeed nothing unusual is occurring at school, insist that the child attend. Truancy cannot be tolerated. The underlying concern, overdependency on caretakers, is the problem that needs attention. Frequently the caretaker (primarily the mother) is overprotective and conveys a sense of uncertainty to the child, who reacts by not wanting to leave home. Rectifying this condition might require the assistance of a mental health worker or psychiatrist.
Sprain *Sprain:* Traumatic wrenching or twisting of a joint, causing injury to the ligaments and/or tendons.	Sprains can occur to any joint but the most common site is the ankle. Partial or total tearing of the ligaments may result.	Children frequently suffer the following sport injuries: 1. Muscle strains (overstretching of a muscle). 2. Sprains (a sudden, painful twist or wrench of a joint, involving injury to the ligaments). Strains are painful, but rarely is there swelling or discoloration.

HEALTH PROBLEM	HEALTH CARE GUIDELINES	HELPFUL HINTS

Sprain—cont'd

Following are signs and symptoms of sprains:
1. Pain (usually quite severe).
2. Swelling (immediate).
3. Discoloration (ranges from red to blue, depending on the amount of red blood cell rupture and/or subcutaneous hemorrhage).
4. The degree of disability depends on the severity of the injury (amount of tear).

Sprains require the following emergency medical management:
1. Rest, avoid all weight bearing.
2. Elevation of the foot.
3. Application of cold or ice packs.
4. X-ray examination should be performed to ensure that a fracture did not occur.

Sprains cause immediate pain and rapid swelling of the joint. Sprains often occur at the ankle.

Mild sprains can be treated at home by (1) elevating the foot on pillows and (2) applying ice packs for the first 24 hours.
Swelling usually disappears in 3 to 5 days.
Sprained ankles are often so painful and extensive that the child cannot walk (and should not walk).
Weight bearing can be resumed gradually with care.
Extensive sprains should be immediately immobilized, packed in ice, and the child transported to a hospital for x-ray examination, since fractured bones can accompany sprains.

Tinea pedis (athlete's foot)

Tinea pedis (athlete's foot): A fungal infection that invades the epidermis of the sole of the foot and tissues between the toes. Organisms associated with or identified as the causative factors are *Candida albicans* and *Epidermophyton floccosum.*

Athlete's foot is a common skin condition affecting males and females equally.
Blisters and cracks in the skin occur and are associated with intense itching. Open skin lesions predispose the skin to entrance of bacteria that can lead to secondary infections.
If untreated, athlete's foot can spread to other parts of the body. Early diagnosis and treatment is recommended.
Fungus thrives in damp dark areas. The surfaces between the toes and beneath the toenails are good media for fungal growth.
Diagnosis of the specific causative factor can be made by culturing skin scrapings and microscopic examination.
Prevention of athlete's foot is the best measure and can be accomplished by keeping the feet, especially the area between the toes, clean and dry.

Athlete's foot (tinea pedis) is a fungal infection affecting the skin of the feet. It is frequently found between the toes and is characterized by severe itching and tiny blisters filled with fluid.
Athlete's foot is usually considered more of a nuisance than a serious disease by most caretakers. In fact, some families consider it a natural occurrence.

Athlete's foot should and can be prevented.
In most cases athlete's foot can be easily controlled. The usual episode consists of intense periodic itching followed by raised blebs (blisters) that break when irritated. At times, deep cracks are created.
Children need to be reminded not to scratch or rub the areas because they are easily torn open.
When openings in the skin exist, other organisms can enter and cause a secondary infection.

HEALTH PROBLEM	HEALTH CARE GUIDELINES	HELPFUL HINTS
		Scratching may likewise spread the fungal condition to unaffected areas of the body.
		Others in the family who use the same linen or walk barefoot where the infected individual walked can also pick up the infection.
		The following recommendations may prove helpful in preventing and/or treating athlete's foot:
		1. Wear white cotton socks rather than nylon or dark-dyed socks (nylon and dark-dyed socks do not absorb moisture as do white cotton socks).
		2. Refrain from walking in bare feet.
		3. Wear shoes that are least likely to cause the feet to perspire.
		4. Keep the feet clean and dry especially between the toes.
	Treatment consists of local application of antifungal powders or ointments. Some physicians may suggest that the feet be soaked in a solution of potassium permanganate (1:10,000) to be followed by application of a drying lotion.	Application of over-the-counter powders, lotions, and creams usually keep this infection under control.
		Creams and lotions, if used, should be applied at night and removed by cleansing prior to dressing.
		If the infection is spreading, skin cracks enlarge, or raw bleeding is noticed, seek medical assistance.

Tonsillitis (sore throat)

Tonsillitis (sore throat): Inflammation of the lymphatic tissue of the tonsils (usually palatine but can include lingual and pharyngeal tissues).	The exact functions of the tonsils (spongy masses of lymphoid tissue) are not known. They are believed to filter out bacteria and assist in the formation of white blood cells.	Some children in this age period have repeated colds or sore throats. Recurrent sore throats are frequently related to infected tonsils (tonsillitis). The sore throat can be mild or severe.
	Following are three types of tonsillar tissue:	Occasionally children do not have sore throats, but have such enlarged tonsils and/or adenoids that they interfere with breathing and/or swallowing. These children frequently are mouth breathers and often snore at night.
	Palatine tonsils (frequently referred to as the tonsils) are located at the back of the oral pharynx. They are oval shaped, approximately the size of an almond, and are embedded in the mucous membrane.	
	Lingual tonsils are located at the base of the tongue.	
	Pharyngeal tonsils, commonly referred to as the *adenoids,* are located on the upper rear wall of the pharynx.	

ACUTE TONSILLITIS

Acute tonsillitis is characterized by rapid onset and is frequently accompanied by elevated temperature (up to 105° F; 40.5 C°) and chills.	Associated signs and symptoms could include the following:	Caretakers will frequently comment on how quickly children become ill. "He was playing all day, just came in, I felt his head, it was burning, and he complained of a very sore throat."
	Pain	
	Difficulty in swallowing (due to inflammation and swelling)	Sore throats (tonsillitis) can include the entire back of the throat or be localized. (Frequently the individual cannot describe the exact location.)
	Reddened throat (due to inflammation and swelling)	
	Headache	
	Lethargy	
	Malaise (general weakness)	

HEALTH PROBLEM	**HEALTH CARE GUIDELINES**	**HELPFUL HINTS**
Tonsillitis—cont'd ACUTE TONSILLITIS—cont'd	On examination of the throat, the tonsillar tissue may appear enlarged and reddened with a yellowish exudate or white patchy areas.	Some children only complain of pain on swallowing—others have constant pain. Some children may have headaches that accompany the sore throat. Medical assistance should be sought in the following circumstances: 1. The temperature rises to about 103° F (39.5° C) and stays elevated. 2. The sore throat prevents swallowing or interferes with breathing. 3. The sore throats arise frequently and children spit out (expectorate) thick puslike (purulent) mucus.
CHRONIC TONSILLITIS Chronic tonsillitis is a recurrent sore throat in which the onset may be less rapid. It is accompanied by fever and chills. The fever may be low grade (101° to 103° F; 38.3° to 39.4° C).	Symptoms may be similar to those associated with acute tonsillitis. On examination of the throat, the tonsillar tissue may appear enlarged and reddened, with a whiteish, puslike exudate. Frequently abscess areas can also be identified. Cultures obtained from the exudate of individuals with tonsillitis, examined microscopically, provide health personnel with the causative agent. When the causative agent is found to be group A β-hemolytic streptococcus, the sore throat may also be referred to as a "strep throat." Medical management is directed toward eradication of the causative agent and provision of comfort through antibiotic therapy, gargles (antimicrobial), and rest. If tonsillitis recurs frequently, interferes with breathing and/or swallowing, or the throat becomes abscessed, a tonsillectomy may be necessary.	Children who have recurring sore throats often develop chronic tonsillitis. The tonsils remain enlarged, and abscess formation is common. Removal of the tonsils (tonsillectomy) is often recommended. It may be necessary to obtain a throat culture (swab of the discharge [exudate] from the tonsils) to identify the organism that caused the infection. Knowledge of the causative agent determines the specific medication or gargles prescribed. Young children may need help learning to gargle. Teach them this procedure before they have a sore throat because cooperation is more easily gained when the throat is not painful. Children with tonsillitis are usually more than willing to rest additional periods. Caretakers know immediately when the child is better by the increased liveliness and reluctance to rest. Occasionally children who have been admitted to the hospital for a tonsillectomy have had the surgery cancelled. Surgery cannot be performed if the tonsils show signs of infection. (See Chapter 13, Hospitalization). Following surgery, the child's throat will be very sore. Keeping the back of the throat wet will reduce some of this discomfort. Have the child drink small amounts (two to four swallows) of lukewarm fluid every hour. (Avoid ice cold drinks because the chilling factor increases discomfort.) Success at getting the child to drink immediately after surgery is fostered through preoperative teaching. *The child needs to know that it is going to hurt to swallow but that drinking fluids will help relieve the pain.*
Tonsillectomy: Surgical excision of the palatine tonsils. *Adenoidectomy:* Surgical excision of only the pharyngeal tonsils. *Tonsillectomy and adenoidectomy:* Surgical removal of both tonsils and adenoids.		

HEALTH PROBLEM	HEALTH CARE GUIDELINES	HELPFUL HINTS
Verruca (warts) *Verruca (warts):* A viral infection invading the skin and underlying tissue (dermis, epidermis, and papillae). It can occur anywhere on the skin surface of the body, but most frequently affects the fingers, hands, and soles of the feet.	As the virus becomes lodged in the skin surface, it forms a small hard growth about ¼ inch (0.63 cm) in diameter. Warts can be flat or raised, dry or moist, or rough or smooth. Warts affect males and females equally, although they are more common in children and young adults than in the older individual. Physical discomfort is usually minimal, but the appearance of warts usually causes great concern to both children and adults. Warts that are painless rarely have to be removed. Many warts disappear without any treatment, although they may exist for many months. Plantar warts (located on the sole of the foot) may cause pain. Their location makes them more sensitive to continued irritation from pressure. Warts that are painful, rapidly growing, or bleed require medical management. Medical management may consist of the following: 1. Topical medication (acids) 2. Electrocauterization (burning the wart) 3. Cryosurgery (freezing with liquid nitrogen) 4. Use of x-ray therapy	Warts (verruca) are usually small, hard raised areas found by caretakers on the skin of their children. Although warts can be found anywhere, typically they are seen on the hands, fingers, or soles of the feet. Warts are rarely painful, but when discovered, it is tempting for children to pick at them in an attempt to remove them. Since warts are caused by a virus, dislodging some of the tissue enhances the growth of additional warts nearby and also permits the entrance of other microorganisms. Caretakers frequently purchase over-the-counter remedies of all sorts, only to discover that they do not rid the child of warts, but may cause scarring instead. Discouraging the child from picking or cutting off the top of the wart may be the best remedy, because it often disappears without treatment. Warts that occur on the feet (plantar) may be uncomfortable. Children might complain of a pebble or something in their shoe that hurts when they walk. The terms warts and calluses are often confused. In some instances both can exist. Seek medical management for the care of warts in the following situations: Several new warts emerge. Old warts change in size or consistency. Painful warts. Bleeding warts. A secondary infection is present at the site of a wart.

UNIT FIVE

ADOLESCENCE *establishing identity*

Adolescence is that wonderful age which spans the period from youth to adulthood. Young people in this period are struggling to leave the world of children and enter the world of grown-ups. During adolescence, young persons begin to make choices that will affect their futures.

In the past, most adolescents became independent adults after graduation from high school. They left the family home, established a residence of their own, and entered the world of work and responsibility. Lately, the trend has been to maintain a bond of dependency through the teenage years and into the twenties while preparing for future vocations. Whereas college educations seemed reserved for the wealthy or intelligent, there are now avenues available for advanced education for individuals from all walks of life. Extension of childhood has brought with it advantages and disadvantages.

Adolescence has been described as a period of chaos. Adolescents struggle with many external and internal factors. Although some teens may have strong family bonds, caring family members, and close friends to help smooth the path to adulthood, others do not. A teen's choices and decisions are often influenced by peer expectations and media output.

The 13- through 19-year-old is continuing to grow and develop physically, mentally, and emotionally.

New emotions, changes in body structure, and the lack of control of internal changes all contribute to a sense of uncertainty. Adolescence is a testing period for the development of self-worth, heterosexual relationships, and vocational choice. Energy seems to be diffused in many directions and is no longer controlled or directed as during previous periods of life.

Caretakers sense the need for granting increased independence and responsibility to adolescents. Caretakers do not always sense that adolescents will continue to need structure, discipline, and guidance.

Adolescents spend much of their time away from home. They focus their attention on one or two close friends rather than on groups. During the early years of this period, close friends are usually members of the same sex, but gradually the attachments change to members of the opposite sex.

The desire to be considered an adult coupled with the desire to retain the carefree life of childhood contribute to the growing pains of adolescence. Confusion experienced within the adolescent surfaces frequently and often explosively in the home setting, which strains family relationships. If trust, love, and a sense of humor can be maintained by caretakers and adolescents during this period of upheaval, the adolescent usually emerges with a sense of self-worth and identity and is able to adjust to the world of adulthood.

CHAPTER 15

ADOLESCENCE *13 through 19 years*

Young people 13 through 19 are no longer characterized as endless bundles of energy or as industrious workers, because this is the age of questioning, striving, and searching. The individual is seeking answers to "Who am I?" "Where am I going?" and "What am I to be?"

Body structure closely resembles adult size and proportions (due to both the final growth spurt and the secondary sex characteristics). Caretakers and often the adolescents themselves expect more adult-like behavior. However, new behaviors follow physical changes rather than precede them.

Adolescents continue to develop their physical and mental skills. These increased abilities permit involvement in many more complex projects. They enjoy competitive sports and games, although they question rules or add innovative twists to increase the challenge. Adolescents gain insight into their own unique talents through exposure to games, sports, and other multifaceted projects. These activities also assist in the development of responsibility and the ability to differentiate right from wrong, safe from dangerous, and even wise from foolish.

Adolescents are capable of and can be held responsible for maintaining adequate hygiene, rest, and nutrition. These three topics frequently become sore points between caretakers and adolescents. Often serious differences of opinion exist as to the meaning of "adequate."

Each generation seems to view the newest generation as a breed quite different from its own. These generation gaps may be due in part to the need for group identity that emerges with each successive generation. Fads in the form of foods, dress codes, and music are but a few of the ways in which group identities seem to emerge.

Another bone of contention frequently centers on "friendships." In some instances, close friends chosen by the adolescent may prove difficult for the caretaker to understand. Caretakers often have difficulties in accepting the fact that their children are growing, trying their wings, beginning to date, and preparing themselves to leave the nest. This final period of childhood provides the adolescent with the tools needed for future life.

GROWTH AND DEVELOPMENTAL LANDMARKS	**ANTICIPATORY GUIDANCE**

Biological

WEIGHT

Weight gain during these 6 years is unique to each individual. The total weight depends on factors that include biological makeup, activity, and food intake.

The normal ranges found in most actuarial tables reflect a weight range for sex, age, and height.

Weight change is common in adolescents. Young people who do not eat balanced meals, but snack on foods such as candy or fried chips, while being inactive, gain large amounts of weight quickly.

Young people who eat more balanced meals and are active do not gain as rapidly. (See Chapter 16, Nutrition.)

HEIGHT

Adult height is usually reached by the end of the nineteenth year, although some males continue to grow taller through their early twenties.

Height is unique for each individual.

The growth spurt that usually occurs in late school age or early adolescence may be delayed. Caretakers can provide support for the teenager who remains short when peers and friends seem to be growing taller and are developing adultlike contours.

Children whose parents are tall are more likely to be tall than children whose parents are short. Height cannot be increased by taking hormones, vitamins, or by stretching exercises.

HEART RATE

The range for heart rate will vary. The normal range at rest for females is 55 to 110 beats per minute and for males is 55 to 105 beats per minute.

Heart rates must always be reviewed in relation to the individual's emotional state and/or activities. Individuals who are athletic will frequently have a slower heart rate than those who lead a more sedentary life with short bursts of activity.

The pulse rate is readily obtained at all the usual pulse sites (radial, brachial, femoral, carotid, temporal, and pedal arteries).

The pulse normally is strong, with a regular rhythm. Arrhythmias should be monitored by health personnel.

Adolescents frequently become concerned because they can hear their heart beat or feel a bounding pulse after strenuous exercise. If the heart beat returns to a slower rate with less pounding, it was probably just a temporary adjustment of the heart to an increased work load and nothing to be concerned about.

If the rate remains rapid and/or the character of the beat can consistently be described as bounding, advice should be sought from health personnel.

RESPIRATION

The respiratory rate decreases to the adult range of 16 to 20 breaths per minute.

Normal respiration is usually effortless and quiet with equal bilateral expansion of the chest. Individual respiratory rates must always be evaluated in relation to the circumstances and activities in which that person is engaged.

Labored breathing may indicate the presence of a health problem.

BLOOD PRESSURE

Blood pressure readings reach adult values: 110/66 to 120/76. During adolescence, the systolic value is roughly equivalent to 100 plus the age.

Blood pressure will vary with each individual.

Males usually have higher blood pressure readings than females.

Following are other factors and circumstances that alter blood pressure readings:

1. The time of day. Early morning readings are lower than midday or evening readings.
2. Activity. Strenuous exercise will elevate the systolic reading.
3. Weight. Individuals who are heavy will have higher blood pressure readings than individuals who weigh less. A rapid weight gain will also increase blood pressure readings.
4. Emotional state. Fright, nervous tension, or excitement will elevate the blood pressure temporarily.
5. Race. Hypertension may be found more frequently in one race than another.

Blood pressure readings are now a routine part of the average health conference or health examination.

GROWTH AND DEVELOPMENTAL LANDMARKS	ANTICIPATORY GUIDANCE

TEMPERATURE

Temperature readings stay within the adult range: 97° to 99° F (36.1° to 37.2° C).

Temperature readings are usually lower in the morning than at midday or evening. (The highest temperature is usually reached between 2 and 4 PM.)

Other factors that influence temperature include the following:

1. State of health. Injury, illness, or dehydration will elevate the temperature reading.
2. Emotional state. Excitement, fear, and anxiety elevate the temperature.
3. Food ingestion. Following meals, body temperature will be elevated.

Body temperatures usually vary with the individual's activity, fluid intake, and environmental changes.

Temperatures that exceed 100° F (38° C) for several days or temperatures over 104° F (40° C) should be reported to health personnel.

HEAD

The head now has the size, shape, contours, and features of the adult.

The size and shape of the head are features that rarely cause concern among teenagers.

The features of the face (such as the nose, lips, eyes, eyebrows, and skin), however, create topics for adolescents' conversation and lamentation.

HAIR

The hair color and texture have reached adult characteristics.

Hairstyles are important to all adolescents. Fashion trends and styles that imitate popular figures in the entertainment, sports, or political fields dominate. It is often quite trying for the adult to see their young people dye, frizz, or straighten their hair.

NOSE

The shape, size, and contour of the nose are well established. Functions remain the same: differentiating odors, warming air, filtering foreign particles, and breathing.

Relatives and close friends begin to notice family resemblances based on characteristics of the nose.

The caretaker often loses patience listening to a teenager lament over a nose that is too long, wide, short, stubby, crooked, bumpy, hooked, etc.

MOUTH

The shape, size, and contour of the mouth are well established.

All permanent teeth are in place, with the exception of the second and third molars. The third molars, wisdom teeth, might not emerge until adulthood, and in some instances, they never emerge.

EYES

Binocular vision is well established.

Pupils should be equal in size and accommodate to light and/or distance.

Refractive difficulties peak during this period.

Normal visual acuity is 20/20.

If children blink excessively, hold reading material close to the face, rub the eyes, squint, or complain of discomfort, health personnel should be consulted.

Wearing glasses may be viewed as a deterrent to attractiveness or a nuisance. Emphasize the need for consistent usage. Neglecting to wear glasses can predispose the individual to further damage or deterioration.

Shatterproof glass is recommended in glasses for young people.

Many adolescents prefer to own and wear contact lenses. Hard and soft lenses are available, but require careful management. Recommendations from health personnel (in particular, ophthalmologists) should be scrupulously followed.

EARS

The shape and contour of the ears are well established. Structure and function are well developed.

Hearing should be binauricular.

GROWTH AND DEVELOPMENTAL LANDMARKS	ANTICIPATORY GUIDANCE

Biological—cont'd

EARS—cont'd

Large quantities of cerumen (earwax) may accumulate in the outer ear. Cerumen may interfere with auditory acuity.

Some adolescents complain of earwax (cerumen) and attempt to remove it with all types of small instruments. Avoid vigorous cleansing or the use of blunt instruments inserted into the outer ear because it is easy to damage the eardrum.

Controversy exists about the potential danger to hearing by continued exposure to amplified sounds (such as stereos, discos, or rock concerts).

SKIN

The texture of the skin has adult characteristics. The skin is dryer with less subcutaneous tissue, resilience, and softness.

Overactivity of sebaceous glands plus hormonal changes precipitate skin eruptions. (See Chapter 17, Acne.)

Skin changes are common. Adolescents express concern over every blemish they discover on their face. (See Chapter 17, Acne.)

TRUNK AND EXTREMITIES

The shape and contour of the chest, abdomen, and back reach adult characteristics.

Back

The spinal column should be straight with shoulder height equal on both sides.

Deviations, forward or laterally, in the contour of the spinal column may be indicative of structural deformity. (See Chapter 17, Curvature of Spine.)

Postural defects might be identified by caretakers or school personnel during this period.

If caretakers or others are constantly reminding the youngster to stand straight or put the shoulders back, it might be helpful to examine the child's posture.

Have the child stand straight, arms at the side with the back facing the examiner. If one of the shoulder blades is more prominent than the other or if one shoulder is higher than the other, health personnel should be consulted.

Another easy test is to have the child face the examiner and bend forward at the waist with arms extended to touch the toes. The contour of the back should be equal on both sides. If there is a noticeable deviation, in which one shoulder blade appears higher than the other, seek health personnel evaluation.

Chest

In the female, breast size and shape will vary with each individual.

In the male, musculature and hair growth will be unique to each individual and are determined in large part by genetic influences.

Expansion of the chest on inspiration should be equal bilaterally.

Extremities

The length, shape, and size of the extremities reach adult proportions unique to each individual.

Muscle mass becomes more evident in both males and females, particularly those who are involved in exercise programs and/or sports. Muscle mass is usually greater in males than in females.

Genetic influence is a major determinant in the proportions of the breast.

If there is one portion of the body that causes teens (both male and female) great concern, it is the chest. Females bemoan breasts that are too small or too large. Males believe that a lack of hair on the chest indicates a lack of masculinity.

Males and females frequently engage in exercise programs to attain physical fitness, better body physique, or to increase attractiveness. At one time body building and weight lifting were performed primarily by the male, but today this is no longer true.

GROWTH AND DEVELOPMENTAL LANDMARKS	ANTICIPATORY GUIDANCE
MOBILITY	
Muscle development and coordination reach the maximum level of adult performance.	Some adolescents will spend a great deal of time in physical activities that develop muscles and refine both gross and fine motor skills.
Gross and fine motor skills continue to be refined at greater levels of complexity.	Adolescents continue to test muscle strength, ability, and endurance and will overdo many of their body-building activities or physical fitness endeavors.
Eye-hand coordination permits intricate skills of manual dexterity that were not possible earlier in life.	Injuries to muscles, ligaments, and bones occur most frequently among adolescents involved in contact sports, gymnastic programs, or other strenuous activities.
The agility noticed in preschool and school-age children may be lost, partially through changes in body structure and increased muscle mass.	Clumsiness and awkward movements are characteristic of the young adolescent and are often related to the growth spurt of puberty.
Adolescents are self-assured in their ability to use and control their bodies in all activities of mobility. This overassurance leads them to take chances that may be hazardous.	Frequently activities are selected that provide a sense of accomplishment, such as hiking, mountain climbing, skateboarding, motorcycling, skiing, and driving cars. Many adolescents thrive on adding risk factors to activities.
	It is essential that responsibility and accountability accompany permission to use motorized vehicles. Teenagers need to demonstrate understanding of the rules of the road peculiar to each vehicle.

Psychological

DEPENDENCE-INDEPENDENCE-INTERDEPENDENCE

Adolescents strive to achieve total independence. Some reach their goal only to discover that they dislike the loneliness attached. Interdependence is more to their liking.	Family relationships can foster a blend of dependence, independence, and interdependence to provide a balance for mature relationships in the future.
Some individuals are independent in many areas, but remain financially dependent for many of their needs. This may be due to educational pursuits or other vocational aspirations.	Teenagers can participate with caretakers in greater decision making regarding major purchases, budgeting, and allocation of household chores.
Teenagers often appear self-sufficient and quite mature, but still require guidance, support, and enforcement of the set parameters within which they must operate. Teens can learn that increased independence must be accompanied by increased responsibility and accountability.	As teens obtain permanent employment, they can be expected to contribute to household financial needs on a set basis (weekly, bimonthly, monthly).
	Accountability and responsibility are key factors of every activity in which they become involved. One example focuses on the use of the family car. Guidelines for usage might include the following:
	1. Contributing monthly (or another mutually acceptable basis) to insurance, cost of gasoline, and routine maintenance of the car.
	2. Attaching a set of responsibilities to driving that demonstrate the utilitarian purpose of the vehicle. For example, teenagers who received their drivers licenses in one family were immediately made responsible for the weekly grocery shopping for a family of five. Although help was provided in the form of grocery lists, the new driver became responsible for budgeting a set amount of money and purchasing the needed food. At first the new driver did not mind making several trips to accomplish the task, but the novelty soon wore off, hastened by the discovery of the cost of gasoline. The outcome in each instance was a young person who could shop prudently, manage money, and use time efficiently. Coupled with the pleasure of driving came responsibility.
As dependability becomes increasingly evident, extended parameters should be added. By the time adolescents reach young adulthood, they should be capable of carrying out responsibilities and completing requirements both at home and school.	Deficiencies in meeting obligations by young adults may be related to the fact that they were never expected to develop a sense of responsibility.

GROWTH AND DEVELOPMENTAL LANDMARKS	ANTICIPATORY GUIDANCE

Social

SOCIAL AWARENESS

Adolescents develop a greater social awareness of the needs of others during this period. Although they are quite egocentric and concerned with self within the confines of their homes, they are easily attracted by a variety of "causes" in the community.

By the end of this period, the emerging young adult frequently becomes supercritical of the way in which adults have managed the societal problems of the world.

Caretakers often become annoyed that teens can become involved in the problems of the world, but cannot become involved in the chores at home.

RELATIONSHIPS

Peer group relationships are extremely important to the adolescent, since it is within these groups that they test and refine male/female roles and functions.

Teens still need groups to plan and participate in group activities, but a few close friends become all important.

Special groups called *cliques* emerge from the larger group of peers. Cliques frequently consist of a few close friends with similar interests who do everyting together and exclude others.

Adolescents who have developed a positive sense of self during earlier periods of life may have less difficulty with peer relationships and decision making in this period than adolescents who developed more negative self-concepts.

Invite and welcome the adolescent's friends and peers to the home. This maintains relationships and provides opportunities to maintain communication with the teen and peers.

Heterosexual relationships take precedence over other relationships. This may be based in part on societal trends, media influence, and changes in familial life-styles.

Adolescents imitate caretakers, television idols, stars, performers, and important others while developing their own heterosexual relationships.

Dating during this period changes from parties and group gatherings to double and single dates. This pattern of dating seems to be accelerated. Single dating now occurs early among teenagers. In past generations, single dates were reserved for the older adolescent.

Teens who are just learning about their newly developing bodies, feeling new emotions, and building new roles may have difficulty in handling behaviors associated with heterosexual relationships.

Heterosexual relationships may arouse feelings and behaviors that can lead to pregnancy, venereal disease, and/or emotional trauma.

The term *love* up to this point in life has often had a singular meaning. Within families it has meant sharing and caring about the welfare of others. In adolescence it seems to be related to physical attraction. Girls seem to refer to love in romantic terms, whereas boys refer to love in descriptions of physical acts.

Relationships with adults often change. The adulation of the school-age child for teachers or counselors is seen less frequently. Adolescents are more critical of the actions of all adults.

Relationships with caretakers often become strained. The ability to communicate with them is diminished.

The long-term psychological and social effects of early dating, sexual arousal, and intimate sexual relations has not been established.

190

GROWTH AND DEVELOPMENTAL LANDMARKS	ANTICIPATORY GUIDANCE

LANGUAGE

Teenagers can use language with ease.

They express their thoughts, describe their feelings, and communicate easily with peers.

Vocabulary continues to increase. Word usage seems to be the more noticeable aspect of language development.

Adolescents develop a jargon or dialect that is often difficult for adults to interpret or understand. The words used are words known to adults, but the meaning adopted by the adolescent is often different.

Each generation uses words or phrases in a unique fashion. Older siblings are often as confused as caretakers by the new meanings given to old words.

At times teens use new words inappropriately. It is helpful if caretakers or other adults correct young people, without humiliating them or laughing at the error. Too often, creativity and initiative are squelched or stifled through inappropriate responses.

Avoid jumping to conclusions about the terms young people use. Special meaings attached to the words need exploration by caretakers and youths to achieve common understanding. Communication gaps can be reduced through concerted efforts to increase understanding.

LEARNING

Inquiry and investigation continue to be an impetus for learning. Enthusiasm for learning, if fostered and rewarded in earlier years, usually continues throughout adolescence. Greater depth of learning can occur because young persons have increased abilities in abstract and reflective thinking.

Formal education leading to a high school degree is still a requirement for most adolescents. Experiential learning takes on a more goal-directed focus than in previous periods.

Adolescents choose and begin to prepare for the vocation of their choice. For many adolescents, formal education (whether vocational or academic) continues into young adulthood.

Some young people whose caretakers are avid readers might read more than children who have not had this exposure. Not all children will follow the example set by caretakers.

Forcing children into a particular mold for which they have no desire or talent stifles self-growth and can create unhappiness.

191

CHAPTER 16

HEALTH MAINTENANCE FOR ADOLESCENTS

Young people 13 through 19 are entering the period where they can assume responsibility for their own health maintenance. Some teenagers continue to enjoy good health, whereas others experience infections, diseases, or accidents.

Nutrition, adequate rest, and personal cleanliness continue to be major areas of concern. School, peers, and group activities frequently occupy much of the adolescent's 24-hour day and take precedence over the need for sleep. Often the adolescent is eating hurriedly, choosing junk foods that can be eaten on the run. Personal hygiene may be neglected in the early teen years, but often becomes overemphasized by late adolescence.

Maintenance may be more difficult than in earlier periods of life. Independence and experimentation predispose these youths to circumstances or situations that may be detrimental to their health.

Adolescents become more self-centered, focusing on their changing bodies, seeking control over their own lives, and experimenting with substances that offer new personal experiences. Experimentation with drugs, alcohol, and/or smoking is often fostered unknowingly by caretakers, peers, or significant others.

Role modeling and behaviors of caretakers and significant others are emulated by the adolescent. The caretaker's dependability, accountability, and responsibility within the home and community play a significant part in the adolescent's future behavior.

Health supervision, guidance, and discipline need to be continued by the caretaker. Emphasis is placed on assisting teenagers to become more accountable for their own health. This chapter will focus on areas of concern for the adolescent and provide helpful hints for health maintenance.

AREAS FOR CONCERN	HELPFUL HINTS

Health conference

Health conferences during adolescence are just as important as in earlier years of development. Thirteen- through nineteen-year-olds develop a concern and responsibility for their own health maintenance that will continue throughout their adult years.

Health conferences continue to provide opportunities to assess progress of growth and development and health status and provide counseling and/or teaching opportunities.

During early adolescent years (usually ages 13 through 15) caretakers may be present during the entire health conference and have access to information.

Sixteen- through nineteen-year-olds are frequently viewed as legal adults. Confidentiality of information remains with the adolescent. Adolescents may or may not choose to share this information with caretakers. State laws and regulations may vary, thus health care workers must be familiar with and adhere to those rules and regulations that govern their practice.

The conference usually consists of a health history update, physical examination, immunizations, and health education or counseling as necessary.

Health history (reviewed and updated)

The examiner will direct questions and comments to the adolescent.

Health assessment: physical examination

Physical examinations are continued on an annual basis.

The pattern of the physical examination retains the characteristics of examinations during previous periods of life. Vital signs, temperature, pulse, respiration, blood pressure, height, and weight measurements will be obtained and compared both to the previous records and to the expected norms for the specific age and sex.

Examination of the head will include gross visual and auditory screening tests, as well as direct inspection of eyes, ears, nose, and throat. Many vision or hearing problems will have been identified before the adolescent years.

If examination reveals a new vision or hearing problem, a referral will be made.

Palpation of lymph glands located behind the ears, along the neck, under the arms, and in the groin area will be included. Enlarged lymph nodes may be indicative of a health problem or infection.

A top priority in this examination is evaluation of the skeletal structure with close scrutiny of the curvature of the spine.

Assessment of the skeletal structure will be achieved while the adolescent is in reclining, sitting, and standing positions. The adolescent is requested to perform specific tasks, skills, or body maneuvers.

Helpful Hints column:

Health practices modeled by caretakers are often followed by the adolescent.

By age 16 caretakers need no longer accompany the youth to a health care conference.

Encourage adolescents to jot down questions or concerns they wish addressed during health conferences.

The caretaker or adolescent can provide the health care worker with information related to injuries, illnesses, or stress-related incidents that occurred since the last health conference.

When the caretaker accompanies the adolescent to a health conference, permit dialogue between the youth and examiner. Offer comments only when specifically requested.

A complete thorough physical examination should be performed annually. In some instances, school health screening programs or school admission prerequisites may provide the impetus for the annual physical examination.

Adolescents are usually willing to cooperate with examiners throughout health examinations.

Most adolescents have a general idea of the expected ranges of normal values for each measurement being taken. The information should be shared by the health worker with the youth.

If abnormalities of vision or hearing are noted, referral to specialists in the field occurs.

During examination of the spinal column it will be necessary to expose the back. Females should be given a drape or gown to provide continued privacy of the breast.

AREAS FOR CONCERN	HELPFUL HINTS

Health assessment: physical examination—cont'd

Structural deformities that may be evidenced during this period deal with forward and lateral curvatures of the spine. (See Chapter 17, Curvature of Spine.)

The performance of body maneuvers also provides the examiner with information related to the musculature, eye-hand coordination, and gross and fine motor skills.

Symmetry of the trunk and extremities is also assessed. Muscle mass and reflexes will be noted.

Auscultation and palpation of the chest, back, and abdomen will be performed while the adolescent is both sitting and reclining.

During assessment of the chest and abdomen, the examiner is gathering information related to the development of secondary sex characteristics (and in late adolescence, primary sex characteristics).

Female

Breast examination focuses on symmetry, size, shape, and color changes of nipples and areolar rings. Physical examination of the female is best scheduled following menstruation. Tenderness and engorgement of breast tissue associated with the menstrual cycle may provide misleading information if the examination is performed just prior to menses.

Health personnel should teach the procedure for monthly breast self-examination and emphasize its importance as soon as menses has begun. (See Chapter 18, Breast Self-Examination.)

Assessment of the external genitalia will include examination and separation of the labia majora and labia minora, noting size, symmetry, the presence and distribution of pubic hair, and the presence of any vaginal discharge.

Examination will also include inspection of the clitoris, urethra, and vaginal orifice. The presence or absence of the vaginal hymen will be noted.

Although some females may have a small amount of clear mucoidal vaginal discharge, the presence of large amounts of purulent or discolored discharge may be indicative of an infection or other health problems. Health supervision and treatment are required. (See Chapter 17, Vaginitis.)

Routine physical examinations of the female do not usually include an internal pelvic examination. It is advisable, however, that by late adolescence (15 to 18, or if the adolescent becomes sexually active), pelvic (internal) examinations with Papanicolaou's smear be performed annually.

Digital examination of the rectum may be performed.

Male

A breast examination, checking size, symmetry, color, changes of nipple and areolar rings, as well as the development of muscle mass, may be included during adolescence.

Examination of the external genitalia will include inspection of the penis for size, shape, location of the urethral meatus, and the presence of a prepuce (foreskin). If present, the foreskin should be easily retracted. If retraction is partial or difficult, this may be indicative of phimosis. (See Chapter 5, Phimosis.)

Helpful Hints:

School health personnel or physical education teachers are frequently the first to notice an abnormality of the spine. Recommendations regarding the suspected presence of a structural deformity should be acted on immediately by the caretaker.

Privacy should be maintained and exposure of body parts kept to a minimum. Draping should always be provided for breasts and genitals.

Self-examination of the breasts should be performed monthly by all females after the onset of menses. The best time for the examination is following menstruation. (See Chapter 18, Breast Self-Examination.)

Unnecessary exposure or manipulation of genitalia is to be avoided. The presence of a female during examinations by male health personnel is highly recommended to reduce anxiety on the part of the female adolescent.

The internal pelvic examination often causes anxiety and concern among females. Stress the need for and value of these examinations. Anxiety can be allayed and cooperation secured if privacy is maintained, simple explanations are provided, and the examiner is gentle throughout the procedure. The success of the first pelvic examination sets the stage for acceptance of this procedure in the future.

Some adolescent males may need reassurance that enlarged breasts, noticeable in the early teen years, are temporary.

Privacy should be provided.

Unnecessary exposure or manipulation of external genitalia should be avoided.

AREAS FOR CONCERN	HELPFUL HINTS

The urethral meatus should be centrally located and at the tip of the glans penis. Deviations of placement of the urethral meatus are usually corrected prior to this age. (See Chapter 5, Hypospadias, Epispadias.)

Examination of the scrotum is performed to determine symmetry and the presence of both testes. The left testis usually hangs lower in the scrotal sac than the right. Any swelling or fullness noted in the scrotum requires further examination.

Digital examination of the rectum is common in the physical examination of males.

Privacy should be maintained.

Explanations of the procedure and directions to be followed secure cooperation and enhance relaxation of musculature during examinations of the rectum.

Laboratory tests that might be performed include the following:
  Complete blood count (CBC)
  Rubella titer (among females only)

The adolescent may be asked to bring a urine specimen or provide one while at the office.

Adolescents can cooperate when a specimen of blood is required.

Health assessment: mental and social evaluation

Health conferences provide opportunities for the examiner to determine the progress of mental and social growth as well as physical growth.

Permit and encourage adolescents to express their concerns about their internal and external body changes. Free-flowing dialogue permits underlying concerns to surface that may not otherwise be identified.

Cognitive development is assessed through the adolescent's response to questions posed by the examiner throughout the examination.

Health protection

Adolescents require few if any immunizations. Tetanus or polio boosters might have to be administered.

A knowledge of past illnesses, injuries, and immunizations is needed by adolescents. Their health history is requested for overseas travel, college entrance, and at the time of hospitalization.

Health promotion

As in other age periods, the emphasis in health promotion is dentition, nutrition, elimination, sleep and rest, play and activity, safety, discipline, hospitalization, and sex education.

DENTITION

Dentition is complete, although in some individuals wisdom teeth (third molars) never erupt or emerge.

Dental examinations are usually recommended annually. The examination involves assessment of the number of teeth (extra or missing), presence of stains or caries, and the quality of the bite. It may also include x-ray examination.

Dental caries continue to be a problem.

Dental hygiene needs are well incorporated in the daily activities of every adolescent.

Adolescents can be responsible for making and keeping dental visits as needed to maintain good dental health.

Adolescents can understand the relationship between dental caries and eating foods high in sugar. Dental caries require repair despite discomfort. Neglect in this area can contribute to premature loss of teeth.

Malocclusions of all types have usually been identified prior to adolescence, although oral surgery and/or orthodontia may continue to be needed.

Teens who require orthodontia benefit from additional support and guidance from friends and families. Orthodontia can be quite painful. Teens may need reminders and encouragement to continue thorough oral hygiene when discomfort exists.

AREAS FOR CONCERN	HELPFUL HINTS

Health promotion—cont'd

NUTRITION

Nutritional requirements vary with each adolescent.

Caloric requirements depend on the metabolic, growth, and activity needs of the individual.

During the pubescent growth spurt, both boys and girls require a greater caloric intake than at other times.

Girls usually proceed through the growth spurt at a younger age than boys, thus most girls either plateau in their caloric requirements or begin to decrease their intake by the end of adolescence.

Girls ages 12 to 14 years need approximately 2400 calories.

Girls ages 15 to 19 years need approximately 2100 calories.

Boys continue to require more calories throughout adolescence than do girls because of the growth spurt and development of muscle mass.

Boys ages 12 to 15 years need approximately 2800 calories.

Boys ages 15 to 19 years need approximately 3000 calories.

Daily requirements of protein are 50 to 60 g. This need is attributed to the growth spurt of puberty in males and females, as well as increased muscle growth, particularly in males.

Calcium and iron continue to be necessary components of the diet. Calcium is needed for bone growth for both males and females.

Additional iron is required in females to replace losses during menstruation.

Vitamin C is needed for iron synthesis, cell growth, and tissue healing.

Vitamin A is necessary for tissue growth and vision.

Vitamin C and A are often limited because of the adolescent's preference for "junk foods" over vegetables and fruits.

Vitamin D is necessary for the use of calcium.

Vitamin B is in greater demand for males for muscle development and accelerated energy than for females.

Fluid intake varies with the needs of each individual and is based on activity, climate, illness, or other stressors. The average daily requirement of adolescents falls within the normal range of adult needs, 2000 to 3000 ml/day.

The daily nutritional intake for the adolescent should include selections from each of the four basic food groups. Recommended amounts follow:

Milk and milk products—1 to 1½ pints (0.47 to .71 L) a day and supplemented with cheese or other dairy products.

Individuals in adolescence are aware of, exposed to, and consume more fast foods and junk foods than in earlier periods. Peer pressure often contributes to food fads, crash diets, or erratic eating habits.

Caretakers, aware of the fact that growing teenagers have greater needs for proteins, vitamins, and minerals than younger children, can help their teens obtain the needed nutrients. Some suggestions include provision of daily breakfast, fresh fruits and vegetables for snacks, and involvement in food purchase, meal planning, and preparation.

Be aware that girls' appetites, nutritional requirements, and caloric intake decrease naturally shortly after the growth spurt ends.

Adolescent girls frequently become weight conscious. Noticing deposits of fat in the lower abdomen, pelvic, and hip regions, they will try "crash diets," which may be detrimental to their health. Rapid weight loss is to be avoided because often required nutrients for health are being omitted.

Some young people will refuse to eat or actually vomit that which they have eaten in an attempt to stay thin or lose weight. This can lead to a major health problem, anorexia nervosa (Chapter 17).

Adolescents require 2 to 3 quarts (1.9 to 2.85 L) of fluid per day. Fluid requirements increase with strenuous exercise, illness, stress, or as environmental temperatures rise.

Encourage adolescents to drink milk, water, and juices rather than coffee, tea, and carbonated beverages to meet their daily fluid needs.

Caloric and nutritional requirements of the adolescent vary with each individual, but the fact remains that the daily diet should include selections from each of the four basic food groups.

Milk and milk products are valuable sources of protein and calcium required for long bone growth and muscle mass development. Although milk is a valuable nutrient, it does not provide all the necessary daily requirements needed for growth. Foods high in iron and vitamins are needed as well.

Most teenagers enjoy ice cream and milk shakes. If encouraged or readily available in the home, teens will also eat grilled cheese sandwiches or sliced cheeses of many varieties.

AREAS FOR CONCERN	HELPFUL HINTS

Meats (including lean meat, poultry, fish, eggs, peanut butter, and legumes)—three servings per day.
Serving size:
1. Meat, poultry, or fish, approximately 4 ounces (112 g)
2. Eggs, 2
3. Legumes, 6 to 8 ounces (168 to 224 g)
4. Peanut butter, 2 or 3 tablespoons

The meat group provides calories, proteins, iron, and other minerals as well as some fats. Liver is well known for its iron content and should be included at least once a week. Remember that liver can be served in a variety of interesting fashions: homemade paté (chicken liver), liver stew, or dumplings often are winning entrees for fussy teen eaters.

Eggs, peanut butter, and legumes (dried beans) all contain high protein values and can be used as meat substitutes in the diet.

Vegetables and fruits—four to six servings each day, one of which is a citrus fruit or a vegetable high in vitamin C. It is desirable to include two vegetable servings daily and at least two to four fruits.
Serving size:
1. Vegetables, 4 to 6 ounces or ½ to ¾ cup (112 to 168 g)
2. Fruits, one medium piece or ½ to 1 cup

Fresh fruits still seem to be preferred over canned or cooked varieties. Fruit juice is often a teenager's favorite beverage. Cabbage, raw or prepared as cole slaw, and tomatoes are two vegetables that are high in vitamin C; oranges and grapefruit are fruit sources high in vitamin C. Vitamin C is needed on a daily basis to permit the body to use iron, grow new cells, and heal wounds.

Yellow vegetables and fruits such as carrots, squash, peaches, or apricots are excellent sources of vitamin A, which is needed for cell growth and vision.

Toward the end of adolescence, young people are often more willing to try cooked vegetable combinations. Comments heard frequently by caretakers include "Why didn't somebody tell me earlier, this was good?"

Bread and cereals—four or five servings each day.
Serving size:
1. Bread, 1 slice or 1 ounce
2. Cereal, 1 ounce (28 g) serving (either ready to eat or weight of cooked cereals prior to cooking)

Breads and cereals remain important to the daily diet as basic sources of carbohydrate needed for quick energy. Many breads and cereals are fortified with vitamins.

Most teenagers meet the daily recommendations for this basic food group, since their fondness for sandwiches, pizza, and pastas is well known.

Eating patterns
Early in the adolescent period the family pattern of three meals a day plus snacks is usually retained.

Older adolescents often develop erratic eating patterns—skipping breakfast, eating a partial school lunch, snacking throughout the day, catching meals on the run, frequenting fast food chains, joining friends at their mealtimes.

Eating patterns may reveal caloric intake in excess of growth and energy requirements. Overeating predisposes the adolescent to weight gain and obesity. (See Chapter 17, Obesity.)

Be aware that although sound nutritional practices may be taught in the home and school, the messages may be lost by teenagers whose major interests lie elsewhere. Nutritionally adequate school lunches may be available, but often ignored. Teens prefer foods and snacks of their own choice.

Family meals become more difficult to arrange because scheduled activities of the adolescent frequently conflict with family meals.

Caretakers can neither monitor nor enforce the food intake of the adolescent who spends increased periods of each day away from the home. Young people who developed and practiced good nutrition during earlier stages of life are likely to emerge from this period with similar practices.

The caretakers who notices the teenager (boy or girl) losing weight, tiring easily, or having a lower energy level than formerly, should investigate the teen's eating pattern and daily food intake.

ELIMINATION
Patterns of elimination are well established and unique to each adolescent.

Alterations in bowel or bladder elimination may result from changes in diet, climate, illness, or stressors of any sort. Most alterations are temporary and the cause is easily identified and quickly rectified. These include constipation, diarrhea, and frequent urination. If an alteration persists, health supervision should be sought. Other elimination problems that should receive immediate attention include the following:
Stools—black (tarry), loose, with strands of mucus or bright red blood.
Urine—smoky color, red tinged, or offensive odor.

The patterns of elimination are so well established by this period of life that it is no longer necessary for caretakers to monitor these activities.

Adolescents can be made aware of the ways in which certain foods contribute either to constipation or loose stools. Similarly, most adolescents become well aware of the relationship between intake and output of fluids.

Adolescents can be expected to report or raise questions if they notice anything unusual in their own elimination pattern.

AREAS FOR CONCERN	HELPFUL HINTS

Health promotion—cont'd

SLEEP AND REST

Adolescents require more sleep and rest than the school-age child because of increased growth, muscle mass development, and activities (physical, social, and/or emotional).

Requirements for sleep and rest are still unique for each individual, but 8 to 10 hours per day are highly recommended.

Caretakers might find it necessary to enforce a reasonable bedtime hour, particularly when teens must attend school the next day.

Adolescents frequently pack their days with one activity after another. It may be necessary for caretakers to intervene and set limits.

It is important that caretakers and adolescents realize that growth and changing bodies put new requirements on the body's systems. Adolescents' bodies need quiet times to permit the systems to catch up to the new demands being made.

It is often difficult for adolescents to reach a balance between needs for rest and sleep and desires of work, school, social life, sports, and other activities. Interestingly enough, some caretakers inadvertently foster overinvolvement in their pride and praise of the adolescent's achievements and abilities.

PLAY AND ACTIVITY

Individual pursuits and interests become well defined. Activities are quite goal directed.

Gross and fine muscle coordination will reach the peak of potential unique for each individual by the end of adolescence.

Interests, talents, and abilities will vary among adolescents and help determine the types of activities in which they will be involved.

Free play, toys, or simple games hold little interest for youths of this age. Competitive group or individual sports capture the attention of most adolescents.

Activities in which adolescents become engaged may not match the expectations or desires of caretakers. Youths should be encouraged in those activities in which they excel and provided with opportunities to progress toward their own full potential.

SAFETY

Teens striving to learn the limits of safety and their own capacities often go far beyond both with unfortunate results.

The adolescent is extremely vulnerable to vehicular accidents. State laws permit the young person to obtain operating licenses for most pleasure vehicles.

Young people often feel omnipotent, imbued with strength, courage, intelligence, and rapid reflexes. Caution is rarely an inbred feature of youth, it seems to develop as a result of experience.

Schools and the media provide many sound educational programs focusing on safety. Too many teenagers fail to believe the messages are meant for them. Principles of safety are also stressed in many places of employment.

Many schools and communities offer excellent driver education programs for teenagers. Unfortunately, the incidence of vehicular accidents involving teenage drivers remains high.

Enforce state and community laws. Prohibit driving experiences to those adolescents who are neither old enough nor licensed to drive.

Caretakers can help adolescent drivers develop a sense of caution by teaching and practicing defensive driving techniques. Rules of etiquette and courtesy taught and maintained within home settings have corollary rules for use on the highways. If caretakers adhere to safety standards and rules, the adolescent will have role models to follow that exemplify the practice of safety principles.

Adolescents should be encouraged to take driver education courses because they provide the groundwork for safe practice. (See Chapter 15, Dependence-Independence-Interdependence.)

Lessons on car maintenance may prove helpful to teach adolescents that there is more to driving a car than just filling it up with gasoline. Examples of lessons to consider would include the following:

1. How to change a tire.
2. How and when to check the oil level.
3. How frequently should fluid levels for transmission, radiators, and batteries be checked.
4. How often complete oil changes should be done.
5. Where the air filter is and when it should be replaced.
6. How to use jumper cables.

198

AREAS FOR CONCERN

HELPFUL HINTS

Other topics for operating motor vehicles safely include (1) how to drive on snow or ice and (2) how to push or tow another vehicle.

These are but a few examples to consider. Adolescents will learn accountability from these experiences.

Violations of principles of safety can result in accidents or injuries.

Some teens will be exposed to firearms. A thorough understanding of the operation and power of a gun should precede usage. Provide a role model of the principles of safety while using guns or other firearms. Avoid keeping loaded guns in the home or cars.

DISCIPLINE (LIMIT SETTING)

Basic to personality development is the sense of belonging, love, and security.

Limit setting during teen years fosters and promotes the sense of security that began in infancy.

As adolescents become comfortable and satisfied with themselves, they will gain assurance necessary for accomplishment of responsibilities in future roles.

Adolescents need to know that the caretakers are available to them to discuss their concerns. If relationships and lines of communication exist, adolescents will seek some advice and direction from caretakers.

Suggestions and recommendations made by caretakers are not always eagerly received. Caretakers should continue to offer suggestions, even though the adolescent finds them difficult to accept.

Discipline continues to be necessary. Consistency by caretakers in the expectations of teenagers' behavior is essential.

Adolescents need and want limits set. However, ambivalence is noted because most adolescents complain about the limits and frequently break them.

Acceptance of and adherence to the limits set in the home assist adolescents in the acceptance of and adherence to rules and authority figures in the community.

Limits are set and enforced by caretakers, although the adolescent should be given opportunities for input. Limits that are set should be based on age, independence, trust, and responsibility demonstrated by youths in their activities in the home and community.

Limits provide tangible proof that someone cares and help provide the knowledge of societal expectations for the future. Caretakers can feel comfortable knowing that although teens may complain bitterly about the limits that have been set, they are really needed and wanted.

SEX EDUCATION

Sex education continues throughout adolescence. Questions and concerns must be answered honestly. Center discussions on emotions and feelings as well as the physical aspects of sex. *Sex education should not be viewed as permission to engage in sex.*

Thirteen- through nineteen-year-old males and females must know and understand their own bodies and each others' as well. Sex education in this period of life should clarify and amplify the knowledges gained in previous periods.

Sex education is not a single lecture offered in school or a one-time discussion by caretakers. It is an ongoing development of knowledge and a sharing of concerns, beliefs, and feelings generated by changing bodies and abilities. Individuals fail to recognize that the physical growth of the body usually precedes the emotional maturity needed to use the new capacities with judgment.

Adolescents who know and understand the physiological changes that have occurred or are occurring usually have many questions and concerns about the feelings brought about by the physical changes. These feelings need open, free-flowing discussions. Caretakers, health personnel, teachers, counselors, and ministers are adults who have opportunities to assist adolescents with these concerns.

Being, sharing, caring, and loving are a few of the psychological topics that should be discussed during sex education.

Caretakers should be the primary source of information, providing adolescents with opportunities to discuss their concerns. If they do not, the teenager will discuss the topic with peers and learn about it from magazines, books, movies, television, radio, and other media sources.

If caretakers are comfortable in their own roles, they are able to discuss sexual topics without embarrassment. Finding the "right words" or the "right time" is not nearly as important as feeling comfortable with the topic. Leaving sex education to chance can lead to the development of negative attitudes about sexual relationships and roles.

The adolescent who boasts the most about sexual physical prowess often knows the least and may indeed be seeking knowledge

AREAS FOR CONCERN	HELPFUL HINTS

Health promotion—cont'd

SEX EDUCATION—cont'd

Teens receive mixed messages about the meaning of "love." In the family, it might mean caring, sharing, and being concerned about the welfare of others in the family. The media often present the view that love is synonymous with satisfaction of physical desires.

The word "love" does indeed have different connotations—love for parents, children, or siblings is different from love between males and females.

Love often has different meanings for members of the opposite sex. Females frequently define and describe love from a romantic view of affection, sharing, and caring. Males, on the other hand, view love as physical satisfaction. This may in part be related to the fact that young males often have a physical reaction (erection of the penis) without physical contact. The erection can occur while looking at a magazine or just seeing an attractive female pass by.

It might prove helpful and avoid misinterpretation, if boys and girls discussed "love" and its meaning to them early in a relationship, since girls view love as romance and affection, and boys view love as physical satisfaction.

Help teenagers understand that "sexy" feelings will occur both consciously and unconsciously. These sensations often pass quickly.

Families and health care workers can take more active roles in providing adolescents with opportunities to learn more about the psychological impact of sexual activity. Adolescents are becoming sexually active in their early teens. Little research is available as to the physical and/or emotional trauma that will result from these activities.

Every family has a unique view of appropriate sexual practices for the members of that family. Caretakers act as role models at all times, and their views in relation to sexual permissiveness are usually well known by the adolescent. Societal pressures, media, and peers influence the adolescent's behavior.

If adolescents have learned to accept changes (physical, physiological, and emotional), they should progress into adulthood with positive attitudes.

Caretakers who suspect their adolescent is sexually active should discuss the likelihood of pregnancy and the dangers of abortion. If sexual activity is to continue, information about contraceptives may be necessary. (See Chapter 17, Pregnancy.)

Adolescents who develop positive attitudes about their sexuality understand the relationship between the physical changes of their body and the feelings evoked.

Hospitalization

Adolescents may need to be hospitalized because of accidents, injuries, or sudden acute illnesses.

Most adolescents are well aware of the need for hospitalization. Health personnel and caretakers provide support, reassurance, and explanations throughout the adolescent's period of hospitalization.

Independence in self-care activities can be expected and fostered.

Hospitalization is often an unplanned emergency. If an adolescent has never experienced hospitalization, everything will be new and even frightening. The physical presence of caretakers may be reassuring to the adolescent. Do not be deceived by the outward calm presented by the teenager.

Teens will need support and reassurance but have difficulty voicing this need.

Separate units for adolescents are highly recommended. Adolescent units usually include television, private phones, and bathrooms. The privacy needs of adolescents are more like adults than school-age children.

Conduct an orientation to the unit on admission to the hospital or as soon as feasible. This orientation should include an introduction to roommates, health personnel, and the physical surroundings.

Limits and expectations of acceptable behavior within the unit should be well established and discussed in detail with the adolescent and caretaker.

Visitors to the adolescent unit need copies of the rules and regulations and can be expected to conform to them.

Although many hospitals have units reserved for adolescents with individual phones and televisions, hospitalized adolescents need to realize that a hospital setting is not the place for raucous parties, loud music, smoking "pot," or drinking alcohol.

Maintaining visiting regulations established by the hospital should be supported by both adolescents and caretakers.

Realize that hospitalization is temporary and that recuperation requires rest and a reduction in stress.

The rights and needs of other hospital clients are to be respected and take priority over the desires of a single adolescent.

200

AREAS FOR CONCERN

Adolescents can cooperate, but intrusive procedures are difficult to accept. Physical pain induces tears. Crying in view of other teens and individuals damages the pride of the adolescent. When intrusive procedures are going to be painful and/or prolonged, they should be performed in an area away from other adolescents with privacy ensured.

Adolescents will need reassurance and support during painful procedures. Health personnel should permit and even encourage crying, since it is as essential in this period of life as in any other. Statements such as "Don't be such a baby," "Don't cry," and "Grow up" should not be used.

Confidence and trust between the adolescent and health workers will be established if positive support and reassurance are offered throughout the entire hospital stay.

Management and treatment being considered for the adolescent's health problem should be discussed with the adolescent and caretaker. Truthful explanations, coupled with a willingness to listen to the adolescent's questions and concerns, make the experience of hospitalization more tolerable and less anxiety provoking.

Adolescent fears center around alteration in body image and lack of peer acceptance. Therefore expressing fears and anxieties should be permitted, and reassurance offered to reduce emotional stress.

HELPFUL HINTS

Realize that hospitalization often causes a regression in behavior. Adolescents may retreat to childlike behaviors that brought comfort. Expecting adult behavior at a time of stress is unrealistic on the part of the caretaker. Offering support, providing explanations, and permitting tears enable most adolescents to cooperate and work with health personnel.

Misbehavior such as spitting, biting, punching, cursing, or abusing health personnel during procedures is neither to be expected nor tolerated.

Caretakers can assist teenagers in gaining confidence and trust in health workers if they feel comfortable in these relationships.

Health personnel and caretakers need to remember that adolescents can comprehend subject matter. Permit adolescents to ask for explanations in regard to their health problem as well as be informed of the expected outcomes of the therapies and management being considered.

By late adolescence, individuals may well indeed determine for themselves the appropriate decisions to be made in regard to their health problem.

CHAPTER 17

HEALTH PROBLEMS OF ADOLESCENTS

The health problems of the 13- through 19-year-old change from the problems found in earlier periods of childhood. Accidental injuries continue to be a major health problem for adolescents. The injuries sustained are more frequently associated with vehicular accidents than with sports or other causes.

Immunization programs provide protection from many communicable diseases. However, immunization against communicable venereal diseases does not exist. Venereal diseases occur frequently among adolescents.

Nutrition continues to be a primary factor in the maintenance of healthy adolescents. Eating patterns of adolescents may be one of two extremes, overeating or undereating. Obesity is common in both males and females.

Health problems in this period of life are often associated with or fostered by hormonal changes. Females frequently experience alterations in menstrual cycles, such as irregularity and/or discomfort. Adolescents sometimes have health problems that are related to structural changes of the body.

This chapter will focus on the common health problems of adolescents, although it will not repeat discussions of conditions presented in previous chapters.

HEALTH PROBLEM	AREAS FOR CONCERN	HELPFUL HINTS
Acne *Acne vulgaris:* A skin condition associated with increased production of sebum from the sebaceous glands and characterized by comedones (blackheads), papules (whiteheads), and pustules (pimples).	Acne is the most commonly encountered skin condition of adolescents and is found in both males and females. Acne lesions occur most frequently on the face, neck, upper trunk, shoulders, and back.	Acne is an extremely common skin condition seen in adolescents (both male and female). Blackheads (comedones) and pimples (pustules) are other terms used to describe the lesions that occur. The lesions are found most often on the face and neck, although it is not unusual to find them on the chest, shoulders, or back. Lack of cleanliness was once believed to be the major cause of acne. Although cleanliness is important to reduce additional problems associated with acne, it is no longer believed to be a causative factor. Acne is a result of many interrelated factors, such as increased activity of glands associated with physical growth and reproduction, nutrition, and even additional stress.
	During adolescence there is an increased production of sebum that is directly related to increased glandular and hormonal activity. Hair follicle openings that are too small or narrow become plugged with sebum produced by sebaceous glands. The sebum at the surface of the skin turns black from exposure to the air, producing the comedone (blackhead). If the sebum plug exists entirely beneath the skin, a bump or papule forms with a whitehead at the tip. When this whitehead ruptures (either naturally or through aggravation) the sebum is released. Fatty acids contained in the sebum are irritating to the skin and cause inflammation and redness. Whiteheads that break naturally and are not further irritated, heal quickly without scarring.	The blackhead is so named because a fatty substance (sebum) is overproduced by the oil glands (sebaceous glands) of the skin, forming a plug. That portion of the sebum plug which becomes exposed to the air turns black—it is not dirt! If the sebum plug does not reach the skin surface, a raised whitehead is produced. This closed whitehead is characteristic of acne lesions. Eventually the whitehead breaks, and the sebum (fatty substances) is released onto the skin. This fatty substance is often irritating to the skin, causing redness and swelling. The area usually heals without scarring. The appearance of new lesions is often associated with menstrual cycles of females.
Acne conglobata: A staphylococcal infection of the skin that leads to pustules and abscesses.	The open acne lesion, however, becomes a portal of entry for pathogens and the formation of a pustule (pimple). If whiteheads are aggravated by squeezing and pushing, the sebum plug may be forced deeper into the dermal layers of the skin, predisposing it to the formation of abscesses. Abscesses and pustules can lead to permanent scarring. The occurrence or exacerbation of acne lesions may be related to ingestion of certain foods (chocolate, nuts, sharp cheeses, and foods high in fat), emotional stress (worries, fears, and anxieties), or contact with particular chemicals (tars and hydrocarbons).	Open acne lesions can become infected. Scarring can occur if the whitehead is overmanipulated (such as through squeezing or forcing it to break). Overmanipulation can cause an infection to occur, with development of a pimple (pustule), or force the plug deeper into the skin tissue, thus leading to the formation of an abscess. Squeezing blackheads, whiteheads, and pimples with the fingers and great force is to be discouraged at all times because it leads to new problems. Blackheads may be removed through the use of a comedone extractor, but caution should be exercised to avoid deep sustained pressure. Follow removal by careful application of a 70% alcohol solution to the exposed lesion. Acne should never be taken lightly.

HEALTH PROBLEM	AREAS FOR CONCERN	HELPFUL HINTS
Acne—cont'd	Medical management should be sought when acne is excessive or lesions go beyond the blackhead or whitehead stage.	When pimples (pustules) follow blackheads (comedones) or whiteheads (papules), health personnel should be consulted.
	Management is directed toward eradication of causative factors, control of papules, comedones, pustules, and abscesses and prevention of scarring.	
	Each individual reacts differently to medical management.	Each individual responds differently both in the development and control of acne.
	Local treatment may include thorough cleansing of the skin two or three times a day with mild soap and warm water. (Soap substitutes containing sulfur and salicylic acid may be recommended.)	Overall cleanliness and additional thorough washing of the face and affected areas are usually recommended.
		Perfumed soaps are omitted; mild soaps or soap substitutes are often used.
	Application of ointments and/or drying lotions is sometimes suggested.	Ointments and lotions are more frequently applied at night. New preparations should be tried on only half of the affected area at first to help determine effectiveness.
	Other aspects of medical treatment might include ultraviolet therapy, the use of antibiotics (tetracycline), or dermabrasion.	Adolescents might notice fewer acne lesions during the summer than in the winter. Related factors contributing to this reduction of lesions might include reduced stress and exposure to the ultraviolet rays of the sun. Exposure to ultraviolet ray lamps should never be attempted without medical supervision and direction.
Anorexia nervosa (self-starvation)		
Anorexia nervosa: Loss of appetite not associated with a physical disease that is characterized by excessive weight loss.	Anorexia nervosa is of unknown etiology. The health history does not usually reveal a previous physical or emotional disorder. The individual's perceived body image, family relationships, and self-control or will power are important factors.	Self-starvation (anorexia nervosa) often seen among adolescents is quite upsetting to caretakers. The caretaker cannot understand the teenager's sudden aversion to food. Even more perplexing is that anorectic adolescents are typically bright, intelligent, and well-behaved, with few previous problems.
	Anorexia nervosa occurs more frequently in females than males and is commonly identified during adolescence.	Caretakers who respond to the weight loss by urging teenagers to eat or by making negative comments about their appearance only compound the problem.
	Although loss of appetite and drastic weight loss (25% or more of total body weight) are the most striking features, excessive exercise, lanugo, and amenorrhea (in females) are often evident.	
	Anorectic individuals, if forced to eat, often induce vomiting.	
	Medical management is difficult and will vary with each person. Therapeutic counseling combined with weight gain and a return to a sound nutritional status are the basic components of the medical regimen.	Adolescents usually cannot stop the self-starvation on their own; counseling should be sought.

HEALTH PROBLEM	AREAS FOR CONCERN	HELPFUL HINTS

Appendicitis

Appendicitis: Inflammation of the appendix.

Appendicitis is one of the more common illnesses of children during school age and adolescence.

The appendix (a pouchlike appendage attached to the cecum and located within the lower right quadrant of the abdomen) has no known function.

For reasons not fully understood, inflammation of the appendix often follows a gastrointestinal tract infection. Inflammation also occurs when fecal material is blocked at the junction of the cecum and appendix.

Characteristics of appendicitis include abdominal pain, nausea (with or without vomiting), low-grade fever, and constipation or diarrhea.

Initially, abdominal pain is generalized, increases in severity, and gradually becomes localized in the lower right quadrant. (Young children may be unable to pinpoint the exact location of the pain.)

The fever may range from 99° to 102° F (37.2° to 38.9° C).

The discomfort of appendicitis is similar to the discomfort experienced in many other illnesses, such as mittelschmerz (ovulation), pelvic inflammatory disease (PID), gastroenteritis, or Meckel's diverticulum. Differentiation is sought through physical examination and laboratory tests.

Laboratory tests reveal an elevated white blood cell count exceeding 12,000 cells per milliliter of blood.

Physical examination is performed with the child lying flat on the back. The child with appendicitis will pull the right leg up toward the abdomen to relieve muscle tension at the right lower quadrant, and marked tenderness can be noted over the right rectus muscle (McBurney's point).

When appendicitis is suspected, hospitalization is required.

Medical management is often a waiting period until a definitive diagnosis is obtained. In some children, the appendicitis attack is mild, making a definitive diagnosis difficult. Hydration is usually maintained parenterally with intravenous fluids. Antibiotics may be administered parenterally.

Surgical intervention is performed as soon as the diagnosis has been established to prevent rupturing of the appendix and potential complications of abscess formation and/or peritonitis.

Appendicitis is sometimes referred to as a severe stomachache. This is misleading, since the appendix is located in the lower abdomen on the right side, and the stomach is in the upper left portion of the abdomen.

Children who complain of abdominal pain or cramping, accompanied by nausea, vomiting, diarrhea, or even constipation should be suspected of having an inflamed appendix. Although the child states, "I have not had a bowel movement," *do not give enemas or laxatives until the cause of the abdominal pain has been identified.*

The application of heat or hot water bottles is to be avoided if appendicitis is suspected, since this can hasten the rupture of the appendix.

Medical advice should be sought when the child complains of nausea, generalized abdominal pain, tenderness of the lower right side of the abdomen, and has a slightly elevated temperature. If indeed the child has appendicitis, surgery is necessary.

Inform adolescents of the reasons for all aspects of the management being carried out. (See Chapter 16, Hospitalization.)

HEALTH PROBLEM	AREAS FOR CONCERN	HELPFUL HINTS

Appendicitis—cont'd

If the severe pain disappears quickly, it is likely that the appendix has ruptured.

If the appendectomy is performed before rupture occurs, recovery is relatively rapid with few aftereffects.

Children whose appendix ruptured before surgery will have a longer convalescent period and a greater chance of complications.

Curvature of spine

Curvature of spine: Alteration in the normal curvature of the spine (Fig. 17-1).

During pubescence and adolescence, abnormal spinal curvatures are often identified.

Adolescents frequently develop abnormal curvatures of the spinal column. These curvatures can be caused by poor posture, congenital defects, or conditions that cause pain on weight bearing.

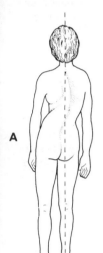 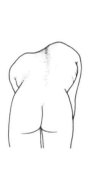

A

B 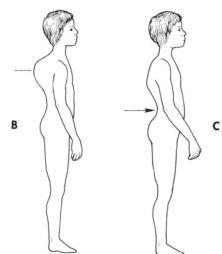 C

Fig. 17-1. Curvatures of spine. **A,** Scoliosis. Lateral curvature of spine. **B,** Kyphosis. Posterior or backward curvature of spine. **C,** Lordosis. Anterior or forward curvature of spine.

SCOLIOSIS

Scoliosis: Lateral curvature of the spine. Usually two deviations (curves) are present (S shape). The second curve develops as compensation for the first.

Although the exact cause is unknown, scoliosis can be classified as follows:

1. Congenital—malformation in the structure of the spine or rib cage.
2. Compensatory—deviation because of unequal leg length or pain on weight bearing.
3. Postural—consistent slumping when sitting or standing.

Scoliosis is much more common in females than in males.

A high familial tendency is noted with scoliosis. If the condition is found in one family member, other family members should be examined.

S-shaped curves (scoliosis) are lateral curves of the spine.

Scoliosis is frequently found in more than one family member.

HEALTH PROBLEM	AREAS FOR CONCERN	HELPFUL HINTS
	Alterations in spinal curvature are insidious because they do not cause pain or discomfort. The deviation remains unnoticed until the curvature is quite pronounced.	
	Scoliosis can be detected during the physical examination. Observation of the adolescent standing erect with arms at the side or bending forward at the waist will reveal the following disparities:	Caretakers become aware that something is wrong when hem lines hang lower on one side, pant legs need to be shorter on one side, or tight fitting shirts or jackets tend to pucker or gather more on one side.
	1. Uneven shoulders, scapulae, or hips. 2. Greater space between the arm and body on one side than the other.	Gym teachers may detect uneven shoulder or hip heights when the adolescent is performing stretching or bending exercises.
		School nurses and health personnel will frequently identify this problem in similar fashion and through more thorough physical examinations.
	Instructing the adolescent to stand straight will not eliminate the deviation.	If curvature of the spine is well established, admonitions from caretakers to "sit up" or "stand straight" cannot be followed by the adolescent.
	Once scoliosis is detected, medical management is required. Management is unique for each individual and depends on many factors, including the age of discovery and severity of the curvature.	Medical management is required.
	If the defect is identified early or the curvature is slight, a brace (Milwaukee) can provide correction. The Milwaukee brace is initially worn for 23 hours a day. As improvement takes place, the length of time the brace must be worn is decreased until it is worn only at night and finally not at all.	A brace may be ordered. Adolescents need to know that the brace is not uncomfortable to wear. They must be willing to wear the brace for the prescribed periods of time to benefit from this treatment. It does not take long before they realize they are more comfortable with the brace on than off.
		The brace is not easily hidden by clothing, and adolescents often rebel against wearing it. Patience and understanding by caretakers and peers will help support the adolescent.
		Adolescents need encouragement (even though the brace must be worn) to stay active in as many activities as possible and continue peer relationships.
	Surgery may be necessary if the spinal curvature is severe or structural. One method may be the use of Harrington rods (metal rods) inserted and attached to the vertebral column by means of clips.	
	Spinal fusion is another surgical method used to correct the deformity.	
	Surgical intervention, whether spinal fusion or the use of Harrington rods, is followed by casting and/or braces. External supports such as casts or braces are worn for at least 6 to 8 months following surgery. (See Chapter 18, Cast Care.)	

HEALTH PROBLEM	AREAS FOR CONCERN	HELPFUL HINTS
Curvature of spine—cont'd KYPHOSIS (HUMPBACK OR HUNCHBACK) *Kyphosis:* Abnormal posterior or backward curvature of the spinal column.	Kyphosis may accompany scoliosis. The causative factor is commonly faulty posture. Other factors may include congenital anomalies, compression fractures, rickets, and arthritis. If the causative factor is faulty posture, exercise programs that strengthen the shoulder, back, and abdominal muscles are instituted.	Humpback (kyphosis) is a backward curvature of the upper spine. Girls encourage the development of kyphosis (humpback) by walking with their shoulders slumped and arms pulled forward. This posture is often assumed as adolescents develop breast tissue. Exercise programs are helpful if the defect is due to faulty posture. Activities such as swimming, dancing, acrobatics, weight lifting, and bowling assist adolescents in the further development of the desired muscles. *Exercise programs are helpful only if followed on a daily basis.*
LORDOSIS *Lordosis:* Abnormal anterior or forward curvature of the spinal column.	Lordosis may accompany scoliosis.	
Drug abuse *Drug abuse:* Any substance taken in excess for the effect it produces.	Drug abuse is a major health problem of adolescents with many causes or contributing factors. Peer pressure, escapism, depression, and the desire for new experiences are among the more common causative factors. Substances commonly used by adolescents include depressants (barbiturates and tranquilizers), stimulants (amphetamines and cocaine), alcohol, marijuana, narcotics (opiates), glue, and LSD (lysergic acid diethylamide). The substances are taken orally, parenterally, or inhaled. Almost every drug has a number of popular or slang names. These slang (street) names change frequently. Each person reacts uniquely to the ingredients used. Some can tolerate large amounts of potentially dangerous substances for long periods of usage, whereas others become physically and/or psychologically dependent on these substances quite rapidly.	The excessive use of any substance (drugs, alcohol, cigarettes) for the effect it produces is considered drug abuse. Many adults do not realize that they provide the role model for drug abuse, since many adults smoke, drink, or take drugs in excess of their physicians' orders. Often, adolescents turn to drugs when they are under stress, find too much conflict in the home, or believe they can no longer communicate with the adults in their environment. Caretakers frequently overreact or panic when they learn that an adolescent is using/trying drugs such as marijuana, LSD, narcotics, depressants, or stimulants. Yet, caretakers often condone the use of alcohol. It is essential that caretakers and adolescents realize that the use of alcohol is extremely dangerous and perhaps more damaging to the body than some of the other substances that people try. The street, or popular, names of drugs and the drugs that are available to young people vary with the times. It would be helpful for caretakers to keep abreast of new terms or names of drugs as well as the effects of drugs.

HEALTH PROBLEM	AREAS FOR CONCERN	HELPFUL HINTS
		Adolescents' friends might think it funny to add a drug to a drink or food at parties. Some drugs, particularly LSD, can cause violent mind transformation or body reactions.
		Drugs and alcohol should never be used together, since they can cause irreversible damage to body organs, coma, and even death.
		Knowing the typical behavior of the adolescent and maintaining open lines of communication are often key factors in identifying potential drug problems.
		The use of drugs changes an individual's behavior in a variety of ways.
		Drug abuse might be suspected if an adolescent becomes withdrawn, changes friends, turns away from activities once enjoyed, demonstrates marked changes of mood, or school grades drop.
Addiction: An overwhelming compulsion or need to take a substance, usually in increasing amounts. Can lead to physical and/or psychological dependence.	Physical dependence exists when physical signs or symptoms appear when the drug is withheld.	Many drugs can cause physical and/or psychological dependency needs (addiction).
	Psychological dependence exists when individuals believe they must have the substance to function effectively.	
	Drug abuse can usually be detected through laboratory tests, although some drugs or substances leave no evidence.	Addiction does not always occur with frequent or sustained use of a drug, although conversely, addiction can occur quickly in some people who only try the drug a few times.
	Individuals who are addicted usually need medical treatment and psychological counseling.	Treatment is usually quite prolonged and requires counseling. Often the entire family needs professional help.
Hepatitis (liver disease)		
Hepatitis: Inflammation of the liver.	Inflammation of the liver (hepatitis) is usually caused by a virus. Toxic substances such as poisons or certain drugs can also cause hepatitis.	Hepatitis is sometimes referred to as *yellow jaundice* or *liver disease.*
	Acute hepatitis is seen more frequently than chronic, although both are prevalent.	
Type A is infectious hepatitis (IH) which is transmitted orally or parenterally with a 2- to 6-week incubation period.	The IH virus (infectious hepatitis) can be found in the feces or body fluids such as blood, saliva, urine, or semen of infected individuals. Transmission occurs through contact with any of the body fluids or feces of the infected individual.	There are two basic types of hepatitis commonly found in adolescents: infectious hepatitis, which easily spreads from one person to another, and serum hepatitis, which is spread only by the transfer of infected blood from one person to another.
Type B is serum hepatitis (SH), which is transmitted parenterally with a 6-week to 6-month incubation period.	The SH virus (serum hepatitis) is found in only the blood of infected individuals. Transmission occurs through blood or plasma transfusions (using blood from infected individuals) and contact with contaminated needles or other instruments.	Infectious hepatitis can be spread through direct body contact such as kissing, intercourse, handling linen contaminated with the feces or urine of an infected person, or by contact with the blood or blood products of an infected person.
		Infectious and serum hepatitis can both be spread to an uninfected person through injections with contaminated needles.

HEALTH PROBLEM	AREAS FOR CONCERN	HELPFUL HINTS
Hepatitis—cont'd	Hepatitis is characterized by a variety of signs and symptoms, often beginning with malaise, fever, or vague complaints of abdominal discomfort. Fever, when present, ranges from 100° to 103° F (37.8° to 39.4° C). The malaise and discomfort suddenly changes to nausea, vomiting, abdominal pain, or the onset of jaundice. Jaundice occurs more often in adults than children. Jaundice (yellow discoloration) is first noticed in the sclera of the eye, followed by a change of skin color. The intensity of the jaundice is often indicative of the severity of the hepatitis. Jaundice remains visible from 1 to 6 weeks and gradually recedes. Complete recovery usually requires 4 months or more. Medical management is required. Rest and adequate nutrition are key ingredients for recovery. Antibiotics are not useful in hepatitis. Drug therapy is kept to a minimum because drug detoxification by the liver is altered by the disease.	The early symptoms of hepatitis are often similar to those of so many other communicable diseases: vague complaints of being tired, abdominal discomfort, loss of appetite, headache, or low fever. The symptoms intensify to nausea and vomiting, abdominal pain, and the appearance of a yellow tinge first seen in the white of the eye (sclera) and later in the skin and urine. This yellow color (jaundice) may be mild, moderate, or severe. The amount of jaundice often indicates the severity of the illness. Even though the jaundice disappears within 6 weeks, recovery from the disease is not complete. Hepatitis requires medical supervision and often hospitalization for prolonged periods. Blood studies differentiate the types of hepatitis. Isolation is not required for serum hepatitis. Infectious hepatitis requires isolation of the infected individual for at least 1 to 2 weeks after the onset of the jaundice to protect others from contracting the disease. Many adolescents can be cared for in the home quite well.
	Bed rest is recommended until all symptoms have disappeared, then a gradual increase in activity is begun. Adequate nutrition reflects selections from the basic four food groups with an emphasis on caloric requirements needed for the age, sex, and height of the individual and additional vitamins (especially vitamin B complex). Alcohol of any type is forbidden. Individuals usually recover from acute hepatitis and develop immunity to future infection by that virus.	Bed rest and good nutrition are absolute requirements for recovery. The diet should include foods from all four basic food groups and contain enough calories needed for the specific age and height. (See Chapter 16, Nutrition.) Four or five light meals plus two snacks might be better tolerated than three large meals. Like so many other communicable diseases, active immunity to the hepatitis virus often exists after the illness. Presently there is no active immunization available.
	Gamma globulin given following exposure to individuals with infectious hepatitis has proven to minimize the effects, although it does not prevent the illness per se. Research is ongoing to produce a vaccine that will provide effective immunity.	Gamma globulin given to exposed individuals may reduce the impact of the illness.
Infectious mononucleosis (glandular fever, "kissing disease") *Infectious mononucleosis:* Acute infectious disease primarily affecting lymphoid tissue.	Infectious mononucleosis is seen in adolescents and young adults and is believed to be caused by a virus (Epstein-Barr).	Infectious mononucleosis is a common adolescent health problem frequently referred to as "kissing disease," "mono," "infectious mono," or "gland fever."

210

HEALTH PROBLEM	AREAS FOR CONCERN	HELPFUL HINTS
	The exact period of incubation is unclear, although it can range from 1 to 7 weeks. Typically, symptoms appear within 2 weeks.	This illness is believed to be spread through direct contact such as mouth to mouth (thus the name, "kissing disease").
	Symptoms of the infection may not be evident in some individuals but they may harbor the virus in the upper respiratory tract (mouth and throat). Carriers of the infectious virus transmit the disease primarily through mouth-to-mouth contact.	
	The severity of infection will vary in each individual. Some will have a subacute form (minimal manifestations) of the disease, but more typically the acute form is characterized by the following: 1. Fever (100° to 102° F; 37.8° to 38.9° C) 2. Sore throat (resembling that of "strep throat") 3. Headache 4. Enlarged lymph nodes (over entire body)	Some individuals may notice nothing more than feeling weak and tired. For those who experience a full-blown illness it will typically begin with overall feelings of weakness and being tired. The fatigue and weakness increase and are accompanied by fever, sore throat, enlarged lymph glands, and often a headache. The person complains of "feeling lousy" and wants nothing more than to stay in bed and sleep.
	A generalized weakness and complaint of being tired are common findings.	Since this illness can have serious ramifications, it is important that the diagnosis be made by health personnel.
	There may also be a skin rash resembling that of rubella (measles), liver involvement with slight jaundice, and/or splenomegaly (enlarged spleen).	
	During the acute stage of the illness, individuals willingly confine themselves to bed. It is not uncommon for the fatigue and malaise (both physical and mental) to persist for several weeks.	
	Diagnosis by laboratory examination will often reveal abnormal white blood cells with a single nucleus. The Paul-Bunnell agglutination test demonstrates the presence of specific antibodies.	
	No specific treatment exists. Supportive therapy is directed toward comfort and rest. Warm water gargles and aspirin prove helpful for sore throats.	Treatment is usually managed in the home and consists of prolonged bed rest; aspirin to reduce fever and pain; and increased amounts of fluid.
	Antibiotics are rarely given, since they are ineffective against the virus.	
	Infectious mononucleosis seems to be a self-limiting disease with complete recovery. During the convalescent period, however, relapses can occur. After recovery, recurrence is unlikely.	Recovery is usually complete. Individuals begin to feel better and must be cautioned against overdoing because relapses (return of symptoms) can occur during the recovery stage. A gradual increase of activities (both physical and mental) is advised.
	Although all signs and symptoms have disappeared, the infected individual may harbor and pass the virus on to others for periods extending beyond 1 year.	Even after all signs and symptoms have disappeared, the disease can still be transmitted to others. The virus can be harbored in the throat of the adolescent for as long as 1 year after the infection.

HEALTH PROBLEM	AREAS FOR CONCERN	HELPFUL HINTS
Mittelschmerz		
Mittelschmerz: Painful ovulation (release of ovum from ovary).	Mittelschmerz, painful ovulation, occurs in some females before menses establishes a regular cycle.	Painful ovulation (mittelschmerz) occurs in some adolescents, particularly before a regular pattern of menstruation is established.
	The low abdominal pain resembles that of appendicitis and may also be accompanied by nausea and/or vomiting. The abdominal pain never localizes to the lower right quadrant but is more prominent on one side than the other. Discomfort usually disappears within 48 hours.	Discomfort rarely exceeds a day or two.
	No medical or surgical treatment is necessary.	
Obesity (corpulence, fat)		
Obesity: An abnormal amount of body fat.	Obesity exists when body weight exceeds 20% of normal ranges for sex, height, and age.	The terms fat, fatty, or fatso are frequently used to describe the child/adolescent who is grossly overweight (obese). Other terms exist that are even less kind. There are periods in life when individuals are extremely vulnerable to gaining weight. One of those vulnerable ages happens to be adolescence when body structures change, hormones behave differently, and activity patterns are altered.
	Obesity results when more calories are ingested than are used by the individual. The causes of obesity are many and complex. Following are some causative factors:	The most common cause of obesity (gross overweight) is consistently eating more food than is necessary for the body needs and activities.
	1. Sex—obesity is more common in females.	A myth exists that it is fine for early teenagers to have some "baby fat" because this fat is needed for the rapid growth spurt of the later teen years. Eating habits established during childhood and maintained in adolescence will also be retained during adult life.
	2. Hereditary or familial tendencies.	
	3. Age.	
	a. Early infancy—growth needs.	
	b. Early pubescence—growth spurt and hormonal changes.	The greatest key to prevention of obesity in adults is to prevent it in children and adolescents.
	c. Pregnancy—increased nutritional needs.	Although overeating is the greatest causative factor, other factors such as activity, stress, and the individual's sex can also contribute to weight problems. It will be no comfort for adolescent girls to know that almost three times as many girls as boys gain weight in excessive amounts during adolescence.
	d. Middle age—hormonal change and decreased activity.	
	4. Activity—as activity decreases, dietary intake remains the same.	
	5. Cultural—family patterns may stress food.	
	6. Psychological—food becomes a substitute for gratifying unmet needs.	Contrary to public opinion, few individuals have physical problems, such as underactive glands, that cause weight gain.
	7. Physiological—endocrine or metabolic disorders such as hypothyroidism or adrenal malfunction affect use of calorie intake.	Excessive weight gain can cause emotional stress and contribute to the development of a poor body image and negative self-concept. When this occurs, adolescents often retreat into themselves and become less active and less outgoing, causing a vicious cycle.
	Excessive amounts of body fat predispose individuals to the following health problems:	
	Structural—increased strain on joints and ligaments such as pes planus (flatfoot), genu valgum (knock-knee), and slipped femoral epiphysis.	

HEALTH PROBLEM	AREAS FOR CONCERN	HELPFUL HINTS

Psychological—poor body image, limited self-concept, loneliness, and introversion.

Heart—enlargement because of overwork and strain.

Circulatory system—blockage, either partial or complete, leading to atherosclerosis and hypertension.

If a physiological problem exists, it must be corrected. Medical supervision and intervention may be required.

Weight loss is achieved by reducing dietary intake below the calories required for physiological needs and activities.

Weight reduction programs must maintain nutritional requirements from the four basic food groups. Diets should be geared to achieve a weight loss of 1 or 2 pounds a week. Counseling, support, and reeducation to new patterns of eating should be included in the reduction program. Losing weight is usually only a part of the problem. Keeping it off might be a lifetime challenge.

Consistent obesity can contribute to physical problems in adolescence and health problems in the future, such as an enlarged heart, high blood pressure (hypertension), and poor circulation (atherosclerosis).

Adolescents who are fat need and usually want help. When physical problems for weight gain have been eliminated, weight loss can be achieved by reducing food intake below the amount the individual is accustomed to eating.

First determine how much food is being eaten. Keep a 2- or 3-day food diary and add the calories for each food item to determine the total calories consumed each day.

Second, determine how much you should weigh. Following is a good rule of thumb for the lowest weight for a particular height:

1. a. For girls 14 years old and over: 100 pounds (45 kg) for 5 feet (150 cm) plus 5 pounds (2.27 kg) for each additional inch.
   b. For boys 14 years old and over: 110 pounds (49.5 kg) for 5 feet (150 cm) plus 5 pounds (2.27 kg) for each additional inch.
2. Then multiply this amount by 10 calories for each pound (only while losing weight).
   a. A girl 14 years old whose height is 5 feet, 4 inches (160 cm), should not weigh less than 120 pounds (54 kg) and can eat 1200 calories/day. The amounts are obtained using the formulas: 100 pounds for the first 5 feet plus 4 inches times 5 pounds (100 + 20 = 120 pounds), 120 pounds × 10 calories equals 1200 calories (120 × 10 = 1200 calories).
   b. A boy 5 feet, 6 inches (165 cm), should not weigh less than 140 pounds and can eat 1400 calories/day. The amounts are obtained using the formulas: 110 pounds for the first 5 feet plus 6 inches times 5 pounds (110 + 30 = 140 pounds), 140 pounds × 10 calories equals 1400 calories (140 × 10 = 1400 calories).

HEALTH PROBLEM	AREAS FOR CONCERN	HELPFUL HINTS

Obesity—cont'd		3. Compare these calorie amounts to those which you are presently eating and to the typical amounts expected during this age period. (See Chapter 16, Nutrition.) Usually there is between a 600- and 1000-calorie difference, which will provide a weight loss of 1 to 2 pounds (0.45 to 0.9 kg) a week.
		4. Avoid fad diets or crash diets. Invariably they leave out needed nutrients, or the diet becomes boring too soon.
		5. Obtain a copy of a weight loss program you can follow (check with the school nurse, family physician, parents, and books).
		6. *Start.*
		  a. Be sure to include 3 meals a day (do not skip meals).
		  b. Select food from all four food groups.
		  c. Provide snacks for yourself (raw fruits or vegetables).
		  d. Try out new foods and recipes on your own.
		7. Weigh yourself once a week. Body weight changes daily, but it goes up as as well as down—do not get discouraged.
		8. Seek support from friends and relatives.
		9. Add activities to your life such as an exercise program, walking, hiking, biking, bowling, tennis, or swimming. Avoid sitting around feeling sorry for yourself.
		10. When you reach your goal, add foods back carefully. Continue to weigh yourself once a week, and cut back immediately if you gain 2 to 3 pounds (0.9 to 1.35 kg).

HEALTH PROBLEM	AREAS FOR CONCERN	HELPFUL HINTS

Pregnancy (parturition)

Pregnancy· The growth and development of a fetus (baby) in the female body, following the uniting of an ovum (egg) and a spermatozoon (sperm).

The incidence of pregnancy both preceding and during the adolescent years is increasing.

Pregnancy in the preadolescent and/or adolescent girl is often the result of antisocial behavior, rebellion against parents, search for affection, or the inability to control new sexual feelings.

There are many potentially dangerous aspects associated with pregnancy in females under 15 years of age. Lack of physical maturity (both physical structure and reproductive organs) and inadequate nutrition predispose the adolescent to toxemias of pregnancy, premature labor, or other complications.

Health professionals are often the first to learn of or confirm that a pregnancy exists. Nonjudgmental trusting relationships need to be established and maintained with the adolescent who often is beset with anxieties and fears. Following are issues that must be faced, and difficult decisions that must be made:

Informing the sex partner
Marriage
Informing parents
Remaining at home
Leaving the community
Natural termination of the pregnancy
Abortion
Keeping the child
Placing the child for adoption
Returning to school

Because each adolescent is unique, so too are the resolutions or decisions that are made.

The adolescent will require support and counseling during and after the pregnancy.

If the decision is to proceed with the pregnancy, then prenatal care is essential.

Prenatal care focuses on the following issues:
1. Maintenance of health
2. Adequate nutrition
3. Pregnancy
4. Preparation for labor and delivery
5. Future decisions related to the infant: keeping the baby or adoption
6. Care of the infant
7. Family planning

Pregnancy, the bearing of a child, in preadolescent or adolescent girls is rarely a planned undertaking.

Like so many other health problems of adolescence, pregnancy is the outcome of behavior brought about as a result of adolescents' search for identity, their need to feel wanted and trusted, broken lines of communication with family members, and experimentation with new experiences.

Teenagers may be unaware of the fact that they are pregnant because menstrual cycles are still irregular.

Early signs of pregnancy may include tenderness and swelling of the breasts, persistent nausea (with or without vomiting), and frequency of urination.

Pregnant adolescents need persons in whom they can confide and who will offer support through this difficult time of fears, anxieties, and decisions.

Hot lines or crisis centers exist in many communities. Adolescents frequently call these facilities for information and guidance.

Adolescents who are unable to communicate with their parents will often confide in someone else.

Decision making is difficult and frequently involves the pregnant adolescent, sex partner, families of each, and community services.

In some communities, confidentiality of the adolescent is maintained, and parents will not be informed by the health personnel or community agency.

Prenatal care is important for the pregnant adolescent, since more risks are associated with teenage pregnancy than with pregnancy in later years.

Prenatal care is necessary for the following reasons:
1. Monitoring the course of the pregnancy
2. Detecting impending difficulties for the mother or child (e.g., rise in blood pressure, change in kidney function, or change in fetal heart rate or activity)
3. Assisting the adolescent in decision making

HEALTH PROBLEM	AREAS FOR CONCERN	HELPFUL HINTS
Pregnancy—cont'd	Postpartal care focuses on restoration of the mother's health, maintenance of the infants's health, and family planning.	4. Providing a knowledge base in regard to pregnancy, labor and delivery, and care of the mother and infant after birth. Adolescent nutrition is frequently poor, and pregnancy compounds the problem. Some teenage girls may believe that failure to eat will bring about an abortion. This, however, is not the case.
Suicide *Suicide:* Self-inflicted loss of life.	Suicide is a frequent cause of death among adolescents. Suicide occurs more often among males than females. Factors associated with suicide include depression, excessive stress, sustained periods of anxiety, or crisis situations. The suicidal adolescent often retreats inward, severing close family relationships and lines of communication. Suicide terminates adolescents' efforts to communicate their confusion, guilt, and sense of hopelessness with others.	Caretakers find it difficult to believe that adolescents would take their own lives (commit suicide) when they have so much to live for. Changes in adolescent's patterns of behavior, eating, dressing, and/or sleeping may provide clues of existing emotional stress. Young people who are loners, act on impulse, are moody, become depressed easily, or talk about death a great deal may also be sending out signals that they need help. *Threats of suicide should always be taken seriously.* The adolescent's need to communicate and to be taken seriously are paramount issues. The need for strong family relationships and open lines of communication cannot be overemphasized. Hot lines and suicide prevention centers are available in many areas and provide immediate counseling or referral opportunities for troubled youths.
Sunburn *Sunburn:* Burning of the skin through overexposure to the ultraviolet rays of the sun.	Sunburn, a common occurrence among teenagers, can range from a mild first-degree burn to a serious second-degree burn, requiring medical attention. Fair-skinned, blue-eyed individuals are more prone to develop sunburns than are olive or swarthy-skinned individuals. Exposure to the sun may be dangerous for individuals who are ill or taking certain medications. Physiological changes resulting from a disease or drug may predispose these individuals to severe sunburn. Sunburn can also result from overexposure to a sunlamp or welder's arcs.	Sunburn often occurs among adolescents who are trying to achieve the "perfect" suntan. Sunburn can and should be prevented. Severe sunburns can be dangerous. Some family members, usually blue eyed and fair skinned, are more prone to sunburn than others. It is important for adolescents and caretakers to know precautions to use with drug therapies, since some medications can predispose individuals to severe sunburn. Likewise, some illnesses alter the body's response to ultraviolet rays, and exposure to the sun may cause additional health problems. Teach children early in life that they can become burned even on overcast, cloudy days because clouds do not filter out the ultraviolet rays that burn the skin.

HEALTH PROBLEM	AREAS FOR CONCERN	HELPFUL HINTS
	Mild and moderate sunburns rarely require medical management. Skin heals without difficulty. Cool tap water compresses applied for 20 minutes, three to four times a day, followed by ointments or lotions provide comfort and hasten healing.	If adolescents insist on suntanning, gradual exposure to the sun is encouraged. Acclimating the skin to increased periods of sunbathing provides a tan quickly and reduces the chance of burning. Start with 20 to 30 minutes of sunning the first day and increase both the length of time and number of exposures each day to help the body adjust without burning. If it is necessary to be outside for longer periods of time, shirts, pants, and a hat will provide some protection. Certain lotions provide some protection from burning but cannot prevent a burn if the individual remains exposed to the sun. Sunbathing on beaches or on boats increases the chances of burning because the ultraviolet rays rebound off the sand and water onto the skin. If a sunburn occurs, applying cool wet compresses three or four times a day for 20 to 30 minutes provides some relief. Certain over-the-counter sprays, ointments, and lotions also provide relief of pain, but should be used cautiously because some individuals react negatively to them.
	Medical management may be needed for severe sunburns. Local anesthetic sprays might be recommended, although some individuals are sensitive to these products. Analgesics such as aspirin or acetaminophens might be offered to reduce pain. Nausea or vomiting accompanying the sunburn, may indicate fluid and electrolyte imbalance.	If blisters develop, care should be taken to prevent secondary infections. When blisters develop, this indicates a more severe burn and may be a clue that the individual is also suffering loss of fluid (dehydration). Clear liquids, such as tea, soda, gelatin water, or apple juice should be taken frequently in small amounts. If nausea and vomiting accompany the blisters and pain of a severe burn, health personnel should be consulted. When fluids can be tolerated, clear liquids should be offered.
Vaginitis *Vaginitis:* Inflammation of the vagina.	Vaginitis can result from excessive irritation such as douches that are too strong, a foreign body, or infectious organisms. The most common causes of vaginitis include *Escherichia coli, Candida albicans* (moniliasis), and *Trichomonas vaginalis.* Other causes can include venereal diseases or streptococcal or staphylococcal infections.	Severe itching at and a thick copious discharge from the vaginal area indicate an infection of or swelling of the tissues of the vagina (vaginitis). Vaginitis is a fairly common occurrence in females of all ages. It occurs most often because of inadequate hygiene or from incorrect wiping following a bowel movement. Although vaginitis can be due to venereal disease or contracted through intercourse, these are not typical causes.

217

HEALTH PROBLEM	AREAS FOR CONCERN	HELPFUL HINTS
Vaginitis—cont'd	Vaginitis is characterized by pruritus (severe itching), vaginal discharge (sometimes white and cheesy, often purulent), and frequency of urination. Inspection of the vagina will reveal reddened mucous membranes.	Most females become aware of the inflammation or infection quickly because of the severe itching noticed throughout the perineal area (around the vagina and rectum), the discharge (ranging from thick milky white to purulent green), and the discomfort associated with urination (burning and frequency). Vaginitis does not disappear without treatment.
	Treatment is based on identification of the organism through microscopic examination of a vaginal smear. Specific jellies, ointments, creams, or douches may be prescribed.	Jellies, ointments, or creams that have been prescribed are inserted into the vagina through the use of special applicators or plungers. Medicated douches may be needed when an infection exists. Once the infection is gone, douches are no longer necessary or recommended as a part of normal perineal hygiene.
Venereal disease (VD) *Venereal disease:* Disease contracted as a result of sexual contact, usually intercourse.	Venereal diseases are highly communicable diseases, usually transmitted directly through sexual person-to-person contact. Although many diseases are categorized as being venereal diseases, the most commonly encountered are gonorrhea and syphilis. They will be discussed in detail. An alarming increase in the incidence of venereal diseases among adolescents and young adults has been noted. *Neisseria gonorrhoeae* infect males and females. There is no immunization available.	Venereal disease is often referred to as *VD*. The most common venereal diseases are lues (syphilis) and clap (gonorrhea). Syphilis and gonorrhea are most often transmitted through sexual intercourse. There seems to be a greater number of cases of gonorrhea among adolescents than ever before.

CHANCROID
   Chancroid: Highly infectious venereal ulcer caused by *Haemophilus ducreyi.*
HERPES GENITALIS:
   Herpes genitalis: Infectious herpetic lesions of the external genitalia caused by a herpes virus.
GONORRHEA (CLAP)
   Gonorrhea (clap): Contagious, purulent inflammation of the genital mucous membranes caused by the gram-negative *Neisseria gonorrhoeae.*
	Immunity is not attained as a result of having had the disease, thus reinfection is common.
	Gonorrhea spreads primarily through direct contact (sexual), although can be contracted indirectly through contact with contaminated linen or toilet facilities.
	The incubation period for gonorrhea ranges from 2 to 21 days (with an average of 3 to 5) after contact. The infection can be transmitted before symptoms appear and until the disease is treated.
	The major characteristics of the illness differ for males and females.
		Immunization is not available against this disease.
		
		When one family member has gonorrhea, it is possible for other members to develop it also through contact with soiled bed linens or the use of common toileting facilities.

HEALTH PROBLEM	AREAS FOR CONCERN	HELPFUL HINTS
	In the male symptoms usually appear within 72 hours after infection. Males complain of burning on urination, followed by a thin watery secretion that gradually becomes thicker and purulent. Males usually seek treatment quickly because the discharge is noticeable, and the discomfort is severe. If untreated, the infection progresses, and ulcerations can occur.	Infected males usually seek treatment quickly, because they experience pain or burning when they urinate, or they notice a discharge from the penis.
	In females, the signs and symptoms are less apparent. Treatment is not sought, and the disease progresses through several stages. The female becomes a reservoir or an unknowing infected carrier of the disease. Infected females experience burning on urination and a slight vaginal discharge. The discomfort is rarely severe, and the discharge disappears without treatment. The disease, however, does not disappear; instead, the gonorrhea organism invades the Bartholin's glands and Skene's ducts and ascends the cervical canal. Abscess formation can occur. Erosion of the endometrium is possible, with further extension of the disease to the fallopian tubes and ovaries.	Girls who are infected, rarely have severe enough signs or symptoms to cause them to seek treatment. Girls with gonorrhea may notice a slight vaginal discharge that disappears or a slight burning on urination, but these signs are similar to other transient female irritations. It is important that adolescent females realize how dangerous gonorrheal infections can be! *Gonorrhea does not disappear.* Indeed, this venereal disease progressively attacks the various female reproductive organs. If untreated, the girl can become sterile or require major surgery. Meanwhile this infected individual continues to infect sex partners and/or family members.
	Gonococcal infection in the pregnant woman can be transmitted to the infant at birth by passage through the infected birth canal. The infection usually affects the infant's eyes (ophthalmia neonatorum). A preventive measure at birth is the instillation of penicillin or a silver nitrate solution into the conjunctival sac of all newborns. Abdominal discomfort can accompany the inflammation of the pelvic organs. If left untreated, surgical removal of the reproductive organs (uterus, ovaries, and fallopian tubes) may be necessary.	If by chance the female with gonorrhea is pregnant, it is entirely possible to pass the illness on to the baby at birth. Gonorrhea damages the baby's eyes and can cause permanent blindness.
	Laboratory tests (serological) are needed for diagnosis of this condition. Treatment is required. Penicillin is the drug of choice.	Males and females who suspect they may have gonorrhea or any venereal disease should seek immediate treatment! This disease does not just go away. Having had the illness once *does not* provide immunity. It is totally possible and probable to contract gonorrhea again if exposed to an infected individual.
SYPHILIS (LUES VENEREA) *Syphilis (lues venerea):* An infectious (often chronic) venereal disease that can cause lesions in any tissue or organ of the body caused by the spirochete *Treponema pallidum.*	There is an alarming worldwide increase in the incidence of syphilis that is particularly noticed in adolescents and young adults. Syphilis can occur at any age and in every culture, race, and geographical point in the world.	Another infectious communicable venereal disease is known as *lues* (syphilis).

HEALTH PROBLEMS	AREAS FOR CONCERN	HELPFUL HINTS
Venereal disease—cont'd SYPHILIS—cont'd	The organism is transmitted almost entirely through direct sexual contact. The spirochete (*Treponema pallidum*) can survive outside the human body for only a few minutes at most, virtually eliminating transmission of the disease by indirect methods. The spirochete usually enters the body through a break in the skin or mucous membrane, although it can also invade intact tissue. Once the infectious organism enters the body, it can affect every tissue and organ. Syphilis progresses through three stages, primary, secondary, and tertiary (latent).	Syphilis is almost always spread through direct sexual contact. Syphilis can be spread through kissing, particularly if the lips or mouth come in contact with the primary or secondary lesion of an infected individual. A single contact can spread the infection from one person to another. The infection races throughout the newly infected individual in a matter of days.
1. *Primary stage*. A painless lesion (a sore) called a *chancre* appears at the site of invasion.	After infection, the incubation period can range from 10 to 90 days although the normal range is typically 2 to 3 weeks. Characteristically, a single painless lesion (chancre) appears at the site of invasion. At one time the most common sites of occurrence for this firm papular sore (chancre) were the head of the penis in males and the external genitalia of the female. Chancres are now frequently found on the lips, tongue, fingers, or anal areas. The chancre frequently has a crusty or ulcerated top. Syphilis is highly infectious in this primary stage. The primary lesion of syphilis heals with or without treatment in 4 to 6 weeks.	A painless sore (chancre) develops during the first stage of syphilis. Adolescents should know that a single painless sore which lasts 2 to 3 weeks and causes no discomfort or pain may be the only sign they have of the presence of a venereal disease. This painless sore is most often found on the genitalia, but may be found elsewhere on the body. When a chancre appears on the lips it may resemble a cold sore (i.e., raised lump with crusty top). The chancre, however, is more firm and neither itches nor causes discomfort. Chancres are visible up to 6 weeks. Cold sores or other nonvenereal lesions rarely last 2 to 3 weeks, thus differentiating them from the syphilitic chancre. Although the chancre disappears without treatment, the disease progressively becomes worse. Syphilis is a dangerous, highly infectious illness, and, if suspected, medical treatment must be sought.
2. *Secondary stage*. A generalized reaction that is usually accompanied by a rash or lesions.	If treatment is sought during this stage, the organism can be identified through microscopic examination (dark field) of material taken from the lesion. Penicillin is the drug of choice. The secondary stage of syphilis is usually reached about 6 weeks to 6 months after the disappearance of the primary lesion (chancre). The secondary stage is not characterized by one single typical response. Some individuals may have a slight rash that causes no distress and disappears quickly. Some individuals may have a generalized macular-papular rash that is also found on the palms of the hand and soles of the feet.	Approximately 2 to 3 months after the single painless sore (chancre) disappears, new signs appear. Often there is a generalized rash that involves the soles of the feet and palms of the hands. The rash can be mild or severe. It can be everywhere on the body or in localized areas. It neither itches nor causes pain.

HEALTH PROBLEMS	AREAS FOR CONCERN	HELPFUL HINTS
	Some individuals may have moist papules called *condylomata lata* located on the external genitalia, anal area, or other moist skin surfaces. Some individuals may have mucous patches that are located in the mouth, throat, and lips. Some individuals may develop alopecia (hair loss), particularly around the occipital area of the scalp and eyebrows. Some individuals may develop nonpainful lymphadenopathy (swollen glands). Although the signs and symptoms vary, certain common features stand out; the rashes or lesions do not itch, nor are they painful, and the swollen glands (lymphadenopathy) are not tender. The individual is highly infectious. The signs and symptoms of this second stage disappear with or without treatment in 2 to 12 weeks.	Some people may develop wartlike lesions (called *condylomata lata*) on the perineum, vagina, or near the rectum that are painless but highly infectious. Some people develop white patches in their throats. These patches cause no discomfort and disappear within a few weeks. Some people may notice loss of eyebrows or the development of bald spots (alopecia) on back of the head. As in the first stage of syphilis, the signs and symptoms will disappear on their own without treatment. When signs and symptoms are present, the person is highly infectious to family, friends, and sex partners.
	If treatment is sought, the disease can be identified through serological tests or microscopic examination (dark field) of the material from the lesions. The treatment of choice is penicillin. If untreated, syphilis can now go into a latent phase lasting from 2 to 15 years (or longer). The latent stage is asymptomatic, although serological examination of the blood would disclose the presence of the disease. During this latent period the disease is not usually infectious, although a pregnant woman could pass the illness onto her unborn child. The child would exhibit a congenital form of syphilis.	Treatment is imperative to avoid future serious complications. Medical supervision and management should be sought. In some individuals the infection may seem to be over. This venereal disease enters a latent phase (tertiary stage) whereby the infected person has no clues or symptoms that the disease continues to progress. This latent, or "quiet," period can last for several years.
3. *Tertiary stage (late syphilis, lues, paresis).* Lesions known as *gumma* that develop in and interfere with the function of the internal organs, cardiovascular system, or central nervous system.	The lesions of the tertiary stage can make their appearance shortly after the lesions of the second stage disappear, although in most instances, these third-stage manifestations do not occur until 15 to 20 years after the initial syphilitic infection. A gumma (soft gummy tumorlike lesion) can affect any organ, bone, or skin tissue, but most frequently interferes with the functions of the cardiovascular or central nervous systems.	The last stage (tertiary) of syphilis causes the greatest amount of damage to the individual. The lesions found in this period can attack the skin, bone, or any organ or body system. Ulcers, blindness, damaged hearts, partial paralysis, loss of intellectual abilities, coma, and even death can occur in this stage. Pain, discomforts of all sorts, and often invalidism accompany these ailments.

221

HEALTH PROBLEMS	AREAS FOR CONCERN	HELPFUL HINTS
Venereal disease—cont'd SYPHILIS—cont'd	Tertiary syphilis is not considered infectious to others, although pregnant women can pass syphilis on to their unborn children. Tertiary syphilis is dangerous, however, to the infected individual because it can produce skin and bone ulcers, blindness, weaken the heart and major vessels, and cause paresis (degeneration of the central nervous system, resulting in progressive loss of physical and mental abilities), or even death. Diagnosis is obtained through serological laboratory tests. Treatment is prolonged and often the disease cannot be cured.	The infected individual is not considered infectious, although pregnant women can pass the disease on to their unborn children. When detected, treatment with penicillin is started, but there is no guarantee that the illness can be cured or that the damage can be overcome.

TECHNIQUES AND HELPFUL HINTS

CHAPTER 18

TECHNIQUES AND HELPFUL HINTS

Procedures and techniques used in the maintenance and promotion of health for children can be used by caretakers in the home. Health care workers often assume that caretakers or other health care workers know how to take a temperature, bathe babies, give medication, or do a number of other relatively easy procedures.

Some of the most common procedures have been selected and described in this chapter. Easy-to-follow instructions are included. Helpful hints and the rationale for performing the procedure in certain ways

are provided. Accompanying illustrations demonstrate how to prepare and handle equipment, as well as how to hold or immobilize children when performing the procedure.

A child's ability to cooperate is usually enhanced if clear concise directions or explanations are offered in words that are easily understood while the procedure is being performed. Although particular equipment and methods have been suggested, it may be necessary to alter the procedure to meet the needs of the child or environment.

PROCEDURE	HELPFUL HINTS

Administration of oral medications

Purpose: To give medications by an oral route.
Materials
Medicine
Spoon, nipple, dropper, or small cup
Bib

Household devices such as measuring cups or spoons are ideal utensils for measuring and giving medications.

1. Wash hands before starting.
2. Apply a bib.
3. Measure out or pour the desired amount of medicine.
  a. Check the label carefully.
  b. Pour only the desired amount.
    (1) Liquids can be measured and administered using a dropper, spoon, or cup.
    (2) Tablets require crushing for infants. Dissolve them in the smallest amount of water possible. (If a tablet is unpalatable, mix it with honey, syrup, or jelly.)

Tablets are easily crushed between the bowls of 2 teaspoons. Children (babies included) will often take medicine dissolved only in water. At times it may be necessary to disguise distasteful medicine. Avoid using foods such as applesauce or other fruits, since the child may refuse these foods in the future. Small amounts of honey, syrup, or jelly have proved effective.

LIQUIDS
1. Hold the infant as for feeding.
2. Place the liquid medicine into the mouth.
  a. Nipple
    (1) Put the nipple into the mouth.
    (2) Add the medicine to the nipple.
    (3) Allow the infant to suck.

Babies under 4 months take liquid medications easily through the nipple method.

  b. Spoon
    (1) Place the spoon with the medicine above the tongue.
    (2) Allow the infant to suck it off.
    (3) Offer an older child the opportunity to take the medicine from the spoon on his own.

Caretaker holding the spoon and guiding medicine into mouth works well through infancy and into toddlerhood.
Older children (toddlers, preschoolers, and older children) frequently take medicine best when allowed to do it on their own under supervision.

  c. Dropper (plastic droppers are safest).
    (1) Place the dropper in the infant's mouth. The infant will automatically suck. (Droppers are most useful in infancy.)

Many oral medications come in bottles with droppers attached.
Infants usually enjoy liquid vitamins.

  d. Cup
    (1) Place the cup with the medicine to the lips and permit the child to suck or drink slowly.

Plastic cups that are flexible are more useful with babies, since cup can be shaped to contour of mouth.
Older children prefer to hold and drink medicine without help.

    (2) If the quantity is large, straws can be used for older toddlers and children. (Some liquid medications can discolor the teeth and must be taken using a straw).

If a straw is used, cut the straw in half to decrease the distance the medication must be drawn up to the mouth. Be sure the entire amount of medication is swallowed.

PILLS, TABLETS, CAPSULES
1. Set out the correct number of pills, tablets, or capsules.

Many medications come in liquid form or chewable tablets, but some do not.
Toddlers and older children can be taught to take pills, tablets, and capsules.

2. Have the child place the medicine (one at a time) on the back of the tongue.

Placing medicine at the back of the tongue serves two purposes. First, placement assists in the swallowing process, and, second, there are fewer taste buds at the back of the tongue, thus decreasing the taste factor.

3. Have the child drink water to assist in swallowing the medicine.

Avoid milk or soda as the liquid used for taking medicine.
  1. Milk stimulates mucus production, and often children develop a future dislike for milk when milk is used as the beverage to take "hated" medicines.

PROCEDURE	HELPFUL HINTS

2. Carbonated beverages often dissolve the medicine before it can be swallowed.
3. Carbonated beverages have an effervescence that frequently prevents the child from taking enough liquid with which to swallow the pill, tablet, or capsule.

4. Repeat the process until all medicines are taken.
5. Offer a fluid of choice after the medication is taken, particularly if the medicine had an unpleasant taste.

Administration of suppository

Purpose: To stimulate intestinal peristalsis or introduce medication when other routes are not feasible.

Materials
   Medicine (suppositories are usually stored in the refrigerator)
   Petroleum jelly, KY Jelly, or other petrolatum product
   Finger cot or rubber glove
1. Wash hands before starting.
2. Set out the suppository. Apply a lubricant to the tip. Place the finger cot on the index finger.

3. Remove the diaper or pants.
4. Place the child on the abdomen.
5. Separate the buttocks and expose the anus.
6. Place the rounded tip of the suppository at the anus.

7. Insert the suppository into the rectum by applying firm pressure with the index finger.
8. Maintain pressure with the index finger until the rectal ring closes down on the finger behind the end of the suppository. The suppository is in place when it moves away from the end of the index finger, and the rectal sphincter can be felt closing down tightly.

9. Remove the finger and pinch the buttocks folds tightly together for a few moments to ensure retention of the suppository.
10. Replace the diaper or panties.

Suppositories are often stored in the refrigerator, since they might lose their firmness and shape at room temperature.

Avoid taking out the suppository too long before use.

Infants are placed on the abdomen. Older children need only be turned on their sides.
Many suppositories will melt quickly from the warmth of the hand, so quick action is necessary.

Be sure that suppository is inserted completely. *There should be no discomfort.*
Sometimes a child will defecate (have a bowel movement) as soon as a suppository is inserted. If this is not the purpose of the medicine, wait until the bowel movement has ended and repeat the procedure.
Maintaining the buttocks close together for a few moments helps the older child understand the need to retain the medicine.

Bathing an infant

Purpose: To cleanse skin surfaces and provide comfort.

Materials
   Plastic tub (or bathinette)
   Washcloth
   Bath towel (two for an infant)
   Bath blanket (receiving blanket)
   Cotton balls (cotton swabs)
   Mild soap
   Water
   Baby oil or lotion
1. Wash hands before starting the bath.
2. Have equipment assembled near the tub.
3. Place the tub on a flat surface (preferably at waist level).

4. Place a bath blanket (opened) next to the tub (this provides a soft surface on which to lay the infant).

The type of tub to be used for bathing will be different for each caretaker. It does not matter which type is used. Some will have a bathinette, others will use small plastic tubs, whereas others may use the kitchen sink.

Placing the tub on a surface area (such as table or counter) eliminates the need for the caretaker to reach or stretch and makes it easier to hold and handle the baby during the bath.

227

PROCEDURE

HELPFUL HINTS

Bathing an infant—cont'd

5. Place a towel (opened) on top of the bath blanket.
6. Fill the tub one third full with warm water. The water temperature should be warm to touch (test with elbow or wrist).

A caretaker's elbow and wrist are more sensitive to temperature changes and are more reliable indicators of heat than the fingers or hand.

7. Place a small towel in the bottom of the tub.

A towel in the bottom of the tub lessens the chance of the baby slipping. Placing the towel in the tub is recommended until the baby is over 6 weeks old.

8. Bring the infant to the table and place on back on a towel that has been placed over the blanket.

Caretakers must have one hand on the baby at all times. As babies grow they become more active and can roll off of table or counter surface or bathinette.

9. Undress the infant, except for the diaper.

Leaving the diaper on eliminates the possibility of the caretaker's clothing being soiled by urine or feces while the infant is being held for the shampoo.

10. Wash the infant's face with clear water (this eliminates getting soap in the eyes, which is irritating and uncomfortable).

When attempting to wash the face, the caretaker will find it necessary to hold the baby's head steady with one hand while washing with the other hand.

a. Starting with the eyes, wash each one separately, wiping from inner canthus to outer canthus. Cotton balls moistened with water may be used (Fig. 18-1).

Wring excess water out of the washcloth before wiping the baby's eyes because this will be less startling.

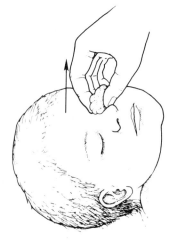

Fig. 18-1. Cleansing eye.

b. Cleanse the nasal orifice of any dried mucus. A moistened cotton swab may be used if necessary (Fig. 18-2).

Dried mucus can be cleared from the nose by wiping with a washcloth. If cotton swabs are used, moisten them with water, and gently remove the mucus from the outer nostril. *Caution:* Do not insert the cotton swab up into the nose, since this may traumatize the mucous membrane or force dried mucus further into the nostril.

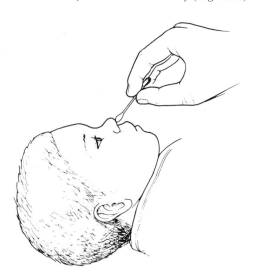

Fig. 18-2. Cleansing nose.

PROCEDURE	HELPFUL HINTS

c. Wash behind the ears. The skin surface behind the ears may become irritated where two skin surfaces rub together. (See Intertrigo, Chapter 6.)

d. Cleanse the external portion of the ear using a moistened cotton swab or cotton ball (Fig. 18-3). *Do not insert the cotton swab into the ear canal.*

Turning the baby's head to one side will expose the ear to facilitate cleansing. *Caution:* If it is necessary to use a moistened cotton swab, do not insert it beyond the external portion of the ear. Trauma to eardrum may result from any vigorous effort to cleanse the ear canal.

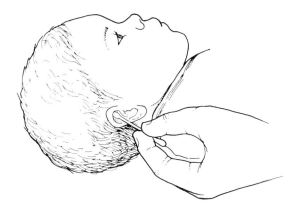

Fig. 18-3. Cleansing outer ear.

e. Wash the remainder of the infant's face and neck folds.

11. Holding the infant in a football hold, tilt the head downward over the tub (Fig. 18-4, *A*).
12. Wash the scalp well with soapy water, paying special attention to the fontanels (soft spots).
13. Rinse soapy water from the scalp and pat it dry.

Special attention should be given to the folds of the neck because food, formula, and perspiration accumulating between the skin folds will cause irritation.

The football hold enables the caretaker to have the baby securely immobilized when washing the baby's head.

Special attention should be given to wash the soft spots (fontanels) well. NOTE: This is an area often avoided because of fear on part of caretaker of injuring the child.

Washing the soft spots (fontanels) with soap and water will not hurt the baby.

The soft spots (fontanels) are where cradle cap often is seen because caretakers do not wash this area. Cradle cap is an accumulation of secretions from hair follicles and sweat glands that become dry and scaly.

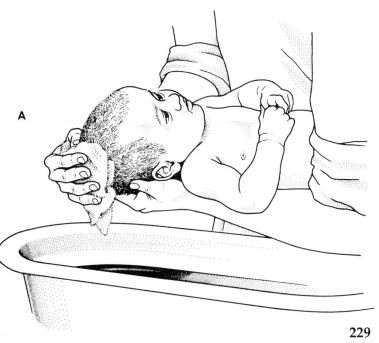

A

Fig. 18-4. Bathing infant. **A,** Use of football hold to bathe infant's scalp.

PROCEDURE

HELPFUL HINTS

Bathing an infant—cont'd

14. Remove the infant's diaper (if pins are used, close them and place them out of the infant's reach).
15. Place the infant in the tub, supporting the body at the hip, shoulders, and head (Fig. 18-4, *B*).

Safety in regard to safety pins cannot be overemphasized. Pins should never be placed in the blanket or left open and lying where the baby can reach them. Remember, whatever babies get in their hands will be put in their mouths.

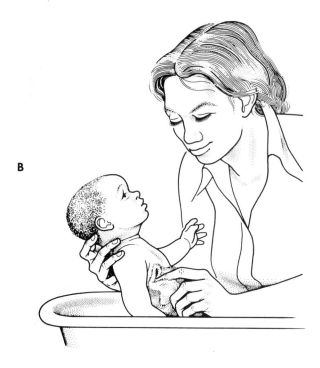

B

Fig. 18-4, cont'd. **B,** Placement of infant in tub.

16. Support the shoulders and head of the infant with one hand while washing the rest of the body with the other hand.
    a. Wash the shoulders, arms, trunk, and abdomen. First soap, then rinse.
    b. Tilt the infant forward on the opposite hand and wash the shoulders and back. The infant's head can be supported by the upper portion of the hand with the infant's chin resting over the thumb and index finger of the caretaker.
    c. Tilt the infant back, provide support with the other hand, and wash the legs and genitalia.
17. Remove the infant from the tub and place on a towel (with a blanket beneath it).
18. Pat the infant dry. A small towel may be placed over the infant to prevent chilling.

To support the baby securely when in the tub, it will be helpful to have the baby's head and shoulder cradled in the caretaker's palm with the little finger under the baby's arm. It is important that the caretaker have a firm grasp of the baby to maintain a secure hold.

Tilting the baby forward is not necessary while the baby is very small. It is possible to wash the baby's back by elevating the head and shoulders to allow access to the back area.

As babies grow older and are able to sit without support, small water toys can be added to provide diversion and fun during bath time.

PROCEDURE	HELPFUL HINTS

19. Inspect the genitalia. Additional cleansing may be necessary.
    a. For females, spread the labia with the index finger and thumb. Cleanse from the top surface of the labia toward the anus (this prevents contaminating the vaginal orifice or urethral meatus with fecal material) (Fig. 18-5).

Cleansing of the genitalia is important for both infant girls and boys because secretions from glands can accumulate, causing irritation and even blockage to urine flow.

Infant girls often have a creamy white mucous discharge that is easily removed by washing. NOTE: Always wash from the front to back to prevent bowel movement from the anal area (rectum) entering the vagina or urethra.

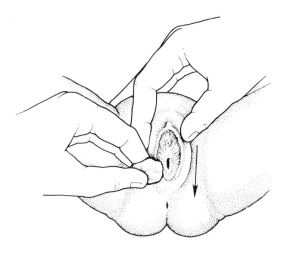

Fig. 18-5. Cleansing female genitalia.

b. For uncircumcised males, retract the foreskin, exposing the tip of the penis. Cleanse the area around and at the tip of the penis.

Infant boys will also have glandular secretions that should be cleansed away to prevent the obstruction of urine flow.

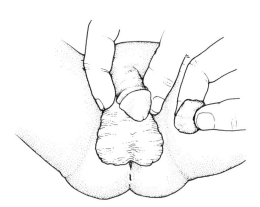

Fig. 18-6. Cleansing male genitalia.

c. For circumcised males, cleanse the tip of the penis. The urinary meatus can become blocked by accumulated or dried secretions (Fig. 18-6).
d. Cleanse the anal area and between the cheeks of the buttocks.

20. Apply baby oil or lotion to the skin folds of the groin and buttocks. *Caution:* Do not use powder and oil at the same time. This makes small curds that are more irritating than nothing at all. When using powder *do not* shake it over the infant, since it can be inhaled and cause irritation to the mucous membrane of the respiratory tract. Place a small amount of powder in the palm of the hand and apply it with the fingertips of the opposite hand.

21. Redress the infant. NOTE: Bath time is a good time to inspect the infant's skin from head to toe. At this time, any irritations or reddened areas may be detected.

Dried secretions, urine, and bowel movement may accumulate between the buttocks and should be removed to prevent irritation.

When using baby oil, apply only a thin layer to those skin folds where irritation is likely to occur, such as the groin, buttocks, and neck folds.

Bath time can be a pleasant and enjoyable time for both the infant and caretaker, even though it may take a few weeks for the infant to adjust to this procedure.

<table>
<tr><td align="center">PROCEDURE</td><td align="center">HELPFUL HINTS</td></tr>
</table>

Breast self-examination

Purpose: To examine the breasts for deviations from normal.

Breast self-examination is most reliable if performed 1 week after menstruation because breasts are not usually tender or swollen at this time. The method of approach, similar to that suggested by the American Cancer Society, is as follows:

Breast self-examination is a must for good health care practice.

Examining the breasts at the same time each month and a few days after the menstrual period will eliminate possible misinterpretation of the examination.

1. Examine the breasts during a bath or shower.
   a. Keep the fingers flat and move them gently over the entire breast.

   The fingers will move easily over a wet surface, decreasing the resistance on pressure.

   b. When examining each breast, extend the arm, on that same side, over your head.

   Placing the arm over the head will expose the entire breast and facilitate a more complete examination by elevation of breast tissue.

   c. Examine the left breast with the right hand and the right breast with the left hand.
   d. Check for the presence of lumps or hard tissue.

   If a lump is discovered, seek medical advice.

2. Examine breasts standing in front of mirror.
   a. Note the size and shape of each breast while holding the arms at the side.

   Inspection of your breasts on a regular schedule provides information regarding breast size and shape. This makes it easier to determine any abnormalities.

   b. Raise the arms over the head and note any change in the contour of the breasts.

   Breast size will often be unequal.

   c. Rest the palms on the hips and press down firmly to tighten the chest muscles.

   Dimpling of skin or a change in breast and nipple shape or size should be reported to a physician.

3. Examine the breasts lying down.
   a. Place a small pillow under the shoulder of the breast to be examined.
   b. Elevate the arm on this same side behind your head.

   Placing the arm behind the head permits breast tissue to be more evenly distributed on the chest.

   c. With the opposite hand and fingers flat, press gently in a circular motion, starting at the top of the breast and moving clockwise around the outer portion of the breast.

   At the lower curve of each breast, there will be a firm ridge. This is normal.

   d. Then place the examining fingers 1 inch (2.5 cm) toward the nipple and circle the breast again. Continue this process until the entire breast and nipple have been examined. Repeat the procedure on the opposite side.

   Any alteration in breast size or tissue consistency that appears abnormal should be brought to the attention of a physician.

   Normally there is no discharge from the nipple. If a discharge is evident, notify a physician.

PROCEDURE	HELPFUL HINTS

Cast care

PETALING THE CAST (Fig. 18-7)

Purpose: To maintain the integrity of the cast and prevent skin irritation under the cast.

Petaling reduces the chance of the cast edges flaking or crumbling. Pieces of cast that reach the skin are quite irritating.

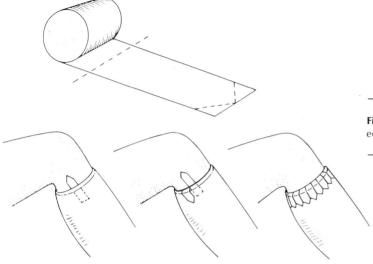

Fig. 18-7. Cast care. Petal tape and roll length of tape over edge with cut edge on inner surface of cast.

Materials

    Waterproof adhesive tape (½ to 1 inch [2.5 cm] wide tape, depending on amount of cast to be covered)

    Scissors

Waterproof tape is recommended to reduce the chance of the tape dislodging due to perspiration or liquid spills.

1. Wash hands before starting.
2. The cast must be dry before the petaling can be applied.
3. Excess batting that extends beyond the cast must be trimmed off.
4. Cut the tape into 2- to 3-inch (5- to 7.5 cm) lengths, depending on the area to be covered.

Cut several pieces before beginning the procedure. Approximate the number needed and cut about six extra.

5. Cut the corners of one end of each piece of tape (Fig. 18-7).
6. Place the uncut edge of the tape on the outside of the cast.
7. Roll a length of the tape over the edge of the cast, ending with the cut edge under the cast. (Placing the cut edge under cast reduces the chance of curled edges or ridges of tape.)
8. Overlap each piece of tape by approximately ¼ to ½ inch (0.6 to 1.3 cm).
9. Proceed around the entire opening in this fashion.

Petaling reinforces the edges of the cast and presents a uniform finished appearance.

CAST CLEANLINESS

Purpose: To prevent soiling of the body cast from urine and feces.

    Materials

    Plastic wrap

    Waterproof tape

    Scissors

Body casts (particularly in infants and toddlers) may require special precautions to prevent cast breakdown or odors.

1. Wash hands before starting.
2. Cut pieces of plastic wrap that will fit the cast opening to be protected.

Plastic wrap is best applied after the cast has been petaled.

3. Tuck one end of the plastic wrap under the cast for the entire length of the opening to be protected.
4. Roll the plastic wrap over the outer edge of the cast and secure it with strips of adhesive tape.
5. Replace the plastic wrap when necessary.

It may be necessary to cut more than one piece of plastic wrap. Molding of the wrap may be necessary around the opening. *Avoid creasing the plastic under the cast because creases are extremely irritating to the skin.* Folds and overlaps can best be accommodated on the outer aspect of the cast.

PROCEDURE

Feeding techniques

Purpose: To provide nourishment.

BREAST-FEEDING (Fig. 18-8)
Materials
    Washcloth
    Towel
    Soap and water

HELPFUL HINTS

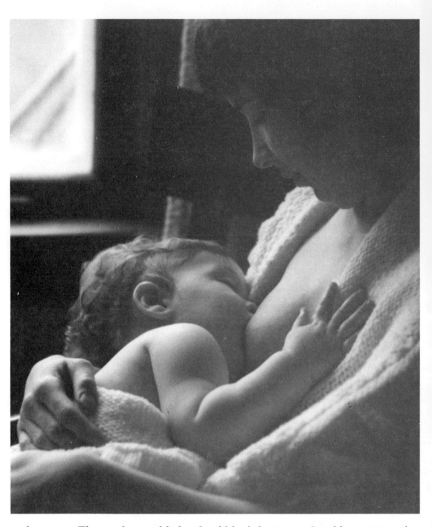

Fig. 18-8. Breast feeding. Comfortable position while breast feeding infant. (Courtesy La Leche League International, Franklin Park, Ill.)

1. Wash hands before starting
2. Wash breasts with soap and water.
3. Rinse them thoroughly.
4. Dry well.
5. Choose a comfortable position.
    a. Sitting in an armed chair (to provide support to the arm holding the infant).
    b. Lying in bed, propped on one side with the head slightly elevated.
6. Bring the infant to the breast (if the mother's nipple is flat, it may be helpful to stroke the nipple or areolar tissue gently to stimulate an erectile position).
7. Touch the infant's cheeks gently with the nipple. The infant will turn toward the nipple and open the mouth to grasp it.

8. The infant may appear to lose the nipple when in fact, he might be trying to place the nipple above the tongue and farther into the mouth. Mothers can help by gently cupping the breasts, particularly the nipples and areolar tissues, to permit the infant to obtain a better grasp.

The mother and baby should both be in comfortable positions that can be easily maintained for the feeding period (10 to 20 minutes).

It is not necessary to force the baby to nurse. If the rooting reflex (Chapter 1, Face) is well developed, the baby will turn his head in the direction of the nipple that is brushing the cheek. A major error is stroking the cheek away from the nipple, which causes the baby to turn away from the breast. The more the mother pushes on the cheek, the harder the baby struggles away from the breast.

While repositioning the nipple be careful to avoid stroking the infant's cheeks because this signals a move of the head away from the breast. If baby has a good grasp of the nipple, the jaws will move regularly up and down. Sucking and swallowing movements are readily seen in the cheeks and throat.

If sucking and swallowing are not evident, the baby probably does not have a good grasp.

PROCEDURE	HELPFUL HINTS

9. Nursing time usually ranges from 5 to 20 minutes, which provides sufficient time to empty the breast and sufficient stimulation for further milk production. Some authorities recommend shorter nursing periods when the infant is very young to permit the mother and infant time to adjust and to prevent the mother's nipples from cracking.

If breast tissue obstructs breathing, the mother can gently move the breast tissue away from the nose, with the index finger, being careful not to disengage the nipple from the baby's mouth.

The length of nursing time will differ for each baby. A regular pattern is quickly established.

10. Alternate breasts at feeding times. (Some mothers use both breasts at each feeding, particularly when establishing breast-feeding).

11. Bubbling is usually performed only at the end of the feeding.

Frequent bubbling is unnecessary with breast-fed babies, because they swallow little air. (See Vertical Support.)

12. Place the infant on either the right side or abdomen after feeding.

Placing the baby on the right side or abdomen facilitates digestion as well as reduces the potential danger of choking should the baby regurgitate or vomit. (See Chapter 5, Regurgitation.)

BOTTLE FEEDING (Fig. 18-9)
Materials
    Bottles: Plastic, glass
    Nipples (variety of types)
    Formula
    Bib

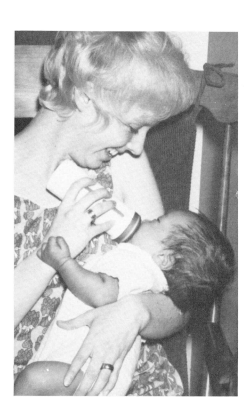

Fig. 18-9. Bottle feeding. Comfortable position for bottle feeding infant. (From Chinn, P.L.: Child health maintenance: concepts in family-centered care, ed. 2, St. Louis, 1979, The C.V. Mosby Co.)

1. Wash hands before starting.
2. Warm the formula if necessary.
3. Be sure the infant is dry and comfortable.
4. Apply the bib.

It is not necessary to heat the formula unless it has been refrigerated or stored in a very cold place. Test the warmth by placing a few drops of the formula on the inner aspect of the wrist. Formula should neither burn nor chill the skin.

PROCEDURE	HELPFUL HINTS

Feeding techniques—cont'd

BOTTLE FEEDING—cont'd

5. Choose a comfortable position. Sit in a chair with arms to provide support to the arm holding the infant.

The caretaker and infant should both be in a comfortable position to facilitate feeding and a feeling of relaxation.

It is possible for the caretaker to feed the infant while reclining in bed as with breast-feeding.

6. Hold the infant in a cradle position close to the body.

Cradling the infant close to the body provides security, comfort, and warmth.

7. Place the nipple at the infant's lips.

Gently touching the lips stimulates the mouth to open.

8. As the infant opens the mouth, insert the nipple, making sure that the nipple is above the tongue.

If the baby does not begin to suck, stroking the cheek gently with a finger may elicit the sucking reflex.

Ensuring placement of the nipple above the tongue permits compression of the nipple and release of the formula into the mouth when the baby sucks. If the nipple is under the tongue, either the nipple holes will be obstructed by the undersurface of the tongue, or the formula, when released, will drool out of the mouth because the baby does not have the ability to channel the fluid to the back of the mouth. As a result, the baby becomes frustrated and restless.

9. Observe the infant for sucking and swallowing movements.

If the baby has a good grasp of the nipple, the jaws will move up and down regularly. Sucking and swallowing movements are readily seen in the cheeks and throat. Bubbles rising from the nipple may be seen with some feeding equipment. Compression of the plastic liners may be seen with other equipment.

Swallowing hard or choking during feeding may indicate that the nipple holes are too large and formula flows too rapidly.

Babies who fall asleep before feeding is completed may indicate that nipple holes are too small, formula flows too slowly, and the infant tires before finishing.

10. Bubble the infant frequently. (See Lifting and Holding the Infant.) Young infants should be bubbled after 1 to 1½ ounces, older infants every 3 to 4 ounces.

All babies are unique in their needs for bubbling. Some may require frequent bubbling, whereas others might complete a feeding before bubbling. Excessive swallowing of air might be a factor in the development of colic for some babies (See Chapter 5, Colic.)

11. The feeding time usually ranges from 10 to 20 minutes.

The length of feeding time is unique for each baby. A regular pattern is quickly established.

12. The feeding schedule and amounts will vary with each infant. (See Chapter 4, Nutrition.)

13. Place the infant on either the right side or abdomen after feeding.

Placing the baby on the right side or abdomen facilitates digestion as well as reduces the potential danger of choking should the baby regurgitate or vomit. (See Chapter 5, Regurgitation.)

SOLIDS (Fig. 18-10)
Materials
  Dish
  Spoon

  Food

  Bib

It is desirable to use a small-bowled spoon for easy entrance to the baby's mouth.

When giving solid foods for the first time, the consistency of the food should be similar to that of formula.

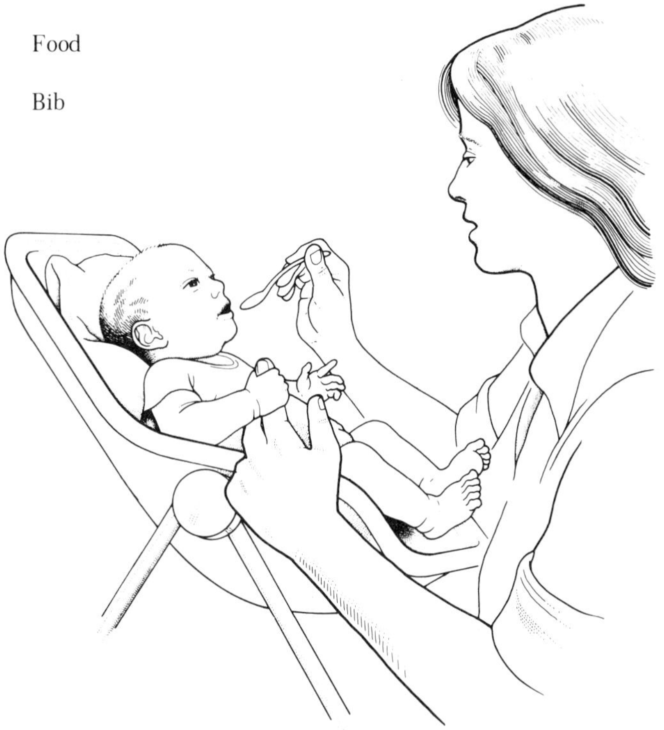

Fig. 18-10. Feeding solids. Spoon feeding infants with use of infant seat.

1. Wash hands before starting.
2. Warm the food slightly.
3. Ensure the proper consistency.
   a. Commercially prepared vegetables, meats, and fruits are usually the desired consistency.
   b. Meats, vegetables, and fruits prepared in the home require pureeing or blending to reach the desired consistency.
   c. Formula is added to dry cereals until the desired consistency is obtained. Rice cereal is the initial cereal of choice for infants, since rice is less likely to cause allergic responses.
4. Place the desired quantities and types of food in the dish.
5. Be sure the infant is dry and comfortable, with the bib in place.
6. Choose a comfortable position. Sit in a chair with arms to provide support to the arm holding the infant.
7. Cradle the infant close to the body.
8. Facilitate feeding by controlling the infant's arms.
   a. Tuck the infant's arm closest to your body behind your back.
   b. Hold the other arm with the hand encircling the infant's body.
9. Place the infant in a seat or high chair. (Use a safety strap to secure child.)
10. Sit facing the infant.
11. Place a small amount of food on the tip of the spoon.
12. Insert the spoon into the infant's mouth.

The amounts and frequency of feedings are listed for each age in Chapters 5 and 8, Nutrition.

It is not necessary to heat foods unless they have been stored in the refrigerator or other cold place. (Test the warmth of prepared foods by placing a small portion on the inner aspect of the wrist, as with a bottle feeding. The food should neither burn nor chill the skin.)

Avoid adding solid foods to the bottle feedings because babies need to learn to eat solids.

PROCEDURE	HELPFUL HINTS

Feeding techniques—cont'd

SOLIDS—cont'd

13. The spoon must be on top of the tongue and far enough back in the mouth that infant can obtain the food through a sucking motion. Food placed at the tip of the tongue will be pushed out of the mouth by the forward thrust of the tongue.

Remember that young babies must learn to eat from a spoon. At first, they will use the sucking reflex to eat solids. The sucking reflex will permit them to take the food from the spoon and swallow it, but in very young babies the forward action of the tongue will often push the solids out of the mouth. When this happens, continue to feed solids but insert spoon farther into the mouth and be sure the spoon is on top of the tongue. As the baby grows older, tongue control develops and feeding becomes easier.

14. Continue the process until the feeding is completed.
15. Solids should be offered before formula or breast-feeding.

If the baby drinks formula or is breast-fed before solids, hunger is satisfied, and the baby will either go to sleep or refuse solids. There will be times when baby is too hungry or anxious to eat solid foods before milk or formula. When this occurs, give a small portion of formula or breast-feed for a few minutes, then quickly switch to solids.

Immobilizing the infant: mummy restraint (Fig. 18-11)

Purpose: To restrain the child safely to facilitate a necessary procedure (eyedrops, eardrops, nosedrops, shampoo)

There are times when a restraint is necessary. Mummy restraints prove useful when unpleasant procedures involving the face or head are necessary.

Material
    Receiving blanket or small sheet
    Safety pins (two or three)

The size of the infant dictates the size of blanket or sheet necessary. Pins are not always needed because the procedure can often be accomplished in less time than it takes to pin the restraint.

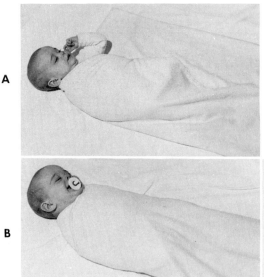

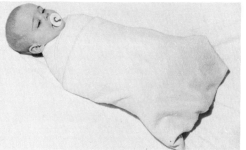

Fig. 18-11. Mummy restraint used to immobilize infant's arms and legs. **A,** Center baby's head at edge of "short side" of open baby blanket or sheet. Place one arm at side and pull blanket snugly over shoulder, arm, and chest and tuck blanket under baby. **B,** Position opposite arm similarly and pull opposite corner over and around baby. **C,** Open out loose end of blanket and bring it up and around baby snugly. (From Ingalls, A.J., and Salerno, M.C.: Maternal and child nursing, ed. 4, St. Louis, 1979, The C.V. Mosby Co.)

1. Wash hands before starting.
2. Place a receiving blanket or sheet opened lengthwise on a flat surface (bed).
3. Place the infant in the center of the blanket with the head extended beyond the edge of the blanket.

PROCEDURE	HELPFUL HINTS
4. Starting at the infant's left side, place the infant's left arm along the side of his body.	
5. Bring the blanket down over the left shoulder across the body and tuck it in firmly under the infant's right side from axilla to toes.	The more firmly the blanket is wrapped around the child, the greater the amount of restraint of arms and torso is achieved.
6. Place the infant's right arm along the side of his body.	
7. Bring the blanket down over the right shoulder across the body and tuck firmly behind the left side.	Talking, cooing, or otherwise soothing the baby while applying the restraint reduces the baby's anxiety and resistance.
8. Use safety pins to secure the blanket in place.	
9. Follow through with the procedure that required this restraint.	Proceed quickly with the procedure that made this restraint necessary.
10. Release the child as quickly as possible after the procedure is finished.	
11. Comfort and reassure the child.	
12. Praise the child for efforts to cooperate. (Even though the child cried and fussed, praise is helpful.)	

Instillation of drops and ointment

EARDROPS

Purpose: Instillation of medication.

Material
   Medication
   Soft tissue
 Position: Sitting or lying down, depending on the child's ability to cooperate
	The medication is frequently supplied in a squeeze bottle with a dropper tip or in a bottle with a dropper attached to the lid. Occasionally a separate dropper is needed. If more than one member of the family is to receive the same medication, individual droppers must be used.

1. Wash hands before beginning.	
2. Have the child lie down or sit with the head turned or tilted to the side so that the affected ear is directed upward.	Children who have frequent earaches quickly learn to cooperate with eardrop instillation because the medication frequently provides instant comfort.
3. For children under two (Fig. 18-12, *A*):	
a. Grasp the earlobe (pinna) firmly between the finger and thumb.	
b. Pull the earlobe *down* and *back* gently so that the external orifice is clear, and the canal is straight.	Caretakers should be taught to pull the earlobe down and back for children under 2 and up and back for children over 2.

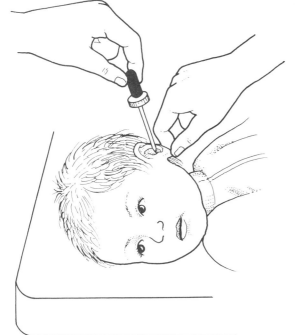

A

Fig. 18-12. **A,** Instillation of eardrops for child under 2 years of age.

|

Instillation of drops and ointment—cont'd

EARDROPS—cont'd

4. For children over two (Fig. 18-12, *B*):

It is helpful to adjust the outer ear as recommended, since this straightens the ear canal, thus enhancing the medication's usefulness.

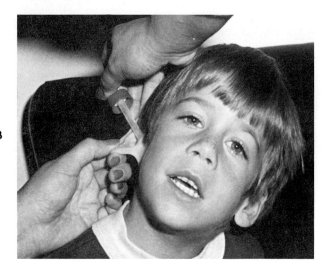

B

Fig. 18-12, cont'd. B, Instillation of eardrops for older child.

   a. Grasp the earlobe (pinna) firmly between the finger and thumb.
   b. Pull the earlobe *up* and *back* gently so that the external orifice is clear, and the canal is straight.
5. Drop the prescribed number of drops directly into the canal.
6. Release the earlobe (pinna) gently.

The outer ear is to be manipulated gently because infected ears are usually quite painful. Additional pain is to be avoided.

7. Maintain a tilted position of the head for a few moments.

Do not plug the ear with cotton or massage it unless directly ordered to do so by health personnel. Maintaining the tipped head position is usually all that is needed to spread the medication evenly.

8. When the erect position is assumed, excess drops may be wiped away with tissue.

NOSEDROPS OR SPRAY

Purpose: To instill medication, loosen mucous secretions, reduce mucosal inflammation, and enhance respiration.

   Material
      Medication
      Tissue

Nosedrops and sprays are frequently used to loosen mucus and clear the nasal passages.

Many nosedrops and sprays are in squeeze-type containers with self-contained tips. If more than one person is using the medication, it is advisable to have separate containers or to wash the tip carefully between applications to prevent the spread of infection.

Children will often accept and cooperate better when nasal sprays are used.

It may be necessary to wipe away or remove excess nasal discharge before administering drops. If mucus is crusted at the nostrils, apply a warm wet washcloth for a few moments to soften and dislodge the crusts, then wipe away gently.

PROCEDURE

HELPFUL HINTS

Procedure for nosedrops
1. Wash hands before beginning.
2. Have the child lie down or sit with the head tilted backward (Fig. 18-13).

Nosedrops must reach the back of the nose; therefore the head must be tilted back during administration. Placing a pillow under the shoulders help maintain the desired position.

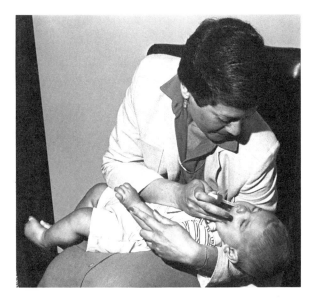

Fig. 18-13. Instillation of nosedrops.

3. Instruct the child to breathe through the mouth.

Children old enough to cooperate should be reminded to breathe through their mouths because this prevents the child from forcefully expelling the drops as they are administered.

4. Drop the prescribed number of drops into each nostril.
5. Sit the child up—do not permit the child to blow the nose, although excess medication may be wiped away gently with a tissue.
6. Instruct the child (if old enough) to expectorate any medication that may have reached the back of the throat.

Children should be encouraged to spit out excess medication that reaches the back of the throat, but discouraged from blowing the nose before the medication can provide relief.

Procedure for nasal spray
1. Wash hands before beginning.
2. Have the child sit or stand.

Nasal sprays are applied in upright positions. Overuse should be avoided.

3. Place the spray tip at the nasal orifice, squeeze the bottle firmly, and have the child inhale.

Children 3 years and older can use these sprays but must be supervised to prevent overuse and assure correct usage.

4. Repeat step 3 with the other nostril.

EYEDROPS AND OINTMENTS

Purpose: To apply medication or lubricant to the eye.

Materials
Gauze squares (or soft tissue)
Eyedropper (unless it is already part of the medicine container)
Medication

Some eye medicines come in squeeze-type containers with a dropper tip. Others may have a dropper attached to the inner surface of the container top or may require a separate eyedropper.

PROCEDURE

HELPFUL HINTS

Instillation of drops and ointments—cont'd

EARDROPS—cont'd

1. Wash hands before eyedrop administration.
2. Check the medication label for the following:
   a. Correct medicine.
   b. Number of drops to be administered.
   c. Eye to be medicated: o.s., left eye; o.d., right eye; and o.u., both eyes.
   d. Frequency of administration.

3. The child can be either sitting, standing, or lying down (depending on ability to cooperate).

4. Tilt the head back and turn to permit the instilled fluid to flow from the inner canthus to outer canthus of the eye (nose toward ear).
5. Using the fingertip, apply gentle pressure on the lower lid, pulling the lid down to form a small cul-de-sac.

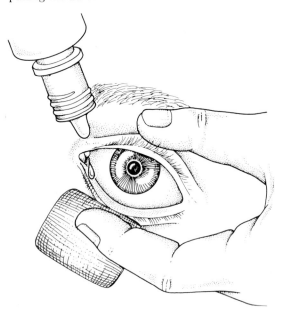

6. Place the eyedropper directly above the cul-de-sac and instill the number of drops required. *Do not touch the eye with the dropper or allow medicine to directly touch the cornea (lens). The cornea of the eye is sensitive and can be easily damaged.*

If more than one person in the family is using the same eyedrops, an individual eyedropper should be used. Individual eyedroppers should be rinsed well under running water for cleansing after each use. *Caution:* Avoid leaving water in the dropper, because this will dilute the potency of the drug.

Be certain you know how the medicine should appear (cloudy or clear) and that it is meant for the eye (optic or ophthalmic solution). *Caution:* Often medicine that becomes cloudy or precipitates is deteriorating and should be discarded.

Eyedrops should be at room temperature before instillation. If they are to be stored in the refrigerator, it will be helpful, prior to administration, to rotate the container between the palms of the hands to bring the medicine to room temperature.

Infants should be lying down with one caretaker restraining the infant's arms and head.

If the caretaker administering the medication stands behind the head, the baby will automatically look up and back, thus providing a natural position for instillation of drops.

Toddlers can be immobilized in a sitting position on the lap of the caretaker with head tilted against the caretaker's body and cradled by the upper and lower arm. The caretaker is able to provide comfort and restraint while administering the drops.

Turning the head sideways permits the medication to flow from the nose toward the ear and prevents administering medication to wrong eye or spreading the infection from one eye to the other.

A gauze square (or soft tissue) can be placed beneath the finger used to retract the eyelid to absorb the overflow of medication (Fig. 18-14).

Older children may wish to hold the tissue and remove the excess medicine on their own.

It is important for children to be instructed not to wipe or rub the eye vigorously, since this may only further irritate the eye or spread the infection to the other eye.

Fig. 18-14. Instillation of eyedrops.

For better control during administration of eyedrops, the person applying the medicine should rest the side of the hand on the child's face or forehead. This reduces the chance of the dropper tip touching the eye or medicine falling directly on the lens (cornea).

PROCEDURE	HELPFUL HINTS

7. If the child is old enough and able to cooperate, instruct the child to look up while the medicine is being administered.

Bringing the dropper toward the eye from behind the head will assist children in looking up and back. After instillation, moving the dropper away from the eye toward the ear often assists moving the eye in the desired direction.

8. Gently release the lower eyelid and instruct the child to blink once or twice. (This ensures better distribution of the medication.) NOTE: Ointments are applied either within the cul-de-sac or along the lower lid, beginning at the inner canthus and ending at the outer canthus.

Infants and toddlers blink the eyes automatically, thus spreading medication. Older children often squeeze the eyelids together tightly, forcing medication out. When instructed to blink, they will follow directions.

Lifting and holding the infant

Purpose: To comfort, feed, bubble, or transport the infant safely.

Until children develop consistent muscle control of the head and back, care must be exercised while lifting, holding, and/or carrying them.

HORIZONTAL SUPPORT (LIFTING)

1. Place your hands so that the forearm of one hand is at the infant's back with the palm of the hand under the buttocks and upper thighs (forming a little seat).
2. The palm of the other hand is placed under the shoulders, neck and back of the head.
3. Lift the baby, maintaining firm support to the head, back, and buttocks.

The buttocks and head are the heaviest portions of the baby's body and require the greatest amount of support.

The baby will feel secure if lifted with assurance, while firm support is maintained.

CRADLING

1. Bring the baby close to your body and while supporting the baby's body next to your own, slide the hand and arm that were supporting the head and shoulders down along the back of the infant until the head rests comfortably near the bend of your elbow, and this hand now extends beneath the buttocks and thighs. The hand (originally) under the buttocks can now be moved (Fig. 18-15).

Bracing the baby's body against your own while shifting arm support maintains the sense of security.

After you have moved your hand to the buttocks area, it is reassuring to grasp one of the baby's thighs in your hand.

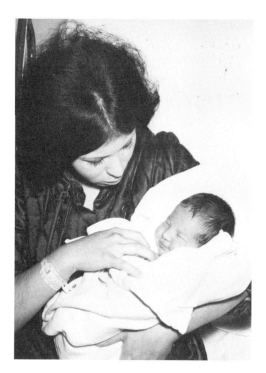

Fig. 18-15. Cradling infant. (From Chinn, P.L.: Child health maintenance: concepts in family-centered care, ed. 2, St. Louis, 1979, The C.V. Mosby Co.)

PROCEDURE	HELPFUL HINTS

Lifting and holding the infant—cont'd

CRADLING—cont'd

2. The infant is held securely by the pressure and support of your body and the arm encircling the infant.

3. Once head and shoulder control are well established in the infant (between the third and sixth month), the amount of support needed decreases.

HORIZONTAL SUPPORT (FOOTBALL HOLD)

1. Follow steps 1 to 3 of horizontal support (lifting).

2. After lifting, rotate the infant's body 90 degrees so that the infant is facing you with feet toward your side. (The arm cradling the infant's head will be fully extended.)

3. Permit the infant's feet and hips to slide next to your body just above your waist. (The elbow of the arm cradling the infant's head will now be flexed and even with the infant's hips).

4. Bring the elbow firmly against the infant's hips, pressing the infant securely against your side (Fig. 18-16).

This position is used most frequently for carrying, feeding, and comforting.

The firmness of your grasp provides security to the baby.

Both the baby and caretaker enjoy this holding position. The baby feels secure and can look at the caretaker. The caretaker has free use of one arm, while maintaining a safe, yet comfortable, grasp of the baby.

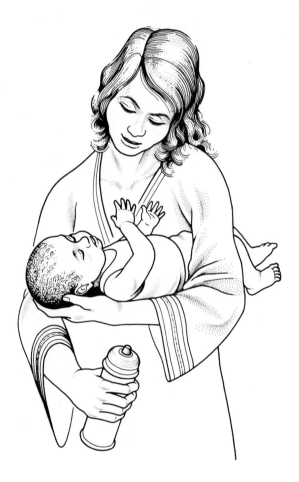

Fig. 18-16. Football hold.

5. Maintain a cradling hold under the head and shoulder.

6. Remove the hand supporting the hips and buttocks. The infant will be supported the entire length of body by your one arm and hand.

This position is useful for shampooing, carrying, and comforting.

PROCEDURE	HELPFUL HINTS

VERTICAL SUPPORT ("BUBBLING" HOLD)

Upright

1. Follow steps 1 to 3 for horizontal support (lifting).
2. Bring the child close to your body while at the same time elevating the child's head and shoulders (Fig. 18-17, *A*). (The child will appear to be sitting in the palm of one hand.)
3. Place the child's head at your shoulder level.

A firm grasp of the baby's buttocks and upper thigh will provide security when the baby is being placed in the sitting position in your hands.

The baby's head may fall forward when being brought against the shoulder. Maintain support to the back of the neck and head.

After the head is stabilized against your shoulder, it is possible to move the hand that provided the support to the head down toward the middle of the back.

This position is useful for bubbling, carrying, or comforting the infant.

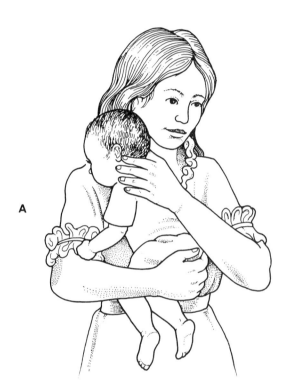

A

Fig. 18-17. Bubbling infant. **A,** Vertical hold. **B,** Lap hold.

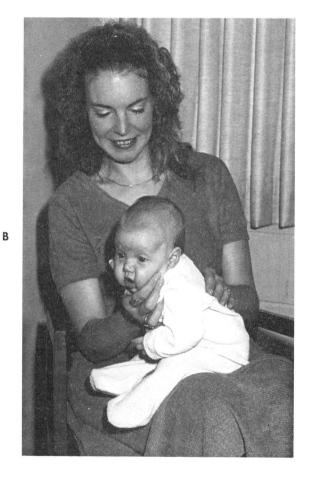

B

4. Support the child firmly against your body by bringing your hand that supported the child's head and shoulders down to the middle of the child's shoulders and back.
5. The hand that is now at the middle of the back can be used to pat the infant or gently rub the back or support the head.

Sitting

1. Follow steps 1 to 3 for horizontal support (lifting).
2. Follow step 1 for cradling.
3. Sit down.
4. Place the infant on your lap.
5. Tilt the infant forward, supporting the chest, neck, and head with the palm of the hand (thumb and index finger encircle chin) (Fig. 18-17, *B*).
6. The free hand can now be used to pat the infant or gently rub the infant's back.

Pinworm diagnosis

Purpose: Collect a specimen that can be used to diagnose the presence of pinworms (Fig. 18-18).

Materials
    Pinworm kits might be available
    Clear plastic tape
    Glass slide (clean)
    Envelope

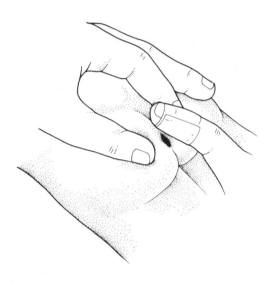

Fig. 18-18. Collecting pinworm specimen.

1. Wash hands before starting.
2. This procedure must be performed in the morning before the child gets up.

Pinworms migrate to the rectum (anal) opening during the night. Specimens collected before the child becomes active are most likely to contain the eggs.
Repeated anal scratching may be indicative of pinworms.

3. Cut 2-inch (5-cm) strip of plastic tape. Place it at the head of child's bed.
4. Remove the diaper or panties.
5. Place the child on the abdomen or side.
6. Roll the tape over the index finger of one of your hands. Be sure the sticky side is out.
7. Separate the child's buttocks with the other hand to expose the anus.
8. Press the taped finger (sticky side out) firmly against the anal opening.
9. Remove the taped finger.
10. Place the tape, sticky surface down, on a clean glass slide.
11. Replace the diaper or panties.
12. Place the slide in an envelope.
13. Mark the envelope with the child's name, date, and time of collection.
14. Give the slide to a physician, nurse, or laboratory as directed.

PROCEDURE	HELPFUL HINTS

Taking temperatures with a glass thermometer

Purpose: To obtain a measurement of body temperature.

Materials
Thermometer
Tissue wipe
Lubricant (for rectal temperature)

1. Wash hands before beginning procedure.
2. Select the correct thermometer. Frequently the oral or axillary thermometer has a longer bulb than the rectal type.
3. Shake the mercury into the bulb end of the thermometer.
   a. Hold the thermometer firmly between the thumb and index finger of the dominant hand.
   b. Bend the arm at the elbow and quickly snap the forearm and wrist in a downward motion.
   c. Repeat until the mercury falls below 95 on the calibrated scale. Hold thermometer at eye level, rotating the cylinder until the mercury line is visible.
4. Position the child for appropriate technique.
   a. Oral—sitting up or lying on back. (Children should be at least preschoolers who will follow directions.)
   b. Axillary—sitting up or lying on back.
   c. Rectal—lying on side or abdomen (Take rectal temperatures on infants and toddlers. If the child resists the intrusive procedure, use the axillary method.)
5. Insert the thermometer.
   a. Oral
      (1) Place the thermometer bulb under the tongue.
      (2) The lips must remain closed.
      (3) Instruct the child not to bite down on the thermometer.
      (4) Leave the thermometer in place a minimum of 5 minutes.
   b. Axillary
      (1) Place the thermometer bulb under the arm.
      (2) Bring the arm alongside the body.
      (3) Hold the thermometer firmly in place a minimum of 10 minutes.
   c. Rectal
      (1) Coat the bulb with petroleum jelly or another lubricant.
      (2) Insert the bulb into the rectum. (Do not insert the thermometer more than 1 inch; 2.5 cm.)
      (3) Hold the stem of the thermometer securely at all times. (Keep the other hand on the child's buttocks to maintain the position.)
      (4) Hold the thermometer in place for a minimum of 3 minutes.
6. Remove the thermometer. Wipe it with a tissue from the stem to the bulb.
7. Read the thermometer.

The state of health is often indicated by the body temperature. When in good health, the body is able to maintain a narrow range of normal temperature (98.6° to 99.5° F; 36.9° to 37.5° C). Normal body temperature fluctuates in relation to the time of day, exercise, food intake, and environmental temperature.

On the market today are several different temperature-taking devices, some of which are disposable. Follow the manufacturer's directions.

Inspect the thermometer before use, ensuring that there are no cracks, the calibrated side is readable, and the mercury is intact.

Stand clear of objects while shaking down the mercury to prevent breaking the thermometer.

Have the child in a comfortable safe position to facilitate the procedure and prevent injury.

The mouth must be kept closed. The child must be able to breathe through the nose. Airflow in the mouth will seriously alter the temperature. (Be sure child has not had anything hot or cold to drink for at least 30 minutes prior to taking the temperature.)

Be sure the child is securely held in one position.

Remind the child not to bite the thermometer because they break easily. (If a thermometer breaks have the child spit out the pieces, rinse the mouth, and spit. *Do not swallow.*)

Instruct the child to open the mouth when you are ready to remove the thermometer to avoid breaking or scraping the teeth.

It is possible to damage the rectum by inserting thermometer too far. Do not be surprised if the child has a bowel movement while having a rectal temperature taken.

Always maintain a hold on the stem of the thermometer, since they do break and can cause extensive damage.

PROCEDURE	HELPFUL HINTS

Taking temperature with a glass thermometer—cont'd

8. Wash the thermometer.
   a. Use cool soapy water.
   b. Rub from the stem to the bulb.
   c. Rinse with cool water.
   d. Dry with tissue from the bulb to the stem.
9. Place the thermometer (bulb end down) in a storage container.

> Avoid using hot water because this will break the thermometer.

> Always store a clean thermometer to prevent future infections.

Urine specimen

Purpose: To provide the health care worker with a specimen of the child's urine.

> Often it is easier to obtain a urine specimen from a child at home than in an office setting.

Materials
   Specimen container (clean glass jar with lid)
   Soap
   Water
   Washcloth

> Specimen containers might be provided by health care workers. If so, use them. (Special specimens, such as a clean-catch specimen, require additional equipment and precautions. Check with health care personnel for additional instructions.)

1. Wash hands before starting the procedure.
2. Cleanse the genitalia.
   a. For boys, wash the penis. Retract the foreskin (if present), wash the glans carefully, rinse well, and dry.
   b. For girls, separate the labia using the index finger and thumb. Wash from top to bottom (pubis to rectum) on each side and down the center. Rinse well and dry.

> Always wash from top to bottom of the genitalia to avoid contamination of the urethra from rectal discharges.

3. Collect the specimen.
   a. For older boys, instruct them to urinate into the specimen container.
   b. For older girls, instruct the child to continue to separate the labia, hold container directly under urethra, and urinate into the specimen container.
   c. Younger children may require special plastic specimen collecting devices that have an adhesive surface to hold the receptacle in place until the child urinates.

> Children 3 years and over are usually capable of following instructions for obtaining urine specimens.

> If a special collection device is used, a diaper is placed over the specimen container to prevent dislodging.

4. Wash hands (both child and caretaker).
5. Place the cover on the container and take the specimen to a health care worker.

APPENDIXES

APPENDIX A

IMMUNIZATIONS

RECOMMENDED SCHEDULE FOR ACTIVE IMMUNIZATION OF NORMAL INFANTS AND CHILDREN*

Age	Immunization recommended
2 months	DTP,† TOPV‡
4 months	DTP, TOPV
6 months	DTP§
1 year	Tuberculin test‖
15 months	Measles, rubella, mumps¶
18 months	DTP, TOPV
4-6 years	DTP, TOPV
14-16 years	Td#—repeat every 10 years

*From American Academy of Pediatrics: Report of the Committee on Infectious Disease, III, 1977. Copyright American Academy of Pediatrics, 1977.
†DTP—diphtheria and tetanus toxoids combined with pertussive vaccine.
‡TOPV—trivalent oral poliovirus vaccine. This recommendation is suitable for breast-fed as well as bottle-fed infants.
§A third dose of TOPV is optional but may be given in areas of high endemicity of poliomyelitis.
‖Frequency of tuberculin testing depends on risk of exposure of the child and on the prevalence of tuberculosis in the population group. The initial test should be at or preceding the measles vaccine.
¶May be given at 15 months as measles-rubella or measles-mumps-rubella combined vaccines.
#Td—combined tetanus and diphtheria toxoids (adult type) for those more than 6 years of age, in contrast to diphtheria and tetanus (DT) toxoids, which contain a larger amount of diphtheria antigen.

PRIMARY IMMUNIZATION FOR CHILDREN NOT IMMUNIZED IN EARLY INFANCY*

Time interval	Age (years)	
	Under 6	6 and older
First visit†	DTP, TOPV, tuberculin test	Td, TOPV, tuberculin test
1 month later	Measles,‡ mumps, rubella	Measles, mumps, rubella
2 months later	DTP, TOPV	Td, TOPV
4 months later	DTP, TOPV§	
8-14 months later		Td, TOPV
10-16 months later or preschool	DTP, TOPV	
At age 14-16 years	Td—repeat every 10 years	Td—repeat every 10 years

*From American Academy of Pediatrics: Report of the Committee on Infectious Diseases, III, 1977. Copyright American Academy of Pediatrics, 1977.
†The sequence of these schedules may be altered if specific infections are prevalent. For example, measles vaccine might be given on the first visit if an epidemic is occurring.
‡Measles vaccine is not routinely given before age 15 months.
§Optional.

APPENDIX B

GUIDELINE FOR ADDITION OF SOLID FOODS TO INFANT'S DIET DURING THE FIRST YEAR

When to start*	Foods added	Feeding
First month	Vitamins A, D, and C in multivitamin preparation (according to prescription)	Once daily at a feeding time
Second to third month	Cereal and strained cooked fruit Egg yolk (at first, hard boiled and sieved, soft boiled or poached later)	10 AM and 6 PM
Third to fourth month	Strained cooked vegetable and strained meat	2 PM
Fifth to seventh month	Zweiback or hard toast	At any feeding
Seventh to ninth month	Meat: beef, lamb, or liver (broiled or baked and finely chopped) Potato: baked or boiled and mashed or sieved	10 or 6 PM

Suggested meal plan for ages 8 months to 1 year or older

7 AM	Milk	8 ounces
	Cereal	2 or 3 tablespoons
	Strained fruit	2 or 3 tablespoons
	Zweiback or dry toast	
12 NOON	Milk	8 ounces
	Vegetables	2 or 3 tablespoons
	Chopped meat or one whole egg	
	Puddings or cooked fruit	2 or 3 tablespoons
3 PM	Milk	4 ounces
	Toast, zweiback, or crackers	
6 PM	Milk	8 ounces
	Whole egg or chopped meat	
	Potato, baked or mashed	2 tablespoons
	Pudding or cooked fruit	2 or 3 tablespoons
	Zweiback or toast	

From Williams, S.R.: Nutrition and diet therapy, ed. 3, St. Louis, 1977, The C.V. Mosby Co.
*Semisolid foods should be given immediately after breast or bottle feeding. One or two teaspoons should be given at first. If food is accepted and tolerated well, the amount should be increased to one or two tablespoons per feeding.
NOTE: Banana or cottage cheese may be used as substitution for any meal.

APPROXIMATE ENERGY VALUE OF COMMON SNACK FOODS OFFERED YOUNG CHILDREN

Food	Portion size	kcal	Food	Portion size	kcal
Cheese cubes	¼ ounce	25	Homogenized milk	3 ounces	60
Hard-boiled egg	½ medium	36	Chocolate milk	3 ounces	80
Frankfurter	1, 5 × ¾ inch	133	Cauliflower buds	2 small	2
Pretzel	3 × ½ inch	20	Green pepper strips	2	2
Potato chip	10	114	Cucumber slices	3 large	2
Popcorn with oil and salt	1 cup	41	Cherry tomato	each	3
Bread stick	1, 4½ inches	38	Raw turnip slices	2	5
Saltines	1	12	Dill pickle, large	⅓	5
Graham cracker	2 squares	55	Apple wedges	¼ medium apple	20
Animal cracker	1	11	Banana	½ small	40
Brownie	1, 3 × 1 × ⅞ inch	97	Orange wedges	¼ medium orange	18
Chocolate cupcake	1	51	Orange juice	3 ounces	35
Vanilla wafer	1	18	Grape juice	3 ounces	60
Yogurt, plain	¼ cup	40	Lemonade	3 ounces	40

From Adams, C.F.: Nutritive value of American foods in common units, Agriculture Handbook No. 456, Washington, D.C., 1975, U.S. Department of Agriculture.

FOOD PATTERN FOR PRESCHOOL CHILDREN*

Food	Portion size	Number of portions advised	
		Ages 2 to 4 years	Ages 4 to 6 years
Milk and dairy products			
Milk†	4 oz	3 to 6	3 to 4
Cheese	½ to ¾ oz	May be substituted for one portion of liquid milk	
Yogurt	¼ to ½ cup	May be substituted for one portion of liquid milk	
Powdered skim milk	2 tbsp	May be substituted for one portion of liquid milk	
Meat and meat equivalents			
Meat‡, fish§, poultry	1 to 2 oz	2	2
Egg	1	1	1
Peanut butter	1 to 2 tbsp		
Legumes—dried peas and beans	¼ to ⅓ cup cooked		
Vegetables and fruits			
Vegetables		4 to 5 to include 1 green leafy or yellow‖	4 to 5 to include 1 green leafy or yellow
Cooked	2 to 4 tbsp		
Raw	Few pieces		
Fruit		1 citrus fruit or other vegetable or fruit rich in vitamin C	1 citrus fruit or other vegetable or fruit rich in vitamin C
Canned	4 to 8 tbsp		
Raw	½ to 1 small		
Fruit juice	3 to 4 oz		
Bread and cereal grains			
Whole grain or enriched white bread	½ to 1 slice	3	3
Cooked cereal	¼ to ½ cup	May be substituted for one serving of bread	
Spaghetti, macaroni, noodles, rice	¼ to ½ cup		
Crackers	2 to 3		
Fat			
Bacon	1 slice	Not to be substituted for meat	
Butter or vitamin A—fortified margarine	1 tsp	3	3 to 4
Desserts	¼ to ½ cup	As demanded by calorie needs	
Sugars	½ to 1 tsp	2	2

From Pipes, P.L.: Nutrition in infancy and childhood, ed. 2, St. Louis, 1981, The C.V. Mosby Co.
*Diets should be monitored for adequacy of iron and vitamin D intake.
†Approximately ⅔ cup can easily be incorporated in a child's food during cooking.
‡Liver once a week can be used as liver sausage or cooked liver.
§Should be served once or twice per week to substitute for meat.
‖If the child's preferences are limited, use double portions of preferred vegetables until an appetite for other vegetables develops.

CALORIE VALUES OF SOME COMMON SNACK FOODS

Food	Weight (g)	Approximate measure	Calories
Beverages			
Carbonated, cola type	180	1 bottle, 6 ounces	70
Malted milk	405	1 regular (1½ cups)	420
Chocolate milk (made with skim milk)	250	1 cup	190
Cocoa	200	1 cup	235
Soda, vanilla ice cream	242	1 regular	260
Cake			
Angel food	40	2-inch sector	110
Cupcake, chocolate, iced	50	1 cake, 2¾ inches in diameter	185
Fruitcake	30	1 piece, 2 by 2 by ½ inch	115
Candy and popcorn			
Butterscotch	15	3 pieces	60
Candy bar, plain	57	1 bar	295
Caramels	30	3 medium	120
Chocolate coated creams	30	2 average	130
Fudge	28	1 piece	115
Peanut brittle	30	1 ounce	125
Popcorn with oil added	14	1 cup	65
Cheese			
Camembert	28	1 ounce	85
Cheddar	28	1 ounce	105
Cream	28	1 ounce	105
Swiss (domestic)	28	1 ounce	105
Cookies			
Brownies	30	1 piece, 2 by 2 by ¾ inch	140
Cookies, plain and assorted	25	1 cooky, 3 inches in diameter	120
Crackers			
Cheese	18	5 crackers	85
Graham	14	2 medium	55
Saltines	16	4 crackers	70
Rye	13	2 crackers	45
Dessert-type cream puff and doughnuts			
Cream puff—custard filling	105	1 average	245
Doughnut, cake type, plain	32	1 average	125
Doughnut, jelly	65	1 average	225
Doughnut, raised	30	1 average	120
Miscellaneous			
Hamburger and bun	96	1 average	330
Ice cream, vanilla	62	3½ ounce container	130
Sherbet	96	½ cup	120
Jams, jellies, marmalades, preserves	20	1 tablespoon	55
Syrup, blended	80	¼ cup	240
Waffles	75	1 waffle, 4½ by 5½ by ½ inch	210

From Williams, S.R.: Nutrition and diet therapy, ed. 4, St. Louis, 1981, The C.V. Mosby Co.

Continued.

Calorie values of some common snack foods—cont'd

Food	Weight (g)	Approximate measure	Calories
Nuts			
Mixed, shelled	15	8 to 12	95
Peanut butter	16	1 tablespoon	95
Peanuts, shelled, roasted	144	1 cup	840
Pie			
Apple	135	4-inch sector	345
Cherry	135	4-inch sector	355
Custard	130	4-inch sector	280
Lemon meringue	120	4-inch sector	305
Mince	135	4-inch sector	365
Pumpkin	130	4-inch sector	275
Potato chips			
Potato chips	20	10 chips, 2 inches in diameter	115
Sandwiches			
Bacon, lettuce, tomato	150	1 sandwich	280
Egg salad	140	1 sandwich	280
Ham	80	1 sandwich	280
Liverwurst	90	1 sandwich	250
Peanut butter	85	1 sandwich	330
Soups, commercial canned			
Bean with pork	250	1 cup	170
Beef noodle	250	1 cup	70
Chicken noodle	250	1 cup	65
Cream (mushroom)	240	1 cup	135
Tomato	245	1 cup	90
Vegetable with beef broth	250	1 cup	80

RULE OF NINES

For children 10 and older, the body surface is basically divided into multiples of nine and expressed in percentages. The percentages break down as follows:

Head = 9% (front = 4.5%, back = 4.5%)

Each arm = 9% (front = 4.5%, back = 4.5%)

Each leg = 18% (front = 9%, back = 9%)

Body (shoulder and hips) = 36% (front = 18%, back = 18%)

Genitalia = 1%

In children under 10 the allocation of percentages is different for the head and legs. *For each year under 10, subtract ½% (0.5%) from each lower limb of the adult percentage and add that number to the child's head percentage.* Thus an infant's proportions would be as follows:

Head = 19% (front = 9.5%, back = 9.5%)

Each leg = 13% (front = 6.5%, back = 6.5%)

A rough estimate of burned surface can be obtained by adding the percentages of involved body parts.

Caution: The rule of nines quickly indicates the amount of surface area involved, but does not determine the extent or depth of the burn.

Other methods of estimating both the extent and severity of burns do exist but require an additional knowledge base and diagrams.

BIBLIOGRAPHY

INTRODUCTION

Bruhn, J.G., and Cordova, F.D.: A developmental approach to learning wellness behavior. Part 1: Infancy to early adolescence, Health Values: Achieving High-Level Wellness **1**:246, Dec., 1977.

Hayman, H.S.: Improving health curriculum scope in the modern world, Health Values: Achieving High-Level Wellness **1**:262, Dec., 1977.

Pender, N.: A conceptual model for preventive health behavior, Nurs. Outlook **23**:385, June, 1975.

Sciarillo, W.G., Jr.: Using Hymovich's framework in the family-oriented approach, MCN **5**:242, July/Aug., 1980.

CHAPTER 1

Alexander, M., and Brown, M.S.: Physical examination. Part 14: Male genitalia, Nurs. '76 **6**:39, Feb., 1976.

Becoming a parent, Columbus, Ohio, 1975, Ross Laboratories, Inc.

Brown, M.S., and Alexander, M.: Physical examination. Part 10: Mouth and throat, Nurs. '74 **4**:57, Aug., 1974.

Brown, M.S., Hudak, C., Brenneman, J., Walsh, K., and Kleeman, K.: Student manual of physical examination, Philadelphia, 1977, J.B. Lippincott Co.

Caring for your baby, Columbus, Ohio, 1978, Ross Laboratories, Inc.

Chinn, P.L.: Child health maintenance: concepts in family-centered care, ed. 2, St. Louis, 1979, The C.V. Mosby Co.

Clark, A., and Alfonso, D.: Childbearing: a nursing perspective, Philadelphia, 1976, F.A. Davis Co.

The first year of life: the first week, Am. Baby **42**:17, Mid-April, 1980.

The first year of life: the first month, Am. Baby **42**:27, Mid-April, 1980.

Guthrie, D., and Guthrie, R.: The infant of the diabetic mother, Am. J. Nurs. **74**:2008, Nov., 1974.

Heagarty, M., Glass, G., King, H., and Manly, M.: Child health: basics for primary care. New York, 1980, Appleton-Century-Crofts.

Klaus, M.H., and Kennell, J.H.: Parent-infant bonding, ed. 2, St. Louis, 1982, The C.V. Mosby Co.

McFarlane, J.: Pediatric assessment and intervention, Nurs. '74 **4**:66, Dec., 1974.

McFarlane, J.M., Whitson, B.J., and Hartley, L.M.: Contemporary pediatric nursing, New York, 1980, John Wiley & Sons, Inc.

Moore, M.L.: The newborn and the nurse. Saunders Monographs in Clinical Nursing, No. 3, Philadelphia, 1972, W.B. Saunders Co.

The phenomena of early development, Columbus, Ohio, 1975, Ross Laboratories, Inc.

Seedor, M.: The physical assessment, New York, 1974, Teachers College Press.

Ziegel, E., and Van Blarcom, C.C.: Obstetric nursing, New York, 1972, Macmillan Publishing Co., Inc.

CHAPTER 2

Becoming a parent, Columbus, Ohio, 1975, Ross Laboratories, Inc.

Brown, M.S., and Alexander, M.: Physical examination. Part 10: Mouth and throat, Nurs. '74 **4**:57, Aug., 1974.

Brown, M.S., Hudak, C., Brenneman, J., Walsh, K., and Kleeman, K.: Student manual of physical examination, Philadelphia, 1977, J.B. Lippincott Co.

Caring for your baby, Columbus, Ohio, 1978, Ross Laboratories, Inc.

Chinn, P.L.: Child health maintenance: concepts in family-centered care, ed. 2, St. Louis, 1979, The C.V. Mosby Co.

The first year of life, Am. Baby **42**:35-63, Mid-April, 1980.

Heagarty, M., Glass, G., King, H., and Manly, M.: Child health: basics for primary care, New York, 1980, Appleton-Century-Crofts.

Klaus, M.H., and Kennell, J.H.: Parent-infant bonding, St. Louis, 1976, The C.V. Mosby Co.

McFarlane, J.: Pediatric assessment and intervention, Nurs. '74 **4**:66, Dec., 1974.

McFarlane, J.M., Whitson, B.J., and Hartley, L.M.: Contemporary pediatric nursing, New York, 1970, John Wiley & Sons, Inc.

The phenomena of early development, Ohio, 1975, Ross Laboratories, Inc.

Seedor, M.: The physical assessment, New York, 1974, Teachers College Press.

Ziegel, E., and Van Blarcom, C.C.: Obstetric nursing, New York, 1972, Macmillan Publishing Co., Inc.

CHAPTER 3

Becoming a parent, Columbus, Ohio, 1975, Ross Laboratories, Inc.

Brown, M.S., and Alexander, M.: Physical examination. Part 10: Mouth and throat, Nurs. '74 **4**:57, Aug., 1974.

Brown, M.S., Hudak, C., Brenneman, J., Walsh, K., and Kleeman, K.: Student manual of physical examination, Philadelphia, 1977, J.B. Lippincott Co.

Caring for your baby, Columbus, Ohio, 1978, Ross Laboratories, Inc.

Chinn, P.L.: Child health maintenance: concepts in family-centered care, ed. 2, St. Louis, 1979, The C.V. Mosby Co.

Erikson, E.: Childhood and society, ed. 2, New York, 1963, W.W. Norton and Co., Inc.

The first year of life, Am. Baby **42**:69-105, 1980.

Heagarty, M., Glass, F., King, H., and Manly, M.: Child health: basics for primary care, New York, 1980, Appleton-Century-Crofts.

Latham, H.C., Heckel, R.V., Hebert, L.J., and Bennett, E.: Pediatric nursing, ed. 3, St. Louis, 1977, The C.V. Mosby Co.

Malasanos, L., Barkauskas, V., Moss, M., and Stoltenberg-Allen, K.: Health assessment, ed. 2, St. Louis, 1981, The C.V. Mosby Co.

Marlow, D.: Textbook of pediatric nursing, ed. 5, Philadelphia, 1977, W.B. Saunders Co.

BIBLIOGRAPHY

McFarlane, J.: Pediatric assessment and intervention, Nurs. '74 4:66, Dec., 1974.

McFarlane, J.M., Whitman, B.J., and Hartley, L.M.: Contemporary pediatric nursing, New York, 1980, John Wiley & Sons, Inc.

Murray, R., and Zentner, J.: Nursing assessment and health promotion through the life span, ed. 2, Englewood Cliffs, N.J., 1979, Prentice-Hall, Inc.

The phenomena of early development, Columbus, Ohio, 1975, Ross Laboratories, Inc.

Scipien, G.M., Barnard, M.U., Chard, M.A., Howe, J., and Phillips, P.: Comprehensive pediatric nursing, New York, 1975, McGraw-Hill Book Co.

Seedor, M.: The physical assessment, New York, 1974, Teachers College Press.

Sutterley, D., and Donnelly, G.: Perspectives in human development, Philadelphia, 1973, J.B. Lippincott Co.

Whaley, L.F., and Wong, D.L.: Nursing care of infants and children, St. Louis, 1979, The C.V. Mosby Co.

CHAPTER 4

Alexander, M., and Brown, M.: Pediatric physical diagnosis for nurses, New York, 1974, McGraw-Hill Book Co.

Alexander, M., and Brown, M.S.: Physical examination. Part 14: Male genitalia, Nurs. '76 6:39, Feb., 1976.

Bates, B.: A guide to physical examination, ed. 2, Philadelphia, 1979, J.B. Lippincott Co.

Becoming a parent, Columbus, Ohio, 1975, Ross Laboratories, Inc.

Benson, E., and McDevitt, J.: Community health and nursing practice, ed. 2, Englewood Cliffs, N.J., 1980, Prentice-Hall, Inc.

Birchfield, M.: Nursing care for hospitalized children based on different stages of illness, MCN 6:46, Jan./Feb., 1981.

Boston Children's Medical Center, and Feinbloom, R.: Child health encyclopedia: the complete guide for parents, New York, 1978, Dell Publishing Co., Inc.

Bowlby, J.: Child care and the growth of love, ed. 2, New York, 1965, Penguin Books.

Brown, M.S., and Alexander, M.: Physical examination. Part 10: Mouth and throat, Nurs. '74 4:57, Aug., 1974.

Brown, M.S., Hudak, C., Brenneman, J., Walsh, K., and Kleeman, K.: Student manual of physical examination, Philadelphia, 1977, J.B. Lippincott Co.

Brown, M.S., and Hurlock, J.: Mothering the mother, Am. J. Nurs. 77:439, March, 1977.

Brown, M.S., and Murphy, M.A.: Ambulatory pediatrics for nurses, New York, 1975, McGraw-Hill Book Co.

Chow, M., Durand, B., Feldman, M., and Mills, M.: Handbook of pediatric primary care, New York, 1979, John Wiley & Sons, Inc.

Clark, A., and Alfonso, D.: Childbearing: a nursing perspective, Philadelphia, 1976, F.A. Davis Co.

Davis, V.: Through the bars of a crib, Am. J. Nurs. 71:1752, Sept., 1971.

Erikson, E.: Childhood and society, ed. 2, New York, 1963, W.W. Norton & Co., Inc.

Feeding your growing baby, Columbus, Ohio, 1978, Ross Laboratories, Inc.

Hanlon, J.J., and Pickett, G.E.: Public health: administration and practice, ed. 7, St. Louis, 1979, The C.V. Mosby Co.

Hardgrove, C., and Rutledge, A.: Parenting during hospitalization, Am. J. Nurs. 75:836, May, 1975.

Heagarty, M., Glass, G., King, H., and Manly, M.: Child health: basics for primary care, New York, 1980, Appleton-Century-Crofts.

Howard, R., and Herbald, N.: Nutrition in clinical care, New York, 1978, McGraw-Hill Book Co.

Hudak, C., Redstone, P., Hokanson, N., and Suzuki, I.: Clinical protocols: a guide for nurses and physicians, Philadelphia, 1976, J.B. Lippincott Co.

Insel, P., and Roth, W.: Health in a changing society, Palo Alto, Calif., 1976, Mayfield Publishing Co.

Isler, C.: The fine art of handling a hospitalized child, RN 41:41, March, 1978.

Kee, J., and Gregory, A.: The ABC's and mEq's of fluid balance in children, Nurs. '74 4:29, June, 1974.

Knofl, K.: Conflicting perspectives on breast feeding, Am. J. Nurs. 74:1848, Oct., 1974.

Lewis, C.: Nutrition: the basics of nutrition, Philadelphia, 1977, F.A. Davis Co.

Malasanos, L., Barkauskas, V., Moss, M., and Stoltenberg-Allen, K.: Health assessment, ed. 2, St. Louis, 1981, The C.V. Mosby Co.

Marlow, D.: Textbook of pediatric nursing, ed. 5, Philadelphia, 1974, 1977, W.B. Saunders Co.

Mayer, J.: Health, New York, 1974, D. Van Nostrand Co.

McCloskey, J.C.: How to make the most of body image theory in nursing practice, Nurs. '76 6:68, May, 1976.

McFarlane, J.: Pediatric assessment and intervention, Nurs. '74 4:66, Dec., 1974.

McFarlane, J.M., Whitson, B.J., and Hartley, L.M.: Contemporary pediatric nursing, New York, 1980, John Wiley & Sons, Inc.

McInnes, M.E.: Essentials of communicable disease, ed. 2, St. Louis, 1975, The C.V. Mosby Co.

McNutt, K., and McNutt, D.: Nutrition and food choices, Chicago, 1978, Science Research Associates, Inc.

Miller, B., and Keane, C.B.: Encyclopedia and dictionary of medicine and nursing, Philadelphia, 1972, W.B. Saunders Co.

Murray, R., and Zentner, J.: Nursing assessment and health promotion through the life span, ed. 2, Englewood Cliffs, N.J., 1979, Prentice-Hall, Inc.

O'Brien, M., Manly, M., and Heagarty, M.: Expanding the public health nurse's role in child care, Nurs. Outlook 23:369, June, 1975.

Otte, M.J.: Correcting inverted nipples—an aid to breast feeding, Am. J. Nurs. 75:454, March, 1975.

Pipes, P.L.: Nutrition in infancy and childhood, ed. 2, St. Louis, 1981, The C.V. Mosby Co.

Schleiher, I.M.: Teaching parents to cope with behavior problems, Am. J. Nurs. 78:838, May, 1978.

Seedor, M.: The physical assessment, New York, 1974, Teachers College Press.

Selekman, J.: Immunization: what's it all about? Am. J. Nurs. 80:140, Aug., 1980.

Sirota, A.: Private care in a public clinic, Am. J. Nurs. 74:1642, Sept., 1974.

Socksteder, S., Gilden, J.H., and Dassy, C.: Common congenital cardiac defects, Am. J. Nurs. 78:266, Feb., 1978.

Taber's cyclopedic medical dictionary, ed. 13, Philadelphia, 1977, F.A. Davis Co.

Thiele, V.F.: Clinical nutrition, ed. 2, St. Louis, 1980, The C.V. Mosby Co.

Tripp, S.: What to ask and what to do when parents call about children's illnesses, Nurs. '74 4:73, June, 1974.

Waring, W., and Jeansonne, L.: Practice manual of pediatrics, St. Louis, 1975, The C.V. Mosby Co.

Wigley, R., and Cook, J.: Community health: concepts and issues, New York, 1975, D. Van Nostrand Co.

Williams, S. R.: Essentials of nutrition and diet therapy, ed. 2, St. Louis, 1978, The C.V. Mosby Co.

Your children and discipline, Columbus, Ohio, 1978, Ross Laboratories, Inc.

CHAPTER 5

Bates, B.: A guide to physical examination, ed. 2, Philadelphia, J.B. Lippincott Co.

Boston Children's Medical Center, and Feinbloom, R.: Child health encyclopedia: the complete guide for parents, New York, 1978, Dell Publishing Co., Inc.

Caldwell, J.: Congenital syphilis: a nonvenereal disease, Am. J. Nurs. **71**:1768, Sept., 1971.

Chow, M., Durand, B., Feldman, M., and Mills, M.: Handbook of pediatric primary care, New York, 1979, John Wiley & Sons, Inc.

Copeland, L.: Chronic diarrhea in infancy, Am. J. Nurs. **77**:461, March, 1977.

Hilt, N., and Schmitt, E.: Pediatric orthopedic nursing, St. Louis, 1975, The C.V. Mosby Co.

Huber, H.: Draining the "fluid ear" with myringotomy and tube insertion, Nurs. '78 **8**:22, July, 1978.

Hudak, C., Redstone, P., Hokanson, N., and Suzuki, I.: Clinical protocols: a guide for nurses and physicians, Philadelphia, 1976, J.B. Lippincott Co.

Isler, C.: Infection: constant threat to perinatal life, RN **38**:23, Aug., 1975.

Maloney, S.: A health care protocol for otitis media, Chapter 15. In Brandt, P.A., Chinn, P.L., Hunt, V.O., and Smith, M.E.: Current practice in pediatric nursing, vol. 2, St. Louis, 1978, The C.V. Mosby Co.

McFarlane, J.M., Whitson, B.J., and Hartley, L.M.: Contemporary pediatric nursing, New York, 1980, John Wiley & Sons, Inc.

McInnes, M.E.: Essentials of communicable disease, ed. 2, St. Louis, 1975, The C.V. Mosby Co.

Miller, B., and Keane, C.B.: Encyclopedia and dictionary of medicine and nursing, Philadelphia, 1972, W.B. Saunders Co.

Moore, M.L.: The newborn and the nurse. Saunders' Monographs in Clinical Nursing, No. 3, Philadelphia, 1972, W.B. Saunders Co.

Taber's cyclopedic medical dictionary, ed. 13, Philadelphia, 1977, F.A. Davis Co.

Test yourself: ear infection, Am. J. Nurs. **78**:229, Feb., 1978.

Thiele, V.F.: Clinical nutrition, ed. 2, St. Louis, 1980, The C.V. Mosby Co.

CHAPTER 6

Brown, M.S., and Alexander, M.: Physical examination. Part 10: Mouth and throat, Nurs. '74 **4**:57, Aug., 1974.

Brown, M.S., Hudak, C., Brenneman, J., Walsh, K., and Kleeman, K.: Student manual of physical examination, Philadelphia, 1977, J.B. Lippincott Co.

Chinn, P.L.: Child health maintenance: concepts in family-centered care, ed. 2, St. Louis, 1979, The C.V. Mosby Co.

Erikson, E.: Childhood and society, ed. 2, New York, 1963, W.W. Norton & Co., Inc.

Heagarty, M., Glass, G., King, H., and Manly, M.: Child health: basics of primary care, New York, 1980, Appleton-Century-Crofts.

Latham, H.C., Heckel, R.V., Hebert, L.J., and Bennett, E.: Pediatric nursing, ed. 3, St. Louis, 1977, The C.V. Mosby Co.

Malasanos, L., Barkauskas, V., Moss, M., and Stoltenberg-Allen, K.: Health assessment, ed. 2, St. Louis, 1981, The C.V. Mosby Co.

Marlow, D.: Textbook of pediatric nursing, ed. 5, Philadelphia, 1977, W.B. Saunders Co.

McFarlane, J.: Pediatric assessment and intervention, Nurs. '74 **4**:66, Dec., 1974.

McFarlane, J.M., Whitson, B.J., and Hartley, L.M.: Contemporary pediatric nursing, New York, 1980, John Wiley & Sons, Inc.

Murray, R., and Zentner, J.: Nursing assessment and health promotion through the life span, ed. 2, Englewood Cliffs, N.J., 1979, Prentice-Hall, Inc.

Scipien, G.M., Barnard, M.U., Chard, M.A., Howe, J., and Phillips, P.: Comprehensive pediatric nursing, New York, 1975, McGraw-Hill Book Co.

Seedor, M.: The physical assessment, New York, 1974, Teachers College Press.

Sutterley, D., and Donnelly, G.: Perspective in human development, Philadelphia, 1973, J.B. Lippincott Co.

Whaley, L.F., and Wong, D.L.: Nursing care of infants and children, St. Louis, 1979, The C. V. Mosby Co.

CHAPTER 7

Alexander, M., and Brown, M.: Pediatric physical diagnosis for nurses, New York, 1974, McGraw-Hill Book Co.

Bates, B.: A guide to physical examination, ed. 2, Philadelphia, 1979, J.B. Lippincott Co.

Benson, E., and McDevitt, J.: Community health and nursing practice, ed. 2, Englewood Cliffs, N.J., 1980, Prentice-Hall, Inc.

Birchfield, M.: Nursing care for hospitalized children based on different stages of illness, MCN **6**:46, Jan./Feb., 1981.

Boston Children's Medical Center, and Feinbloom, R.: Child health encyclopedia: the complete guide for parents, New York, 1978, Dell Publishing Co., Inc.

Bowlby, J.: Child care and the growth of love, ed. 2, Baltimore, 1965, Penguin Books.

Brown, M.S., and Alexander, M.: Physical examination. Part 10: Mouth and throat, Nurs. '74 **4**:57, Aug., 1974.

Brown, M.S., Hudak, C., Brenneman, J., Walsh, K., and Kleeman, K.: Student manual of physical examination, Philadelphia, 1977, J.B. Lippincott Co.

Brown, M.S., and Murphy, M.A.: Ambulatory pediatrics for nurses, New York, 1975, McGraw-Hill Book Co.

Chow, M., Durand, B., Feldman, M., and Mills, M.: Handbook of pediatric primary care, New York, 1979, John Wiley & Sons, Inc.

Davis, V.: Through the bars of a crib, Am. J. Nurs. **71**:1752, Sept., 1971.

Developing toilet habits, Columbus, Ohio, 1977, Ross Laboratories, Inc.

Erikson, E.: Childhood and society, ed. 2, New York, 1963, W.W. Norton & Co., Inc.

Evans, D.W.: Practical advice about a delicate pediatric problem, RN **41**:51, Aug., 1978.

Hardgrove, C., and Rutledge, A.: Parenting during hospitalization, Am. J. Nurs. **75**:836, May, 1975.

Heagarty, M., Glass, G., King, H., and Manly, M.: Child health: basics for primary care, New York, 1980, Appleton-Century-Crofts.

Howard, R., and Herbald, N.: Nutrition in clinical care, New York, 1978, McGraw-Hill Book Co.

Insel, P., and Roth, W.: Health in a changing society, Palo Alto, Calif., 1976, Mayfield Publishing Co.

Isler, C.: The fine art of handling a hospitalized child, RN **41**:41, March, 1978.

Kee, J., and Gregory, A.: The ABC's and mEq's of fluid balance in children, Nurs. '74 **4**:29, June, 1974.

Klein, J.W.: Educational component of day care, Children Today **1**:2, Jan./Feb., 1972.

Lewis, C.: Nutrition: the basics of nutrition, Philadelphia, 1977, F.A. Davis Co.

Malasanos, L., Barkauskas, V., Moss, M., and Stoltenberg-Allen, K.: Health assessment, ed. 2, St. Louis, 1981, The C.V. Mosby Co.

Marlow, D.: Textbook of pediatric nursing, ed. 5, Philadelphia, 1977, W.B. Saunders Co.

McCloskey, J.C.: How to make the most of body image theory in nursing practice, Nurs. '76 **6:**68, May, 1976.

McFarlane, J.: Pediatric assessment and intervention, Nurs. '74 **4:**66, Dec., 1974.

McFarlane, J.M., Whitson, B.J., Hartley, L.M.: Contemporary pediatric nursing, New York, 1980, John Wiley & Sons, Inc.

McInnes, M.E.: Essentials of communicable disease, ed. 2, St. Louis, 1975, The C.V. Mosby Co.

McNutt, K., and McNutt, D.: Nutrition and food choices, Chicago, 1978, Science Research Associates, Inc.

Medenwald, N.Q.: Children's liberation—in a hospital, MCN **5:**231, July/Aug., 1980.

Melichar, M.: Using crisis theory to help parents cope with a child's temper tantrums, MCN **5:**181, May/June, 1980.

Miller, B., and Keane, C.B.: Encyclopedia and dictionary of medicine and nursing, Philadelphia, 1972, W.B. Saunders Co.

Murray, R., and Zentner, J.: Nursing assessment and health promotion through the life span, ed. 2, Englewood Cliffs, N.J., 1979, Prentice-Hall, Inc.

Nolte, D.: Children learn what they live. Living Scrolls, Columbus, Ohio, 1972, Ross Laboratories, Inc.

O'Brien, M., Manley, M., and Heagarty, M.: Expanding the public health nurse's role in child care, Nurs. Outlook **23:**369, June, 1975.

Pipes, P.L.: Nutrition in infancy and childhood, ed. 2, St. Louis, 1981, The C.V. Mosby Co.

Ruble, J.: Childhood nocturnal enuresis, MCN **6:**26, Jan./Feb., 1981.

Schleiher, I.M.: Teaching parents to cope with behavior problems, Am. J. Nurs. **78:**838, May, 1978.

Seedor, M.: The physical assessment, New York, 1974, Teachers College Press.

Selekman, J.: Immunization: what's it all about, Am. J. Nurs. **80:** 140, Aug., 1980.

Sirota, A.: Private care in a public clinic, Am. J. Nurs. **74:**1642, Sept., 1974.

Surgeon General's Report on Health Promotion and Disease Prevention: Healthy people, Washington, D.C., 1979, U.S. Department of Health, Education, and Welfare.

Taber's cyclopedic medical dictionary, ed. 13, Philadelphia, 1977, F.A. Davis Co.

Thiele, V.F.: Clinical nutrition, ed. 2, St. Louis, 1981, The C.V. Mosby Co.

Tripp, S.: What to ask and what to do when parents call about children's illnesses, Nurs. '74 **4:**73, June, 1974.

Walker, J., and Shea, T.: Behavior modification: a practical approach for educators, ed. 2, St. Louis, 1980, The C.V. Mosby Co.

Waring, W., and Jeansonne, L.: Practical manual of pediatrics, St. Louis, 1975, The C.V. Mosby Co.

When your child is contrary, Columbus, Ohio, 1978, Ross Laboratories, Inc.

Wigley, R., and Cook, J.: Community health: concepts and issues, New York, 1975, D. Van Nostrand Co.

Williams, S.R.: Essentials of nutrition and diet therapy, ed. 2, St. Louis, 1978, The C.V. Mosby Co.

Your children and discipline, Columbus, Ohio, 1978, Ross Laboratories, Inc.

CHAPTER 8

Bates, B.: A guide to physical examination, ed. 2, Philadelphia, 1979, J.B. Lippincott Co.

Boston Children's Medical Center, and Feinbloom, R.: Child health encyclopedia: the complete guide for parents, New York, 1978, Dell Publishing Co., Inc.

Bridgewater, S., and Voignier, R.: Allergies in children: teaching, Am. J. Nurs. **78:**620, April, 1978.

Bridgewater, S., Voignier, R., and Smith, C.S.: Allergies in children: recognition, Am. J. Nurs. **78:**615, April, 1978.

Campbell, L.: Special behavioral problems of the burned child, Am. J. Nurs. **76:**220, Jan., 1976.

Chow, M., Durand, B., Feldman, M., and Mills, M.: Handbook of pediatric primary care, New York, 1979, John Wiley & Sons, Inc.

Kinzie, V., and Lau, C.: What to do for the severely burned, Am. J. Nurs. **43:**46, April, 1980.

McFarlane, M.J., Whitson, B.J., and Hartley, L.M.: Contemporary pediatric nursing, New York, 1980, John Wiley & Sons, Inc.

McInnes, M.E.: Essentials of communicable disease, ed. 2, St. Louis, 1975, The C.V. Mosby Co.

Miller, B., and Keane, C.B.: Encyclopedia and dictionary of medicine and nursing, Philadelphia, 1972, W.B. Saunders Co.

Minster, J.: Nursing management of patients with scabies and lice, Nurs. Clin. North Am. **15:**747, Dec., 1980.

Swift, N.: Helping patients live with seizures, Nurs. '78 **8:**24, June, 1978.

Taber's cyclopedic medical dictionary, ed. 13, Philadelphia, 1977, F.A. Davis Co.

Test yourself: ear infection, Am. J. Nurs. **78:**229, Feb., 1978.

Voignier, R., and Bridgewater, S.: Allergies in children: testing and treating, Am. J. Nurs. **78:**617, April., 1978.

CHAPTER 9

Brown, M.S., and Alexander, M.: Physical examination. Part 10: Mouth and throat, Nurs. '74 **4:**57, Aug., 1974.

Brown, M.S., Hudak, C., Brenneman, J., Walsh, K., and Kleeman, K.: Student manual of physical examination, Philadelphia, 1977, J.B. Lippincott Co.

Chinn, P.L.: Child health maintenance: concepts in family-centered care, ed. 2, St. Louis, 1979, The C.V. Mosby Co.

Erikson, E.: Childhood and society, ed. 2, New York, 1963, W.W. Norton & Co., Inc.

Heagarty, M., Glass, G., King, H., and Manly, M.: Child health: basics for primary care, New York, 1980, Appleton-Century-Cofts.

Malasanos, L., Barkauskas, V., Moss, M., Stoltenberg-Allen, K.: Health assessment, ed. 2, St. Louis, 1981, The C.V. Mosby Co.

Marlow, D.: Textbook of pediatric nursing, ed. 5, Philadelphia, 1977, W.B. Saunders Co.

McFarlane, J.M., Whitson, B.J., and Hartley, L.M.: Contemporary pediatric nursing, New York, 1980, John Wiley & Sons, Inc.

Murray, R., and Zentner, J.: Nursing assessment and health promotion through the life span, ed. 2, Englewood Cliffs, N.J., 1979, Prentice-Hall, Inc.

Scipien, G.M., Barnard, M.U., Chard, M.A., Howe, J., and Phillips, P.: Comprehensive pediatric nursing, New York, 1975, McGraw-Hill Book Co.

Seedor, M.: The physical assessment, New York, 1974, Teachers College Press.

Sutterley, D., and Donnelly, G.: Perspectives in human development, Philadelphia, 1973, J.B. Lippincott Co.

Whaley, L.F., and Wong, D.L.: Nursing care of infants and children, St. Louis, 1979, The C.V. Mosby Co.

CHAPTER 10

Alexander, M., and Brown, M.: Pediatric physical diagnosis for nurses, New York, 1974, McGraw-Hill Book Co.

Bates, B.: A guide to physical examination, ed. 2, Philadelphia, 1979, J.B. Lippincott Co.

Benson, E., and McDevitt, J.: Community health and nursing practice, ed. 2, Englewood Cliffs, N.J., 1980, Prentice-Hall, Inc.

BIBLIOGRAPHY

Berner, C.: Assessing the child's ability to cope with stresses of hospitalization, Chapter 10. In Brandt, P., Chinn, P., and Smith, M.E.: Current practice in pediatric nursing, vol. 1, St. Louis, 1976, The C.V. Mosby Co.

Birchfield, M.: Nursing care for hospitalized children based on different stages of illness, MCN **6**:46, Jan./Feb., 1981.

Boston Children's Medical Center, and Feinbloom, R.: Child health encyclopedia: the complete guide for parents, New York, 1978, Dell Publishing Co., Inc.

Brown, M.S., and Alexander, M.: Physical examination. Part 10: Mouth and throat, Nurs. '74 **4**:57, Aug., 1974.

Brown, M.S., Hudak, C., Brenneman, J., Walsh, K., and Kleeman, K.: Student manual of physical examination, Philadelphia, 1977, J.B. Lippincott Co.

Brown, M.S., and Murphy, M.A.: Ambulatory pediatrics for nurses, New York, 1975, McGraw-Hill Book Co.

Chow, M., Durand, B., Feldman, M., and Mills, M.: Handbook of pediatric primary care, New York, 1979, John Wiley & Sons, Inc.

Davis, V.: Through the bars of a crib, Am. J. Nurs. **71**:1752, Sept., 1971.

Developing toilet habits, Columbus, Ohio, 1977, Ross Laboratories, Inc.

Erikson, E.: Childhood and society, ed. 2, New York, 1963, W.W. Norton & Co., Inc.

Evans, D.W.: Practical advice about a delicate pediatric problem, RN **41**:51, Aug., 1978.

Furste, W., and Aguirre, A.: Preventing tetanus, Am. J. Nurs. **78**:834, May, 1978.

Green, C.S.: Understanding childen's needs through therapeutic play, Nurs. '74 **4**:31, Oct., 1974.

Hanlon, J.J., and Pickett, G.E.: Public health: administration and practice, ed. 7, St. Louis, 1979, The C.V. Mosby Co.

Hardgrove, C., and Rutledge, A.: Parenting during hospitalization, Am. J. Nurs. **75**:836, May, 1975.

Heagarty, M., Glass, G., King, H., and Manly, M.: Child health: basics for primary care, New York, 1980, Appleton-Century-Crofts.

Howard, R., and Herbald, N.: Nutrition in clinical care, New York, 1978, McGraw-Hill Book Co.

Insel, P., and Roth, W.: Health in a changing society, Palo Alto, Calif., 1976, Mayfield Publishing Co.

Isler, C.: The fine art of handling a hospitalized child, RN **41**:41, March, 1978.

Kee, J., and Gregory, A.: The ABC's and mEq's of fluid balance in children, Nurs. '74 **4**:29, June, 1974.

Klein, J.W.: Educational component of day care, Children Today **1**:2, Jan./Feb., 1972.

Lewis, C.: Nutrition: the basics of nutrition, Philadelphia, 1977, F.A. Davis Co.

Malasanos, L., Barkauskas, V., Moss, M., Stoltenberg-Allen, K.: Health assessment, ed. 2, St. Louis, 1981, The C.V. Mosby Co.

Marlow, D.: Textbook of pediatric nursing, ed. 5, Philadelphia, 1977, W.B. Saunders Co.

McCloskey, J.C.: How to make the most of body image theory in nursing practice, Nurs. '76 **6**:68, May, 1976.

McFarlane, J.M., Whitson, B.J., and Hartley, L.M.: Contemporary pediatric nursing, New York, 1980, John Wiley & Sons, Inc.

McInnes, M.E.: Essentials of communicable disease, ed. 2, St. Louis, 1975, The C.V. Mosby Co.

McNutt, K., and McNutt, D.: Nutrition and food choices, Chicago, 1978, Science Research Associates, Inc.

Medenwald, N.Q.: Children's liberation—in a hospital, MCN **5**:231, July/Aug., 1980.

Miller, B., and Keane, C.B.: Encyclopedia and dictionary of medicine and nursing, Philadelphia, 1972, W.B. Saunders Co.

Murray, R., and Zentner, J.: Nursing assessment and health promotion through the life span, ed. 2, Englewood Cliffs, N.J., 1979, Prentice-Hall, Inc.

Nolte, D.: Children learn what they live. Living Scrolls, Columbus, Ohio, 1972, Ross Laboratories, Inc.

O'Brien, M., Manly, M., and Heagarty, M.: Expanding the public health nurse's role in child care, Nurs. Outlook **23**:369, June, 1975.

Pipes, P.L.: Nutrition in infancy and childhood, ed. 2, St. Louis, 1981, The C.V. Mosby Co.

Ruble, J.: Childhood nocturnal enuresis, MCN **6**:26, Jan./Feb., 1981.

Schleiher, I.M.: Teaching parents to cope with behavior problems, Am. J. Nurs. **78**:838, May, 1978.

Seedor, M.: The physical assessment, New York, 1974, Teachers College Press.

Selekman, J.: Immunization: what's it all about? Am. J. Nurs. **80**:140, Aug., 1980.

Smith, M.E.: The preschooler and pain, Chapter 12. In Brandt, P., Chinn, P., and Smith, M.E.: Current practice in pediatric nursing, vol. 1, St. Louis, 1976, The C.V. Mosby Co.

Surgeon General's Report on Health Promotion and Disease Prevention: Healthy people, Washington, D.C., 1979, U.S. Department of Health, Education, and Welfare.

Taber's cyclopedic medical dictionary, ed. 13, Philadelphia, 1977, F.A. Davis Co.

Thiele, V.F.: Clinical nutrition, ed. 2, St. Louis, 1980, The C.V. Mosby Co.

Tripp, S.: What to ask and what to do when parent's call about children's illnesses, Nurs. '74 **4**:73, June, 1974.

Walker, J., and Shea, T.: Behavior modification: a practical approach for educators, ed. 2, St. Louis, 1980, The C.V. Mosby Co.

Waring, W., and Jeansonne, L.: Practical manual of pediatrics, St. Louis, 1975, The C.V. Mosby Co.

When your child is contrary, Columbus, Ohio, 1978, Ross Laboratories, Inc.

Wigley, R., and Cook, J.: Community health: concepts and issues, New York, 1975, D. Van Nostrand Co.

Williams, S.R.: Essentials of nutrition and diet therapy, ed. 2, St. Louis, 1978, The C.V. Mosby Co.

Your children and discipline, Ohio, 1978, Ross Laboratories, Inc.

CHAPTER 11

Bates, B.: A guide to physical examination, ed. 2, Philadelphia, 1979, J.B. Lippincott Co.

Boston Children's Medical Center, and Feinbloom, R.: Child health encyclopedia: the complete guide for parents, New York, 1978, Dell Publishing Co., Inc.

Chow, M., Durand, B., Feldman, M., and Mills, M.: Handbook of pediatric primary care, New York, 1979, John Wiley & Sons, Inc.

McFarlane, J.M., Whitson, B.J., and Hartley, L.M.: Contemporary pediatric nursing, New York, 1980, John Wiley & Sons, Inc.

McInnes, M.E.: Essentials of communicable disease, St. Louis, 1975, The C.V. Mosby Co.

Miller, B., and Keane, C.B.: Encyclopedia and dictionary of medicine and nursing, Philadelphia, 1972, W.B. Saunders Co.

Smith, E., Liviskie, S., Nelson, K., and McNemar, A.: Reestablishing a child's body image, Am. J. Nurs. **77**:445, March, 1977.

Taber's cyclopedic medical dictionary, ed. 13, Philadelphia, 1977, F.A. Davis Co.

CHAPTER 12

Alexander, M., and Brown, M.S.: Physical examination. Part 14: Male genitalia, Nurs. '76 **6**:39, Feb., 1976.

Brown, M.S., and Alexander, M.: Physical examination. Part 10: Mouth and throat, Nurs. '74 **4**:57, Aug., 1974.

Brown, M.S., Hudak, C., Brenneman, J., Walsh, K., and Kleeman, K.: Student manual of physical examination, Philadelphia, 1977, J.B. Lippincott Co.

Chinn, P.L.: Child health maintenance: concepts in family-centered care, ed. 2, St. Louis, 1979, The C.V. Mosby Co.

Erikson, E.: Childhood and society, ed. 2, New York, 1963, W.W. Norton & Co., Inc.

Heagarty, M., Glass, G., King, H., and Manly, M.: Child health: basics for primary care, New York, 1980, Appleton-Century-Crofts.

Malasanos, L., Barkauskas, V., Moss, M., and Stoltenberg-Allen, K.: Health assessment, ed. 2, St. Louis, 1981, The C.V. Mosby Co.

Marlow, D.: Textbook of pediatric nursing, ed. 5, Philadelphia, 1977, W.B. Saunders Co.

McFarlane J.M., Whitson, B.J., and Hartley, L.M.: Contemporary pediatric nursing: a conceptual approach, New York, 1980, John Wiley & Sons, Inc.

Murray, R., and Zentner, J.: Nursing assessment and health promotion through the life span, ed. 2, Englewood Cliffs, N.J., 1979, Prentice-Hall, Inc.

Scipien, G.M., Barnard, M.U., Chard, M.A., Howe, J., and Phillips, P.: Comprehensive pediatric nursing, New York, 1975, McGraw-Hill Book Co.

Seedor, M.: The physical assessment, New York, 1974, Teachers College Press.

Sutterley, D., and Donnelly, G.: Perspectives in human development, Philadelphia, 1973, J.B. Lippincott Co.

Whaley, L.F., and Wong, D.L.: Nursing care of infants and children, St. Louis, 1979, The C.V. Mosby Co.

CHAPTER 13

Alexander, M., and Brown, M.S.: Pediatric physical diagnosis for nurses, New York, 1974, McGraw-Hill Book Co.

Alexander, M., and Brown, M.S.: Physical examination. Part 14: Male genitalia, Nurs. '76 **6**:39, Feb., 1976.

Bates, B.: A guide to physical examination, ed. 2, Philadelphia, 1979, J.B. Lippincott Co.

Benson, E., and McDevitt, J.: Community health and nursing practice, ed. 2, Englewood Cliffs, N.J., 1980, Prentice-Hall, Inc.

Birchfield, M.: Nursing care for hospitalized children based on different stages of illness, MCN **6**:46, Jan./Feb., 1981.

Boston Children's Medical Center, and Feinbloom, R.: Child health encyclopedia: the complete guide for parents, New York, 1978, Dell Publishing Co., Inc.

Brown, M.S.: What you should know about communicable diseases and their immunization. Part II: Diphtheria, pertussis, tetanus and polio, Nurs. '75 **5**:56, Oct., 1975.

Brown, M.S., and Alexander, M.: Physical examination. Part 10: Mouth and throat, Nurs. '74 **4**:57, Aug., 1974.

Brown, M.S., Hudak, C., Brenneman, J., Walsh, K., and Kleeman, K.: Student manual of physical examination, Philadelphia, 1977, J.B. Lippincott Co.

Chow, M., Durand, B., Feldman, M., and Mills, M.: Handbook of pediatric primary care, New York, 1979, John Wiley & Sons, Inc.

Erikson, E.: Childhood and society, ed. 2, New York, 1963, W.W. Norton & Co., Inc.

Evans, D.W.: Practical advice about a delicate pediatric problem, RN **41**:51, Aug., 1978.

Green, C.S.: Understanding children's needs through therapeutic play, Nurs. '74 **4**:31, Oct., 1974.

Hanlon, J.J., and Pickett, G.E.: Public health: administration and practice, ed. 7, St. Louis, 1979, The C.V. Mosby Co.

Hardgrove, C., and Rutledge, A.: Parenting during hospitalization, Am. J. Nurs. **75**:836, May, 1975.

Heagarty, M., Glass, G., King, H., and Manly, M.: Child health: basics for primary care, New York, 1980, Appleton-Century-Crofts.

Howard, R., and Herbald, N.: Nutrition in clinical care, New York, 1978, McGraw-Hill Book Co.

Insel, P., and Roth, W.: Health in a changing society, Palo Alto, Calif., 1976, Mayfield Publishing Co.

Isler, C.: The fine art of handling a hospitalized child, RN **41**:41, March, 1978.

Lewis, C.: Nutrition: the basics of nutrition, Philadelphia, 1977, F.A. Davis Co.

Malasanos, L., Barkauskas, V., Moss, M., and Stoltenberg-Allen, K.: Health assessment, ed. 2, St. Louis, 1981, The C.V. Mosby Co.

Marlow, D.: Textbook of pediatric nursing, ed. 5, Philadelphia, 1977, W.B. Saunders Co.

McCloskey, J.C.: How to make the most of body image theory in nursing practice, Nurs. '76 **6**:68, May, 1976.

McFarlane, J.M., Whitson, B.J., and Hartley, L.M.: Contemporary pediatric nursing: a conceptual approach, New York, 1980, John Wiley & Sons, Inc.

McNutt, K., and McNutt, D.: Nutrition and food choices, Chicago, 1978, Science Research Associates, Inc.

Medenwald, N.Q.: Children's liberation—in a hospital, MCN **5**:231, July/Aug., 1980.

Miller, B., and Keane, C.B.: Encyclopedia and dictionary of medicine and nursing, Philadelphia, 1972, W.B. Saunders Co.

Murray, R., and Zentner, J.: Nursing assessment and health promotion through the life span, ed. 2, Englewood Cliffs, N.J., 1979, Prentice-Hall, Inc.

O'Brien, M., Manly, M., and Heagarty, M.: Expanding the public health nurse's role in child care, Nurs. Outlook **23**:369, June, 1975.

Pipes, P.L.: Nutrition in infancy and childhood, ed. 2, St. Louis, 1981, The C.V. Mosby Co.

Seedor, M.: The physical assessment, New York, 1974, Teachers College Press.

Surgeon General's Report on Health Promotion and Disease Prevention: Healthy people, Washington, D.C., 1979, U.S. Department of Health, Education, and Welfare.

Taber's cyclopedic medical dictionary, ed. 13, Philadelphia, 1977, F.A. Davis Co.

Thiele, V.F.: Clinical nutrition, ed. 2, St. Louis, 1980, The C.V. Mosby Co.

Walker, J., and Shea, T.: Behavior modification: a practical approach for educators, ed. 2, St. Louis, 1980, The C.V. Mosby Co.

Waring, W., and Jeansonne, L.: Practical manual of pediatrics, St. Louis, 1975, The C.V. Mosby Co.

Wigley, R., and Cook, J.: Community health: concepts and issues, New York, 1975, D. Van Nostrand Co.

Williams, S.R.: Essentials of nutrition and diet therapy, ed. 2, St. Louis, 1978, The C.V. Mosby Co.

CHAPTER 14

Bates, B.: A guide to physical examination, ed. 2, Philadelphia, 1979, J.B. Lippincott Co.

Benson, E., and McDevitt, J.: Community health and nursing practice, ed. 2, Englewood Cliffs, N.J., 1980, Prentice-Hall, Inc.

Boston Children's Medical Center, and Feinbloom, R.: Child health encyclopedia: the complete guide for parents, New York, 1978, Dell Publishing Co., Inc.

Bridgewater, S., Voignier, R., and Smith, C.S.: Allergies in children: recognition, Am. J. Nurs. **78**:615, April, 1978.

Carroll, C., and Miller, D.: Health: the science of human adaptation, ed. 2, Dubuque, Iowa, 1979, Wm.C. Brown Co., Publishers.

Chow, M., Durand, B., Feldman, M., and Mills, M.: Handbook of pediatric primary care, New York, 1979, John Wiley & Sons, Inc.

Hilt, N., and Schmitt, E.W.: Pediatric orthopedic nursing, St. Louis, 1975, The C.V. Mosby Co.

Insel, P., and Roth, W.: Health in a changing society, Palo Alto, Calif., 1976, Mayfield Publishing Co.

McFarlane, J.M., Whitson, B.J., and Hartley, L.M.: Contemporary pediatric nursing: a conceptual approach, New York, 1980, John Wiley & Sons, Inc.

Miller, B., and Keane, C.B.: Encyclopedia and dictionary of medicine and nursing, Philadelphia, 1972, W.B. Saunders Co.

Smith, E., Liviskie, S., Nelson, K., and McNemar, A.: Reestablishing a child's body image, Am. J. Nurs. 77:445, March, 1977.

Taber's cyclopedic medical dictionary, ed. 13, Philadelphia, 1977, F.A. Davis Co.

Voignier, R., and Bridgewater, S.: Allergies in children: testing and treating, Am. J. Nurs. 78:617, April, 1978.

Wieczorek, R.R., and Horner-Rosner, B.: The asthmatic child: preventing and controlling attacks, Am. J. Nurs. 79:258, Feb., 1979.

CHAPTER 15

Alexander, M., and Brown, M.S.: Physical examination. Part 14: Male genitalia, Nurs. '76 6:39, Feb., 1976.

Brown, M.S., Hudak, C., Brenneman, J., Walsh, K., and Kleeman, K.: Student manual of physical examination, Philadelphia, 1977, J.B. Lippincott Co.

Burton, R., Ramer, B., Thomas, M., and Thurber, S.: Key issues in health, New York, 1978, Harcourt Brace Jovanovich, Inc.

Chinn, P.L : Child health maintenance: concepts in family-centered care, ed. 2, St. Louis, 1979, The C.V. Mosby Co.

Clark, A., and Alfonso, D.: Childbearing: a nursing perspective, Philadelphia, 1976, F.A. Davis Co.

Erikson, E.: Childhood and society, ed. 2, New York, 1963, W.W. Norton & Co., Inc.

Insel, P., and Roth, W.: Health in a changing society, Palo Alto, Calif., 1976, Mayfield Publishing Co.

Malasanos, L., Barkauskas, V., Moss, M., and Stoltenberg-Allen, K.: Health assessment, ed. 2, St. Louis, 1981, The C.V. Mosby Co.

Marlow, D.: Textbook of pediatric nursing, ed. 5, Philadelphia, 1977, W.B. Saunders Co.

McFarlane, J.M., Whitson, B.J., and Hartley, L.M.: Contemporary pediatric nursing: a conceptual approach, New York, 1980, John Wiley & Sons, Inc.

Scipien, G.M., Barnard, M.U., Chard, M.A., Howe, J., and Phillips, P.: Comprehensive pedtriatric nursing, New York, 1975, McGraw-Hill Book Co.

Seedor, M.: The physical assessment, New York, 1974, Teachers College Press.

Sutterley, D., and Donnelly, G.: Perspectives in human development, Philadelphia, 1973, J.B. Lippincott Co.

Whaley, L.F., and Wong, D.L.: Nursing care of infants and children, St. Louis, 1979, The C.V. Mosby Co.

CHAPTER 16

Alexander, M., and Brown, M.S.: Pediatric physical diagnosis for nurses, New York, 1974, McGraw-Hill Book Co.

Alexander, M., and Brown, M.S.: Physical examination. Part 14: Male genitalia, Nurs. '76 6:39, Feb., 1976.

Bates, B.: A guide to physical examination, ed. 2, Philadelphia, 1979, J.B. Lippincott Co.

Blust, L.C.: School nurse practitioner in a high school, Am. J. Nurs. 78:1532, Sept., 1978.

Boston Children's Medical Center, and Feinbloom, R.: Child health encyclopedia: the complete guide for parents, New York, 1978, Dell Publishing Co., Inc.

Brown, M.S., Hudak, C., Brenneman, J., Walsh, K., and Kleeman, K.: Student manual of physical examination, Philadelphia, 1977, J.B. Lippincott Co.

Burton, R., Ramer, B., Thomas, M., and Thurber, S.: Key issues in health, New York, 1978, Harcourt Brace Jovanovich, Inc.

Chow, M., Durand, B., Feldman, M., and Mills, M.: Handbook of pediatric primary care, New York, 1979, John Wiley & Sons, Inc.

Erikson, E.: Childhood and society, ed. 2, New York, 1963, W.W. Norton & Co., Inc.

Hanlon, J.J., and Pickett, G.E.: Public health: administration and practice, ed. 7, St. Louis, 1979, The C.V. Mosby Co.

Heagarty, M., Glass, G., King, H., and Manly, M.: Child health: basics for primary care, New York, 1980, Appleton-Century-Crofts.

Howard, R., and Herbald, N.: Nutrition in clinical care, New York, 1978, McGraw-Hill Book Co.

Insel, P., and Roth, W.: Health in a changing society, Palo Alto, Calif., 1976, Mayfield Publishing Co.

Isler, C.: The fine art of handling a hospitalized child, RN 41:41, March, 1978.

Lewis, C.: Nutrition: the basics of nutrition, Philadelphia, 1977, F.A. Davis Co.

Malasanos, L., Barkauskas, V., Moss, M., Stoltenberg-Allen, K.: Health assessment, ed. 2, St. Louis, 1981, The C.V. Mosby Co.

Marlow, D.: Textbook of pediatric nursing, ed. 5, Philadelphia, 1977, W.B. Saunders Co.

Mayer, J.: Health, New York, 1974, D. Van Nostrand Co.

McFarlane, J.M., Whitson, B.J., and Hartley, L.M.: Contemporary pediatric nursing: a conceptual approach, New York, 1980, John Wiley & Sons, Inc.

McNutt, K., and McNutt, D.: Nutrition and food choices, Chicago, 1978, Science Research Associates, Inc.

Miller, B., and Keane, C.B.: Encyclopedia and dictionary of medicine and nursing, Philadelphia, 1972, W.B. Saunders Co.

Murray, R., and Zentner, J.: Nursing assessment and health promotion through the life span, ed. 2, Englewood Cliffs, N.J., Prentice-Hall, Inc.

Pipes, P.L.: Nutrition in infancy and childhood, ed. 2, St. Louis, 1981, The C.V. Mosby Co.

Schowalter, J.E., and Lord, R.D.: The hospitalized adolescent, Children 18:127, July/Aug., 1971.

Seedor, M.: The physical assessment, New York, 1974, Teachers College Press.

Surgeon General's Report on Health Promotion and Disease Prevention: Healthy people, Washington, D.C., 1979, U.S. Department of Health, Education, and Welfare.

Taber's cyclopedic medical dictionary, ed. 13, Philadelphia, 1977, F.A. Davis Co.

Thiele, V.F.: Clinical nutrition, ed. 2, St. Louis, 1980, The C.V. Mosby Co.

Walker, J., and Shea, T.: Behavior modification: a practical approach for educators, ed. 2, St. Louis, 1980, The C.V. Mosby Co.

Waring, W., and Jeansonne, L.: Practical manual of pediatrics, St. Louis, 1975, The C.V. Mosby Co.

Wigley, R., and Cook, J.: Community health: concepts and issues, New York, 1975, D. Van Nostrand Co.

Williams, S.R.: Essentials of nutrition and diet therapy, ed. 2, St. Louis, 1978, The C.V. Mosby Co.

CHAPTER 17

Anderson, B.: The patient with scoliosis: Carole, a girl treated with bracing, Am. J. Nurs. 79:1592, Sept., 1979.

BIBLIOGRAPHY

Bates, B.: A guide to physical examination, ed. 2, Philadelphia, 1979, J.B. Lippincott Co.

Benson, E., and McDevitt, J.: Community health and nursing practice, ed. 2, Engelwood Cliffs, N.J., 1980, Prentice-Hall, Inc.

Boston Children's Medical Center, and Feinbloom, R.: Child health encyclopedia: the complete guide for parents, New York, 1978, Dell Publishing Co., Inc.

Brown, L.K.: Toxic shock syndrome, MCN **6**:57, Jan./Feb., 1981.

Burton, R., Ramer, B., Thomas, M., and Thurber, S.: Key issues in health, New York, 1978, Harcourt Brace Jovanovich, Inc.

Caldwell, J.: Congenital syphilis: a nonvenereal disease, Am. J. Nurs. **71**:1768, Sept., 1971.

Carroll, C., and Miller, D.: Health: the science of human adaptation, ed. 2, Dubuque, Iowa, 1979, Wm.C. Brown Co., Publishers.

Chow, M., Durand, B., Feldman, M., and Mills, M.: Handbook of pediatric primary care, New York, 1979, John Wiley & Sons, Inc.

Clark, A., and Alfonso, D.: Childbearing: a nursing perspective, Philadelphia, 1976, F.A. Davis Co.

deToledo, C.H.: The patient with scoliosis: the defect, classification, and detection, Am. J. Nurs. **79**:1588, Sept., 1979.

Hanlon, J.J., and Pickett, G.E.: Public health: administration and practice, ed. 7, St. Louis, 1979, The C.V. Mosby Co.

Heagarty, M., Glass, G., King, H., and Manly, M.: Child health: basics for primary care, New York, 1980, Appleton-Century-Crofts.

Hilt, N., and Schmitt, E.: Pediatric orthopedic nursing, St. Louis, 1975, The C.V. Mosby Co.

Insel, P., and Roth, W.: Health in a changing society, Palo Alto, Calif., 1976, Mayfield Publishing Co.

Malasanos, L., Barkauskas, V., Moss, M., and Stoltenberg-Allen, K.: Health assessment, ed. 2, St. Louis, 1981, The C.V. Mosby Co.

McFarlane, J.M., Whitson, B.J., and Hartley, L.M.: Contemporary pediatric nursing: a conceptual approach, New York, 1980, John Wiley & Sons, Inc.

Micheli, L.J., Magin, M.O., and Rouvales, R.: The patient with scoliosis: surgical management and nursing care, Am. J. Nurs. **79**:1599, Sept., 1979.

Miller, B., and Keane, C.B.: Encyclopedia and dictionary of medicine and nursing, Philadelphia, 1972, W.B. Saunders Co.

Murray, R., and Zentner, J.: Nursing assessment and health promotion through the life span, ed. 2, Englewood Cliffs, N.J., Prentice-Hall, Inc.

Smith, E., Liviskie, S., Nelson, K., and McNemar, A.: Reestablishing a child's body image, Am. J. Nurs. **77**:445, March, 1977.

Taber's cyclopedic medical dictionary, ed. 13, Philadelphia, 1977, F.A. Davis Co.

CHAPTER 18

Dison, N.: Clinical nursing techniques, ed. 4, St. Louis, 1979, The C.V. Mosby Co.

Gorman, C., and Kennedy, C.E.: The parient-educator nurse, MCN **5**:277, July/Aug., 1980.

Hilt, N., and Schmitt, E.: Pediatric orthopedic nursing, St. Louis, 1975, The C.V. Mosby Co.

King, E., Wieck, L., and Dyer, M.: Illustrated manual of nursing techniques, Philadelphia, 1977, J.B. Lippincott Co.

INDEX